SPORTS MEDICINE AND PHYSIOLOGY

RICHARD H. STRAUSS, M.D., *Editor*

Ohio State University College of Medicine,
and University of Hawaii School of Medicine

1979   **W. B. SAUNDERS COMPANY**   *Philadelphia • London • Toronto*

W. B. Saunders Company: West Washington Square
Philadelphia, PA   19105

1 St. Anne's Road
Eastbourne, East Sussex BN21 3UN, England

1 Goldthorne Avenue
Toronto, Ontario M8Z 5T9, Canada

Sports Medicine and Physiology   ISBN   0-7216-8592-7

Last digit is the print number: 9   8   7   6   5   4   3   2   1

CONTRIBUTORS

ROBERT B. ARMSTRONG, PH.D.

Associate Professor of Physiology, School of Medicine,
Oral Roberts University

JOHN BERGFELD, M.D.

Head, Section of Sports Medicine,
Department of Orthopedic Surgery,
Cleveland Clinic

ARTHUR L. BOLAND, JR., M.D.

Chief Surgeon for Athletics,
Harvard University;
Clinical Instructor in Orthopedic Surgery,
Harvard Medical School;
Associate in Orthopedic Surgery,
Peter Bent Brigham Hospital, Boston

PETER R. CAVANAGH, PH.D.

Associate Professor of Biomechanics,
Pennsylvania State University

MICHAEL M. DEHN, M.S.

Dallas Cardiac Institute

V. REGGIE EDGERTON, PH.D.

Professor of Kinesiology and Brain Research Institute,
University of California, Los Angeles

JAMES G. GARRICK, M.D.

333 East Virginia Avenue, Phoenix, Arizona;
formerly Associate Professor of Orthopedic Surgery
and Head of the Division of Sports Medicine,
University of Washington School of Medicine

DON W. GRIEVE, M.SC., PH.D.

Reader in Biomechanics, Royal Free Hospital
School of Medicine, London

ROBERT D. GROVER, M.D., PH.D.

Professor of Medicine; Director, Cardiovascular
Pulmonary Research Laboratory, Division of Cardiology,
Department of Medicine, University of Colorado
School of Medicine

DANIEL F. HANLEY, M.D.

Member, Medical Commission,
International Olympic Committee;
College Physician, Bowdoin College, Brunswick, Maine

L. Howard Hartley, M.D.

Associate Professor of Medicine,
Harvard Medical School

Howard G. Knuttgen, Ph.D.

Professor of Physiology,
Sargent College of Allied Health Professions,
Boston University

Lyle J. Micheli, M.D.

Director, Division of Sports Medicine,
and Associate in Orthopaedic Surgery,
Children's Hospital Medical Center, Boston;
Instructor in Orthopaedic Surgery,
Harvard Medical School

Jere H. Mitchell, M.D.

Professor of Medicine and Physiology, University
of Texas Health Science Center at Dallas

Robert J. Murphy, M.D.

Head Team Physician and Associate Clinical Professor
of Medicine, Ohio State University

Ethan R. Nadel, Ph.D.

Associate Professor, Departments of Epidemiology and
Public Health and Physiology; John B. Pierce Foundation
Laboratory, Yale University School of Medicine

Thomas B. Quigley, M.D.

Professor of Surgery, Emeritus, Harvard Medical School;
Surgeon Emeritus, Department of Athletics,
Harvard University; Lecturer in Orthopedic Surgery,
Tufts University School of Medicine

Nathan J. Smith, M.D.

Professor of Pediatrics and Orthopaedics (Sports Medicine),
University of Washington School of Medicine

Thomas P. Stossel, M.D.

Associate Professor of Medicine,
Harvard Medical School; Medical Oncology Unit,
Massachusetts General Hospital, Boston

Richard H. Strauss, M.D.

Assistant Professor of Medicine,
Ohio State University College of Medicine;
Physician, Sports Medicine Clinic,
University Health Service, Ohio State University;
Associate Clinical Professor of Physiology,
University of Hawaii School of Medicine

Ronald L. Terjung, Ph.D.

Associate Professor of Physiology,
Upstate Medical Center, State University of New York,
Syracuse

Clayton L. Thomas, M.D., M.P.H.

Vice President Medical Affairs, Tampax Incorporated;
Consultant in Human Reproduction,
Department of Population Sciences,
Harvard School of Public Health

Joseph S. Torg, M.D.

Professor of Orthopaedic Surgery,
University of Pennsylvania School of Medicine;
Director, University of Pennsylvania Sports Medicine Center

Wayne D. Van Huss, Ph.D.

Professor of Health, Physical Education, and Recreation,
Michigan State University

Jack H. Wilmore, Ph.D.

Professor and Head, Department of Physical Education,
University of Arizona

PREFACE

A basic knowledge of sports medicine is increasingly necessary for persons who work in disciplines related to sports. This book is an overview of sports medicine intended as a text for college students in the fields of physical education, coaching, and athletic training. It may also be of use to others in health-related fields and to individuals with a strong personal interest in sports.

Each chapter is written by an authority in the field. The book can be read from cover to cover but is arranged in four sections to facilitate selective reading by persons with diverse backgrounds. Those who have studied exercise physiology may wish to use Section I, *Basic Physiology of Exercise,* as a review.

Section II is entitled *Advanced Topics in Exercise Physiology and in Medicine.* It contains material which, because of its complex nature, often is not included in texts on exercise physiology. However, such material is presented here for those readers who desire a more complete view of sports physiology.

Section III, *Sports Injuries and Medicine,* contains the core of sports medicine. The goals of this section are to teach the student how to recognize sports medical problems; when to send the athlete to a health professional; what limitations in activity to expect; and how to prevent problems whenever possible.

Section IV, *Special Topics in Sports Medicine,* goes beyond the playing field to discuss the young, the old, heat stress, altitude, diving, nutrition, drugs, and heart disease. These chapters may be read selectively or in total.

Study questions are included at the end of each chapter as an aid to self-evaluation.

RICHARD H. STRAUSS, M.D.

CONTENTS

SECTION 3: SPORTS INJURIES AND MEDICINE

SECTION 4: SPECIAL TOPICS IN SPORTS MEDICINE

BASIC PHYSIOLOGY OF EXERCISE

The material in Section 1 describes the physiological basis for physical activity. Readers who have studied exercise physiology previously may wish to use these chapters as a review.

1. BIOCHEMISTRY: ENERGY LIBERATION AND USE
2. SKELETAL MUSCLE PHYSIOLOGY
3. THE NERVOUS SYSTEM
4. THE RESPIRATORY SYSTEM
5. THE CIRCULATORY SYSTEM
6. PHYSICAL CONDITIONING AND LIMITS TO PERFORMANCE

1

BIOCHEMISTRY: ENERGY LIBERATION AND USE

ROBERT B. ARMSTRONG, Ph.D.

Nearly all the physiological changes that occur in the body during exercise are in some way related to the muscles' utilization of energy to power their contractile processes. During rest, the energy needs of the muscles are relatively low. In a resting man with a total body energy utilization of 1.3 kcal/min (kilocalories per minute), only about 20 per cent of that energy, or 0.26 kcal/min, is used by the muscles. This may be considered relatively low, because muscles make up almost half the body weight and yet use only one-fifth of the energy.

If the same man now begins to exercise vigorously — for example, at a level that he can maintain for only 1 or 2 minutes — there is a drastic alteration in energy utilization by his body. At this exercise intensity the man may expend as much as 35 kcal/min. Moreover, as much as 90 per cent of that total energy requirement is now used by the muscles. Thus, during this exercise the muscles require about 32 kcal/min, representing a 120-fold increase in their energy needs from rest to exercise. This change becomes even more dramatic when we realize that during exercise, some muscles are much more active than others and may actually increase their energy utilization by more than 200-fold above the resting level.

When these tremendous alterations in energy utilization between rest and exercise are considered, it becomes apparent that the muscles must either possess the capacity to store large quantities of energy that can be called upon during periods of muscle activity or be able to produce the energy needed for muscle contraction on very short notice. The purpose of this chapter is to introduce the subject of exercise metabolism, and, consequently, the subject of exercise physiology. The intention is not to present a detailed examination of the biochemical aspects of exercise but rather to give an overview of the major processes involved in energy release and capture in muscle cells and of the regulation of the energy stores in the body.

THE ENERGY SOURCE FOR MUSCLE CONTRACTION: ATP

Although the term "energy" is commonly used in everyday communication and conveys a reasonably clear meaning to the listener, most people would probably have a difficult time defining the word precisely. One hears such statements as "I wish I had

3

her energy" or "That takes a lot of time and energy." What exactly does the word mean?

Energy is defined as the *ability to do work*. Remembering that work is force exerted over a distance, energy can also be thought of as the ability to produce a change. Although there are various types of energy (e.g., mechanical, electrical, chemical) that can be interconverted under the proper conditions, energy can neither be created nor destroyed. This fact constitutes the first law of thermodynamics, which is one of the most important laws in science.

Regardless of its type, energy exists in one of two forms: potential or kinetic. *Potential energy* is the energy stored within a system as a consequence of its position or its internal structure. When this stored energy is released, it results in movement or a change in position, during which it can perform work. This active form of energy is referred to as *kinetic energy*.

The type of energy used by the muscle cell to generate contractile force is chemical; that is, energy that is stored in chemical molecules and transferred among molecules to permit work to be done in the cell. The specific molecule used in muscle cells as the immediate energy source for contraction is *adenosine triphosphate* (ATP). This "high-energy phosphate" molecule is illustrated in Figure 1–1.

When the last phosphate group is split off from the ATP molecule, a large amount of chemical potential energy (about 7.6 kcal/mole ATP) is released from the molecule as kinetic energy, which can be used by the contractile proteins of the muscle cell to generate force. The other products of this chemical reaction are *adenosine diphosphate* (ADP) and inorganic phosphate (P_i):

$$ATP \xrightarrow{\text{ATPase}} ADP + P_i + energy \tag{1}$$

Something else should be noted about this reaction. An enzyme called an *ATPase* is involved in the splitting of the P_i from ATP. Almost all chemical reactions in living cells are *catalyzed*, or helped, by protein enzymes. Enzymes speed up and control reactions in cells without undergoing a net change themselves. Every enzyme is fairly specific for a particular type of reaction. Thus, ATPase enzymes are required to catalyze the breakdown of ATP for energy release.

The specific ATPase that splits ATP to provide energy for muscle contraction is conveniently located on one of the major contractile proteins of the muscle cell, *myosin* (see Chapter 2). Thus, energy released in this particular reaction is directly available to the molecules that generate contractile force in the muscle.

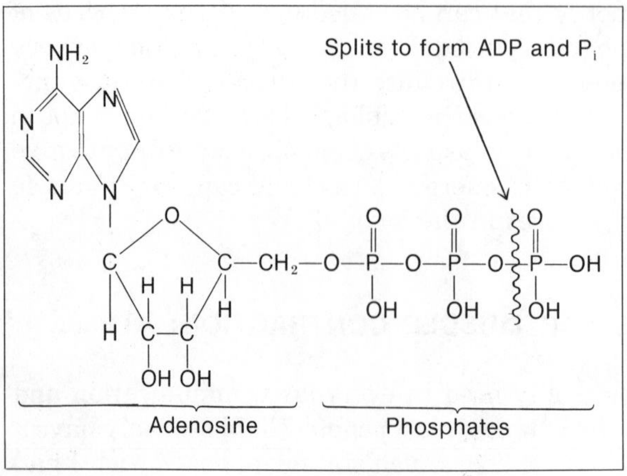

Figure 1–1. Adenosine triphosphate (ATP).

Although this discussion is concerned primarily with the energy that powers muscle contraction, it should be pointed out that ATP also provides energy for a number of other essential processes in the muscle cell. For example, ATP is split for energy for protein synthesis, for active transport of ions (e.g., Na^+, K^+, and Ca^{++}) across membranes, and for activation of some of the metabolic pathways in the cell. However, the large changes in energy use in the muscles during exercise are a result of ATP utilization for contraction.

The fact that the energy requirements of the muscles increase dramatically during exercise has already been discussed. Since this energy comes from ATP, the next question to be answered is: What is the source of the large quantities of ATP that must be available for the muscle during periods of increased contractile activity?

One way of providing the necessary energy would be to store large quantities of ATP in the muscle cell so that an adequate energy reserve would be readily available. However, there is only a small supply of ATP in cells. In fact, during intense muscular contraction, the ATP stored in the cell would be depleted in less than 1 second. (Utilization of the ATP reserve will be discussed at greater length later in the chapter.) Therefore, muscle cells must have a means of rapidly replacing ATP as it is used to power contraction.

ATP RESYNTHESIS BY OXIDATIVE PHOSPHORYLATION (AEROBIC METABOLISM)

Muscle cells cannot obtain ATP from the blood or from other tissues, but they do possess the necessary enzymes for resynthesizing ATP from ADP and P_i using energy from other chemical sources. ATP synthesis is essentially the reverse of ATP breakdown (Equation 1):

$$ADP + P_i + energy \longrightarrow ATP \qquad (2)$$

Thus, the muscle cell must have a means of obtaining energy from some other chemical source to enable the *phosphorylation* of ADP to take place.

Most of the phosphorylation of ADP to ATP occurs in specific cell organelles called *mitochondria* (Fig. 1–2). The mitochondria are conveniently located in the muscle cell immediately adjacent to the contractile strands, or *myofibrils,* that contain the contractile proteins (Fig. 1–3).

Positioned on the *cristae* (Fig. 1–2), or inner membranes of each mitochondrion, are numerous discrete series of molecules, each of which constitutes a *respiratory chain* (or *electron transport system*). The function of the respiratory chain is to accept

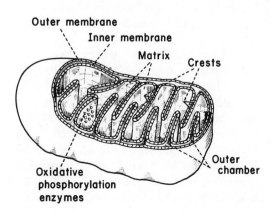

Figure 1–2. Structure of a mitochondrion. (From Guyton, A. C.: *Textbook of Medical Physiology,* 5th ed. Philadelphia, W. B. Saunders Company, 1976.)

Myofibril

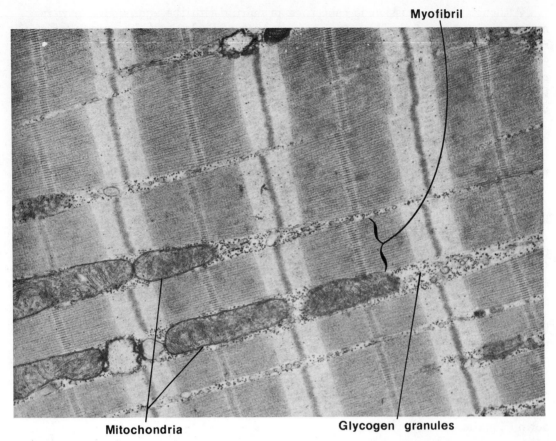

Mitochondria   **Glycogen granules**

Figure 1–3. Electron micrograph of a muscle cell showing the relationship between the myofibrils and mitochondria. (From Guyton, A. C.: *Textbook of Medical Physiology,* 5th ed. Philadelphia, W. B. Saunders Company, 1976.)

pairs of hydrogen atoms (H_2) from other metabolic pathways in the cell and to transfer the H_2 from one molecule to the next in succession. These transfers are called *oxidation-reduction reactions.* Oxidation refers to hydrogen removal from a molecule, reduction to hydrogen gain.

As the H_2 is passed from one molecule in the chain to the next, considerable amounts of chemical energy are liberated. It is this energy that is used to phosphorylate ADP to ATP. Phosphorylation can occur at three different places in the respiratory chain; that is, at three different steps, enough energy is released from the transfer of the H_2 to allow synthesis of ATP to occur (Fig. 1–4).

About half the energy released in the oxidation-reduction reactions of the respiratory chain is captured in ATP. The remainder is given off as heat. The heat cannot be considered entirely as "wasted" energy, since it is important for the maintenance of body temperature.

When the H_2 reaches the end of the respiratory chain, it combines with one atom of molecular oxygen (O_2) to form water, H_2O (Fig. 1–4). When O_2 is not available to the cell, the respiratory chain is unable to discharge its H_2, the chain "backs up," and ATP synthesis in the mitochondrion cannot proceed. This fact is of prime importance in understanding exercise physiology. A large number of the physiological changes that occur in the body when a person begins to exercise have the express purpose of providing the active muscles with O_2 to allow them to resynthesize enough ATP to keep up with the elevated energy needs.

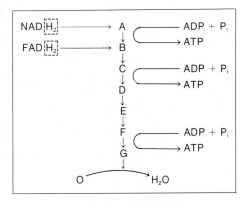

Figure 1-4. Schematic representation of the respiratory chain.

The process of ATP synthesis in the respiratory chain, with O_2 as the final hydrogen acceptor, is called *oxidative phosphorylation*. The term "aerobic metabolism" refers to the production of ATP in the presence of oxygen. Oxidative phosphorylation constitutes the most efficient method available to the cell for resynthesizing ATP from ADP.

In summary, the respiratory chain requires three things for oxidative phosphorylation: (1) ADP (and P_i); (2) oxygen; and (3) hydrogen. ADP is made available to the respiratory chain by the splitting of ATP to provide for the energy requirements of the cell, and oxygen is obtained by simple diffusion into the cell from the circulating blood. What is the source(s) of the H_2?

H₂ PRODUCTION IN THE CELL

H₂ Transfer to the Respiratory Chain

Figure 1-4 shows that H_2 is delivered to the respiratory chain by molecules of NAD and FAD*. NAD and FAD are *coenzymes*: they function as H_2 acceptors and carriers in the cell. The general equation for a *dehydrogenase* reaction may be given as:

$$AH_2 + NAD \xrightarrow{\text{dehydrogenase}} A + NADH_2 \qquad (3)$$

where A is a substrate that is oxidized, with reduction of NAD. The enzyme catalyzing the reaction is a dehydrogenase. Following the reduction of the coenzyme, it transfers the H_2 to the respiratory chain.

Before proceeding with consideration of the sources of H_2 in the cell, two other important points should be made about the two coenzymes. First, the dehydrogenase reactions in the cell are coupled specifically to either NAD or FAD; that is, the two coenzymes are not used interchangeably. Secondly, reference to Figure 1-4 will show that the number of molecules of ATP formed in the respiratory chain from one pair of hydrogen atoms is dependent upon the particular coenzyme that serves as carrier in the reaction: if NAD, three ATP will be synthesized; if FAD, only two ATP are produced. Thus, the ratios of ATP produced per atom of oxygen reduced (P:O ratio) for $NADH_2$ and $FADH_2$ are 3 and 2, respectively.

---

*NAD = nicotinamide adenine dinucleotide; FAD = flavin adenine dinucleotide.

Major Sources of H_2 in the Muscle Cell

NAD and FAD reductions occur in several enzyme pathways in the cell that sequentially break down nutritive molecules derived from the digestion of foods. The two major sources of H_2 for oxidative phosphorylation in muscle cells are *fatty acids* and *glucose* (a sugar). These molecules are illustrated in Figure 1–5. In a later section, the different conditions under which muscles preferentially metabolize one or the other of these two *substrates** for energy will be discussed in some detail. For now, it is sufficient simply to indicate that muscles "prefer" to use fatty acids. When fatty acids and oxygen are available to the muscle cell, fat constitutes the primary substrate for generation of H_2.

FATTY ACID OXIDATION

Muscle cells store some fat that may be used for oxidation, but the primary source of fatty acids is the circulating blood. Fatty acids diffuse freely from capillary blood, through the cell membrane, into the cytoplasm of the cell (Fig. 1–6). The rate of entry of fatty acids into the cell depends on the concentration gradient; thus, increased entry rate can result from (1) increasing the fatty acid concentration in the blood, or (2) increasing their rate of oxidation in the cell. Later in this chapter the first possibility will be discussed: regulation of fatty acid levels in the blood. For now, fatty acid metabolism in the muscle cell will be the main concern.

β-**Oxidation.** Once inside the muscle cell, the fatty acid is enzymatically "activated" with energy derived from ATP (Fig. 1–6). The activated fatty acid is then ready to be metabolized in the mitochondrion to generate H_2. The fatty acid is *catabolized* (broken down) by a sequence of mitochondrial enzymes in a process called *β-oxidation* (beta-oxidation) (Fig. 1–6). The purpose of this group of enzymes is twofold: (1) to oxidize (remove H_2 from) the fatty acid at two different steps, providing two H_2 each time through the pathway; and (2) to sequentially split off 2-carbon fragments, called *acetyl-CoA*, that can be completely oxidized in another metabolic pathway. It can be seen in Figure 1–6 that one H_2 produced in the β-oxidation of fatty acids is picked up by FAD and the other by NAD. The reduced FAD and NAD then transfer their H_2 to the respiratory chain for oxidative phosphorylation.

---

*A substrate is a substance upon which an enzyme acts.

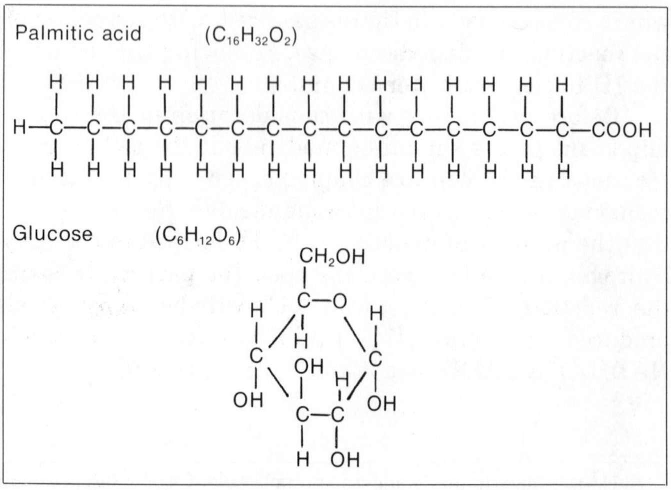

Figure 1–5. Structures of a typical fatty acid (palmitic acid) and glucose.

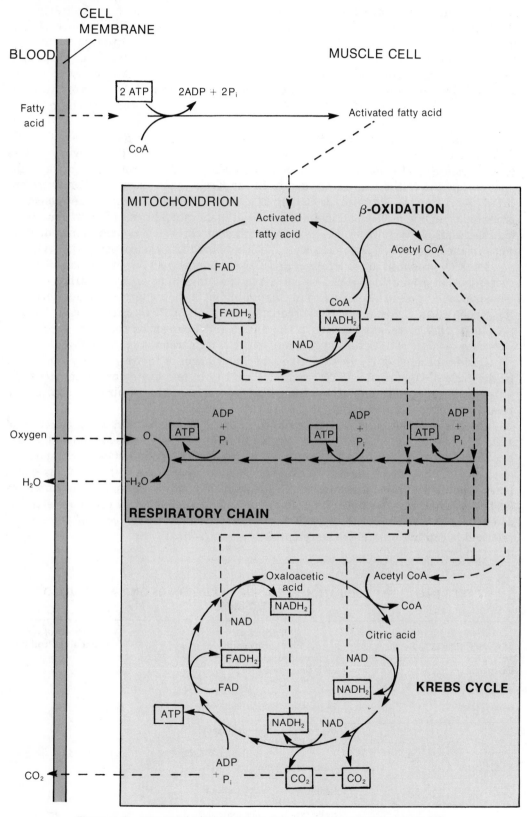

Figure 1-6. Metabolic pathways for fatty acid oxidation in the muscle cell.

If the number of carbon (C) atoms in palmitic acid (Fig. 1–5), a typical fatty acid that muscle cells metabolize, is counted, it can be seen that eight 2-carbon acetyl-CoA molecules can be produced. To completely degrade (break down) the palmitic acid, therefore, it is necessary for the molecule to pass through β-oxidation seven times (the seventh time through, the 4-carbon activated fatty acid is split into two 2-carbon acetyl-CoA molecules). Thus, during β-oxidation of palmitic acid, 14 pairs of hydrogen atoms are picked up by either FAD or NAD for transfer to the respiratory chain (Table 1–1).

Krebs Cycle. The eight acetyl-CoA molecules produced by β-oxidation of palmitic acid are completely oxidized in the *Krebs cycle** (Fig. 1–6). The enzymes of the Krebs cycle are also located in the mitochondrion in close proximity to those for β-oxidation and to the respiratory chain. In the Krebs cycle, each 2-carbon fragment (from acetyl-CoA) is degraded, producing CO_2 and H_2. The eight acetyl-CoA molecules produced from one molecule of palmitic acid will generate 32 pairs of hydrogen atoms for the respiratory chain (Table 1–1). Note that at three of the oxidation-reduction steps in the cycle, NAD is the coenzyme; at the fourth site the coenzyme is FAD.

The CO_2 produced in the Krebs cycle diffuses out of the cell into the blood (down its concentration gradient) so it can be carried to the lungs to be expired. Carbon dioxide transport will be discussed in detail in Chapter 4, but it should be pointed out here that the Krebs cycle is the major CO_2-producing metabolic pathway in the cell. During periods of high metabolic activity in the muscles, it is essential that they receive an adequate blood flow both for oxygen delivery and for carbon dioxide removal.

Besides producing H_2 for oxidative phosphorylation in the respiratory chain, the Krebs cycle also generates ATP from ADP and P_i in one of its enzymatic steps. To differentiate this ATP production from that occurring in the respiratory chain, it is referred to as "phosphorylation at the substrate level" (Fig. 1–6).

Complete oxidation of one molecule of palmitic acid results in the production of 129 molecules of ATP (Table 1–1). A number of different fatty acids are normally used by muscle cells to produce ATP, and the amount of ATP generated depends upon the structure of the particular fatty acid. The various fatty acids differ in their chain length (number of carbon atoms) and in the types of bonds between the carbon atoms (saturated and unsaturated fatty acids), but their metabolism in the muscle cell is essentially the same. As fatty acids are oxidized, about 40 per cent of the energy released is captured as ATP; the remainder is lost as heat.

---

*Also called the tricarboxylic acid cycle or the citric acid cycle.

TABLE 1–1. ATP PRODUCTION FROM THE OXIDATION OF ONE MOLECULE OF PALMITIC ACID

Enzyme Pathway	Method of Phosphorylation	Number of ATP Molecules Produced
Fatty acid activation	ATP consumed	−2
β-oxidation	Respiratory chain oxidation of 7 $NADH_2$	21
	Respiratory chain oxidation of 7 $FADH_2$	14
Krebs cycle	Respiratory chain oxidation of 24 $NADH_2$	72
	Respiratory chain oxidation of 8 $FADH_2$	16
	Substrate level phosphorylation	8
Total		129

GLUCOSE OXIDATION

The other major metabolic substrate used by muscle cells to generate H_2 for oxidative phosphorylation is glucose. As muscles increase their contractile activity, glucose becomes the most important source of energy for the muscle cell. Glucose may be obtained by the muscle either from the circulating blood or from glucose stored in the muscle cell as *glycogen*. The source of the glucose, that is, blood glucose or muscle glycogen, is an important consideration in the metabolic response of the muscle cell to different intensities of exercise. This point will be discussed later in the chapter, but for now glucose oxidation will be considered in general terms.

Ultimately, all the glucose the muscle cell utilizes must come from the blood (Fig. 1–7). Whether it is stored as glycogen or immediately metabolized for ATP production, glucose enters the cell by facilitated diffusion and is phosphorylated, or "activated," to *glucose-6-phosphate* with expenditure of one ATP. The diffusion of glucose into muscle cells (as well as into most cell types in the body) is generally very slow. In fact, under most conditions it is necessary for the hormone *insulin* to be present in the blood for glucose to enter muscle cells in significant quantities. Interestingly, muscle contraction also stimulates glucose entry into muscle cells.

After entering the cell and being phosphorylated to glucose-6-phosphate, glucose is "trapped" in the muscle cell and cannot diffuse back into the blood. Muscle cells do not possess the enzyme necessary for converting glucose-6-phosphate back to glucose. In resting muscles, most of the glucose entering the cells is stored as glycogen, which is simply a polymer, or chain, of glucose molecules with branch points.

Glycolysis. When glucose is needed for ATP synthesis, glycogen is broken back down to glucose-6-phosphate, which is then oxidized in an enzyme pathway referred to as *glycolysis* (Fig. 1–7). In this pathway the glucose-6-phosphate is again phosphorylated and then split into two 3-carbon phosphate molecules. Each of these resulting triose phosphates is oxidized with the production of $NADH_2$. At two succeeding steps in glycolysis, substrate level phosphorylation of ADP occurs. The end products of glycolysis are two molecules of pyruvic acid. Also, during glycolysis of one molecule of glucose from glycogen, nine molecules of ATP are generated (Table 1–2).

Krebs Cycle. Pyruvic acid is completely oxidized in the mitochondrion to CO_2 and H_2O. Following the diffusion of pyruvic acid into the mitochondrion from the cytoplasm, it is oxidized by the *pyruvate dehydrogenase* enzyme complex (Fig. 1–7 and Table 1–2). Also, in the reactions catalyzed by this complex, a CO_2 is removed from each pyruvic acid molecule, and the resulting 2-carbon fragment is combined with CoA to form acetyl-CoA. As previously mentioned, acetyl-CoA is also the end product of β-oxidation of fatty acids (Fig. 1–6). The pathway for the oxidation of carbohydrate and fat is therefore the same from the point at which they are converted to acetyl-CoA. Acetyl-CoA formed from both fatty acids and glucose is fed into the Krebs cycle for complete oxidation (Fig. 1–7).

In summary, complete oxidation of one molecule of glucose derived from glycogen results in the production of 39 molecules of ATP (Table 1–2). As in fatty acid oxidation, about 40 per cent of the energy in the glucose molecule is captured in ATP. The remaining 60 per cent is given off as heat.

Effects of Training on Oxidative Enzymes

The various enzyme pathways in the muscle cell that are involved in oxidative phosphorylation are contained primarily in the mitochondria (except the glycolytic enzymes). One way of increasing the ability of the cell to produce ATP is to increase the number of mitochondria, and, hence, the quantities of the oxidative enzymes. This is precisely what occurs in muscle cells that are utilized during endurance training.

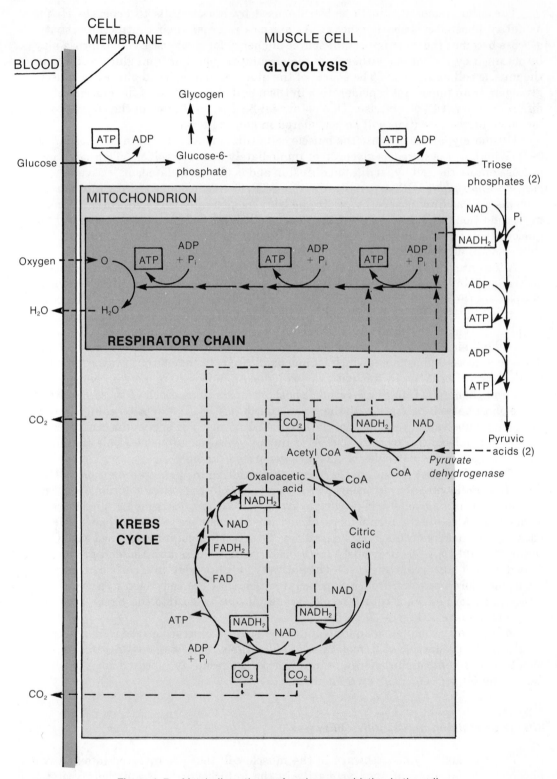

Figure 1–7. Metabolic pathways for glucose oxidation in the cell.

TABLE 1–2. ATP PRODUCTION FROM THE OXIDATION OF ONE MOLECULE OF GLUCOSE STORED AS GLYCOGEN

Enzyme Pathway	Method of Phosphorylation	Number of ATP Molecules Produced
Glycolysis	Respiratory chain oxidation of 2 $NADH_2$	6
	Substrate level phosphorylation	4
	ATP consumed	−1
Pyruvate dehydrogenase	Respiratory chain oxidation of 2 $NADH_2$	6
Krebs cycle	Respiratory chain oxidation of 6 $NADH_2$	18
	Respiratory chain oxidation of 2 $FADH_2$	4
	Substrate level phosphorylation	2
Total		39*

*Complete oxidation of one molecule of glucose obtained from the blood results in a net yield of 38 molecules of ATP because of the consumption of ATP in the step in which glucose is phosphorylated to glucose-6-phosphate (see Fig. 1–7). Furthermore, the value of 39 cannot technically be considered the net yield of ATP from oxidation of glucose from glycogen, since glycogen synthesis from glucose-6-phosphate requires expenditure of ATP. However, when the muscle becomes active and stored glycogen is broken down, the immediate "net" production of ATP is 39 per molecule of glucose.

In training for "aerobic" athletic events (e.g., distance running, swimming, or bicycling), the oxidative capacity of the muscles used in the particular exercise may increase by as much as three to four times. Accompanying this increase in mitochondrial density is an elevation in the number of capillaries supplying blood to the muscle fibers. Thus, endurance training increases the ability of the muscles to obtain blood during exercise and to use the delivered oxygen to resynthesize ATP.

On the other hand, training for strength events (e.g., weight lifting, shot putting, or discus throwing) does not stimulate an increase in mitochondria and capillarization in the active muscles. The effects of training on muscle will be discussed further in Chapter 2.

REGULATION OF OXIDATIVE PHOSPHORYLATION

The biochemical mechanisms that the cell uses to synthesize ATP from ADP and P_i — oxidative phosphorylation and substrate level phosphorylation — have now been discussed. It should be apparent that the ATP and ADP in the cell together constitute an "adenosine phosphate pool"; that is, the basic molecule exists in one or the other of these two forms.* Furthermore, it is reasonable to expect that the cell would attempt to maintain this "pool" primarily in the form of ATP so that energy would always be available to power its energy-dependent processes. On the other hand, it would be wasteful for the resting muscle cell to metabolize large quantities of fat and glucose when little ATP breakdown is occurring. In other words, it is desirable for the cell to carefully synchronize its metabolic processes and its energy requirements.

---

*In actuality, adenosine and adenosine monophosphate (AMP) also are present and play important roles in the cell. However, for this discussion, only the two forms ATP and ADP need be considered.

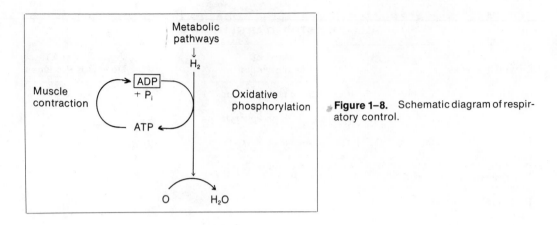

Figure 1-8. Schematic diagram of respiratory control.

This matching of production to need is called *respiratory control* (Fig. 1–8). Phosphorylation of ADP to ATP is "tightly coupled" to oxidation in the respiratory chain. This means that the transfer of H_2 cannot proceed in the chain unless ADP is available. Thus, it is only as ADP becomes available from ATP breakdown in the various energy-requiring processes in the cell that metabolism can proceed.

ANAEROBIC METABOLISM

To this point, the discussion has centered on the biochemical pathways that muscle cells use to maintain ATP levels when oxygen is available. It should be reemphasized that for oxidative phosphorylation to proceed, oxygen must be present in the mitochondrion to serve as the final hydrogen acceptor. When oxygen is not available in sufficient quantities, ADP rephosphorylation in the mitochondrion cannot keep pace with ATP breakdown. Under these conditions, maintenance of ATP levels in the cells must depend upon *anaerobic* (without oxygen) biochemical mechanisms.

The total ATP/ADP pool in the muscle cell is limited. In fact, the maximal amount of ATP present in the cell (about 5 micromoles per gram of muscle) is sufficient to power intensive muscular activity for only a fraction of a second. Therefore, the muscle needs some way to immediately resynthesize ATP from the ADP produced during contraction. This is accomplished through the reaction illustrated in Figure 1–9.

Creatine Phosphate

Creatine phosphate (CP) is a high-energy compound, like ATP, that is present in the muscle cell. Although CP cannot serve as the immediate energy source for muscle contraction, it can readily donate its high-energy phosphate to ADP. Thus, as ATP is

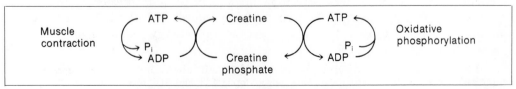

Figure 1-9. Phosphorylation of ADP by creatine phosphate.

broken down during contraction, it can be resynthesized immediately from the resulting ADP and the CP. However, again, the muscle cell contains only limited quantities of CP. There is about five times as much CP in the muscle cell as ATP, so the combined *phosphagen* (ATP and CP) stores in the muscle are sufficient to support intense muscular activity for a maximum of only 3 to 8 seconds.

As indicated in Figure 1–9, the creatine produced in the CP-ADP reaction is rephosphorylated to CP by ATP produced in the metabolic pathways discussed previously. Hence, the muscle cell ultimately depends upon oxidation to maintain its high-energy stores, even though it can support brief bursts of contractile activity with the ATP and CP reserves. As a matter of fact, much of our normal daily activity, as well as a variety of sporting events, consists of brief periods of intense muscular activity interspersed with longer periods of relative inactivity.

Anaerobic Glycolysis

Another important mechanism the muscle uses to produce ATP when oxygen supplies are inadequate is *anaerobic glycolysis* (Fig. 1–10). The substrate the muscle uses for anaerobic glycolysis is stored glycogen. The enzymes that catalyze the breakdown of glycogen in the muscle cell are "activated" by calcium ions (Ca++), as well as by several hormones (see Chapter 9). As will be discussed in Chapter 2, Ca++ serves as the "trigger" for muscle contraction, so it is convenient that it also activates glycogen mobilization in the muscle cell. The cell thus insures itself an immediate energy substrate supply when it begins to contract.

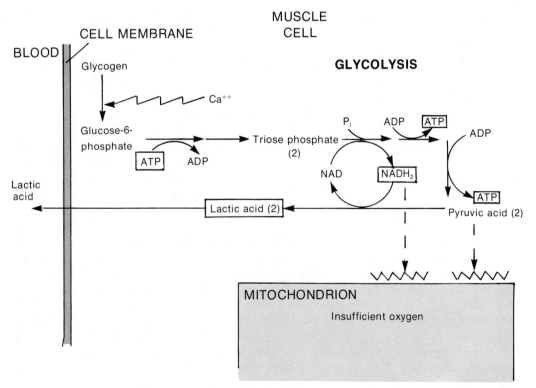

Figure 1–10. Anaerobic glycolysis in the muscle cell.

The glucose-6-phosphate resulting from glycogen breakdown is oxidized to two molecules of pyruvic acid in the pathway of glycolysis as previously described, with a "net" production of 3 ATP through substrate level phosphorylation (Fig. 1–10). It will be recalled that under aerobic conditions (1) the $NADH_2$ produced in glycolysis transfers its H_2 to the respiratory chain for oxidative phosphorylation; and (2) the pyruvic acid molecules enter the mitochondrion and are completely oxidized in the Krebs cycle (Fig. 1–7). However, when oxygen is not available, both these processes are blocked. Thus, under anaerobic conditions when $NADH_2$ cannot transfer its H_2, the NAD in the cell would exist in the reduced form and glycolysis would be inhibited at the enzymatic step in which NAD serves as coenzyme (Equation 3). To circumvent this problem, pyruvic acid can accept the H_2 from $NADH_2$, freeing NAD and forming lactic acid (Fig. 1–10).

Lactic acid production thus allows glycolysis to proceed when anaerobic conditions in the cell retard $NADH_2$ oxidation in the mitochondria. Although only three molecules of ATP are produced from the anaerobic glycolysis of one glucose molecule (compared with 39 during complete oxidation of the same molecule), this mechanism allows the muscle cell to phosphorylate ADP to ATP in the absence of oxygen. It should be pointed out that muscle cells do not undergo aerobic and anaerobic metabolism on an "either-or" basis. In a healthy individual, oxygen is always available to the muscle and there is always an aerobic component to muscle metabolism. The anaerobic component may best be thought of as being "added on" when the aerobic pathways cannot meet the cell's energy needs.

During anaerobic glycolysis, the concentration of lactic acid rises in the muscle cell. The elevated level of this weak acid lowers the pH of the cell (that is, it makes the cell fluids more acidic). The enzymes in the muscle cell are highly sensitive to pH, and as the pH is lowered, the catalytic rates of most enzymes decrease, diminishing the cell's ability to metabolize and produce ATP. Thus, the rate at which lactic acid can be produced in the muscle cell is self-limiting.

These detrimental effects of increased acidity in the cell are countered in two major ways. First, buffers in the cell, particularly the cell proteins, resist changes in pH; second, as the concentration of lactic acid rises in the cell, it freely diffuses out into the blood down its concentration gradient. When blood flow to an active muscle is adequate, anaerobic metabolism in the cells may continue for prolonged periods of time since lactic acid accumulation is prevented.

Several of the major fates of lactic acid after it enters the blood are illustrated in Figure 1–11. The lactic acid produced by anaerobic muscle cells can be utilized as a substrate for oxidation by other, aerobic, muscle cells in the body. These "aerobic" muscle cells may be cells that simply are less active (e.g., arm muscles during bicycling), or muscle cells that have more mitochondria and a more profuse capillary blood supply (see Chapter 2). On the other hand, lactic acid can be used by several tissues in the body, in particular the liver, to resynthesize glucose through an enzymatic process called *gluconeogenesis*.

It was previously indicated that endurance training increases muscular aerobic capacity. It might be expected that high-intensity training (e.g., "sprint" training), would similarly increase the levels of the enzymes involved in anaerobic glycolysis. The fact is that although such changes may occur, they are not of the magnitude of those observed in the oxidative enzymes with endurance training (two- to fourfold). The glycolytic enzymes exist in relatively high concentrations even in untrained muscle, and it appears that even intensive anaerobic training does not markedly increase their activities. However, the experimental evidence for changes in the glycolytic enzymes of human muscles with training is conflicting and awaits further clarification.

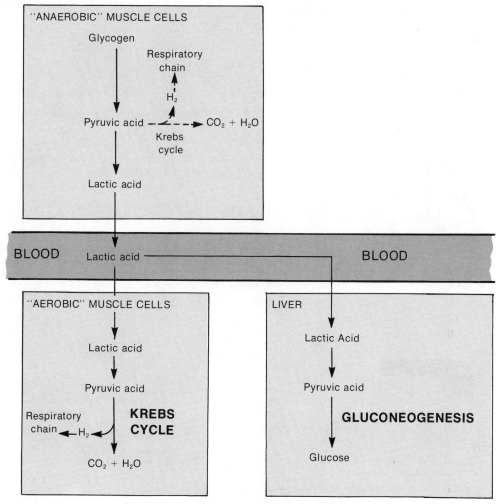

Figure 1–11. Lactic acid removal from the blood.

AEROBIC AND ANAEROBIC METABOLISM DURING EXERCISE

To clarify and to integrate the information that has been presented up to this point, it is helpful to consider the relationship between aerobic and anaerobic metabolism in several generalized exercise situations: (1) during moderately fast walking; (2) during jogging (e.g., at a speed that could be maintained for 15 to 30 minutes); and (3) during running (e.g., at a speed that could be maintained for about 5 minutes).

During walking, the whole-body energy requirements increase above the resting level (Fig. 1–12A). Although elevated heart rate and respiration rate, as well as various other factors, contribute to the increased energy requirements of the body, the primary reason for the elevation is the utilization of ATP by the active skeletal muscles to generate contractile tension. The diagram (Fig. 1–12A) indicates that after the first few minutes of exercise, aerobic metabolism accounts for 100 per cent of the whole-body power output. Why the "lag" in aerobic metabolism at the beginning of the exercise?

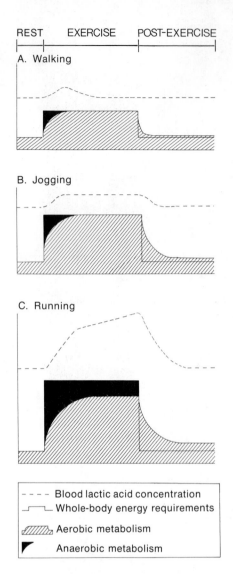

Figure 1–12. Relationship between whole-body power output and power input (anaerobic and aerobic) at rest and during five minutes of exercise at different intensities.

When the muscles first become active, blood flow to muscle is not sufficient to supply the increased oxygen needs for aerobic metabolism. Several minutes are required for the increased cardiac output (see Chapter 5) and the opening of the capillary beds in the muscles to supply the required oxygen. It is necessary for anaerobic mechanisms to make up the *oxygen deficit*. Although the precise temporal relationships among the anaerobic processes is difficult to ascertain, it is probable that during the first few moments of exercise the major anaerobic source of ATP is creatine phosphate. However, anaerobic glycolysis is initiated immediately and after the first few seconds is able to make up the aerobic deficit until the oxidative mechanisms become fully operative. It should be noted that a small rise in blood lactate may occur during the first minutes of low-intensity exercise, but that as exercise continues the blood level returns to the resting value.

During fast jogging (Fig. 1–12B) the energy requirements of the muscles are elevated above those during walking, and therefore the whole-body energy utilization is higher. However, after adjustments in blood flow, the jogger is able to meet whole-body energy needs aerobically, and aerobic metabolism equals the total power output. In this instance, though, the blood lactic acid concentration remains elevated during the exercise. The continued elevation in blood lactic acid concentration after the initial rise indicates that although the body as a whole is completely aerobic, some muscle cells are producing ATP anaerobically (Fig. 1–11). Thus, the level blood lactic acid concentration results from a balance between lactic acid production in some muscle cells and its oxidation in other muscle cells or other tissues.

Figure 1–12C illustrates the relationship between anaerobic and aerobic metabolism when the runner surpasses his maximal aerobic capacity ($\dot{V}_{O_2 max}$). Following circulatory adjustment, the energy requirements of the muscles still exceed what can be provided through oxidative phosphorylation. During this time, the blood lactic acid concentration continues to rise throughout exercise, for there is a net whole-body anaerobic component.

It is important to emphasize that the information contained in Figure 1–12 refers to whole-body metabolism, not to the changes that occur in a single muscle or individual muscle fiber. Thus, even though a person may be able to meet his total energy requirements aerobically (Fig. 1–12A and B), some muscle cells may be relying upon anaerobic glycolysis to meet their energy needs. Note also that the elevated aerobic metabolism continues following the period of exercise in all three cases (Fig. 1–12A, B, and C). This is referred to as the *oxygen debt,* and primarily represents the repayment of the deficit that occurred during the exercise.

REGULATION OF SUBSTRATE UTILIZATION IN MUSCLE CELLS

It has been pointed out several times in preceding sections that fatty acids normally constitute the "preferred" metabolic substrate in the muscle cell when oxygen is available to the cell. The subject of metabolic regulation is exceedingly complex (and not completely understood), but in the following discussion some general principles will be outlined that should help in understanding how substrate utilization in muscles is regulated.

So that the primary purpose of the various controls can be understood, an underlying "reason" for metabolic control should be presented. The principle upon which the description of the regulation of substrate utilization will be based is the *glucose-sparing effect.* In several vital tissues in the body, in particular the brain and other neural structures, glucose is the only substrate that can normally be metabolized for ATP production. Thus, through most of the 24-hour period when glucose is not entering the blood stream from the digestive tract, the body's metabolic strategy is to spare glucose for the vital glucose-dependent tissues through promoting fat oxidation in the other tissues (including muscle). This glucose-sparing effect will be discussed at greater length later in the chapter, but it is important that this underlying concept be understood before the regulation of substrate utilization in the muscles is considered.

Figure 1–13 illustrates a simplified scheme of metabolic control in a muscle cell. When blood flow to the muscle is adequate to provide oxygen and fatty acids, which freely diffuse into the cells, oxidation of the fatty acids tends to inhibit glucose metabolism. This is accomplished primarily through regulation of one of the enzymes in glycolysis — phosphofructokinase (PFK). When blood flow provides adequate oxygen and fatty acids, the cell is able to maintain relatively high levels of ATP. Also, as a result of the high rates of oxidative metabolism, concentrations of the Krebs cycle intermediates are elevated in the cell. One of these intermediates, citric acid, has an inhibitory effect on PFK, and when the concentration of this molecule increases in the cell during aerobic metabolism, glucose oxidation through glycolysis is retarded. This inhibitory effect is enhanced by high levels of ATP.

Blockage of the degradation of glucose in the glycolytic pathway at the PFK step has the effect of increasing the concentrations of the glycolytic intermediates above the reaction, including glucose-6-phosphate (Fig. 1–13). Elevated levels of glucose-6-phosphate in the cell in turn inhibit (1) the reaction in which glucose entering the cell is phosphorylated (which in turn inhibits glucose entry into the cell); and (2) the breakdown of glycogen. Thus, fatty acid metabolism in the cell has the overall effect of retarding glucose metabolism. However, when fatty acid oxidation cannot meet the muscle cell's energy needs, whether because of excessive energy expenditure in the muscle or because of inadequate blood flow, the inhibition on glucose metabolism is removed and glycolysis proceeds.

The values in Table 1–3 show that the muscles obtain increased amounts of fat during prolonged, moderately intense exercise. This is accomplished by (1) an elevation in the concentration of blood plasma fatty acids; and (2) an increase in the blood

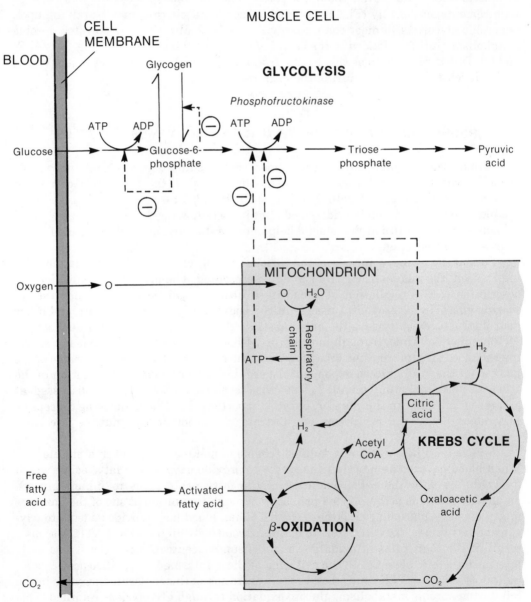

Figure 1–13. Inhibitory effects (⊖) of fatty acid oxidation on glycolysis in the muscle cell.

TABLE 1–3. FATTY ACID DELIVERY TO MUSCLE BY THE BLOOD AT REST AND DURING MODERATELY INTENSE EXERCISE

Variable	Rest	Exercise
Cardiac output (l/hr)	300	900
Muscle blood flow (l/kg/hr)	1.7	20.6
Blood fatty acid concentration (mg/l)	60	200
Fatty acids delivered to muscle (mg/kg/hr)	102	4120

flow to the muscle. Thus, in this particular exercise situation, the amount of fatty acid delivered to the muscle by the circulating blood per unit time increased about 70-fold from rest to exercise. Unlike glucose, which is maintained at fairly constant levels in the blood, the plasma fatty acid concentration may vary over a wide range. During prolonged exercise, the blood level may increase by three or four times (Table 1–3).

One of the major effects of training on skeletal muscles is an increased reliance on fatty acids as the substrate for ATP production during exercise. For example, if muscle substrate utilization is compared during running at the same speed before and after training, the muscles will generate a greater proportion of their ATP from fat than from carbohydrate after the training period. This results primarily from the increase of mitochondria in the trained muscle, which contain the enzymes for β-oxidation of fat, the Krebs cycle, and the respiratory chain. This transition to a greater reliance on fat for energy production has a glycogen-sparing effect and serves as an important adaptive mechanism for increasing the amount of time during which exercise can be performed at a given intensity.

CONTROL OF BLOOD PLASMA FATTY ACID CONCENTRATION

Fat is stored in the adipose tissue cells of the body in the form of *triglycerides*. A triglyceride molecule has a *glycerol* backbone with three fatty acids attached to it (Fig. 1–14). In Figure 1–14, all three fatty acids are palmitic acid molecules, but triglycerides may contain mixtures of the various fatty acids. The formation of triglyceride from *α-glycerophosphate* and fatty acids is called *esterification.** The degradation of triglyceride to glycerol and fatty acids is referred to as *lipolysis* (Fig. 1–14).

Esterification and lipolysis proceed simultaneously in fat cells, so that triglycerides are continuously being built up and broken down by separate enzyme systems. By affecting the balance between these two processes, the plasma fatty acid concentration can be finely regulated (Fig. 1–15). One of the major regulators of fatty acid release from fat cells is the availability of glucose to the cell. For fatty acids to be reesterified to triglyceride, α-glycerophosphate must be made available to the cell. The source of α-glycerophosphate is glucose; α-glycerophosphate is produced from one of the intermediates in glycolysis (dihydroxyacetone phosphate). When glucose entry into the fat cell is low, α-glycerophosphate levels fall and reesterification of triglycerides declines. Therefore, fatty acid levels increase in the fat cell from continued lipolysis, increased amounts of fatty acids diffuse into the blood down their concentration gradient, and the plasma concentration of fatty acids is elevated.

---

*An ester is formed when water is removed during bond formation between an alcohol and an acid.

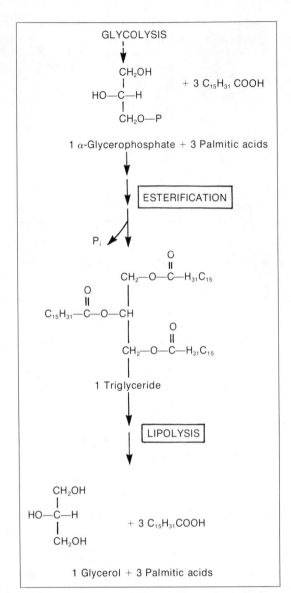

Figure 1–14. Esterification and lipolysis of triglyceride (fat).

Also, as indicated in Figure 1–15, glucose entering the fat cell can be converted to fatty acids, which in turn can be esterified for storage as fat. Thus, both of the precursors for triglyceride synthesis (i.e., α-glycerophosphate and fatty acids) can be produced by fat cells from glucose. Note that the fat cell cannot convert the glycerol released during lipolysis to α-glycerophosphate. The glycerol formed during lipolysis in the fat cell diffuses into the blood, and most of it is carried to the liver where it is metabolized.

Included in Figure 1–15 are several of the hormones that affect fatty acid mobilization. Insulin is necessary for glucose to enter the fat cell and therefore is important in promoting esterification, while several other hormones are effective in increasing fat mobilization. These hormonal effects will be discussed at greater length in Chapter 9. However, it should be pointed out that during exercise insulin levels in the blood decrease, whereas the plasma concentrations of epinephrine, norepinephrine, glucagon, and growth hormone (as well as other lipolytic hormones) increase. Thus, hormonal alterations during exercise favor lipolysis and have the effect of mobilizing fatty acids for the muscles to oxidize.

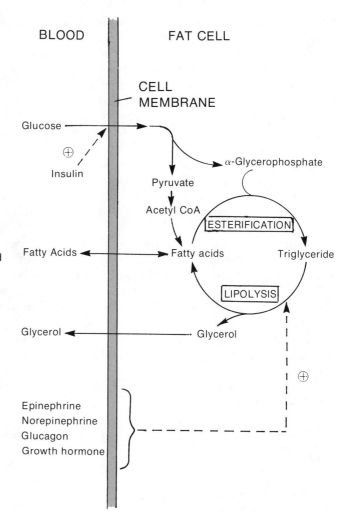

Figure 1–15. Regulation of fatty acid release from the fat cell.

REGULATION OF WHOLE-BODY METABOLISM

In the preceding sections, reference was made to the importance of the hormone insulin in the regulation of substrate utilization in the body. To conclude the discussion of metabolism, it is appropriate to summarize the overall effects of insulin on the body's metabolism and the major factors that control the release of insulin into the blood.

Two general metabolic conditions in the body can be described: (1) the *absorptive state,* during which glucose (from starches and sugar), amino acids (from protein), and fatty acids (from triglycerides) are being absorbed into the blood stream from the digestive system following a meal; and (2) the *postabsorptive state,* in which nutritive substrates are not entering the blood from the digestive system and energy must be supplied from the body stores.

During the absorptive state, in which digested food is being absorbed into the blood, the overall metabolism of the body is directed primarily toward storage of the absorbed energy substrates (i.e., glucose and fat) (Fig. 1–16). The major regulator of these "storage processes" is insulin. When the glucose concentration in the blood is elevated following ingestion of dietary carbohydrate, cells in the pancreas (β-cells) are stimulated to release insulin into the blood stream.* Insulin has a variety of effects on many tissues, but one of its major roles is to increase glucose diffusion into muscle and fat cells (Fig. 1–16). The overall effect of insulin on muscle cells is to stimulate glycogen production, whereas in fat cells it stimulates triglyceride synthesis. Also, when blood glucose levels are elevated during the absorptive state, the liver stores glucose as glycogen and converts excess amounts of glucose to fatty acids, which can then be stored as triglycerides in the adipose tissue. Insulin also facilitates amino acid uptake by muscle cells and thus stimulates protein synthesis. However, excessive amounts of amino acids in the diet are simply converted by the liver to fat, which is subsequently stored in the adipose tissue.

Thus, during the absorptive state, which generally exists for several hours following the consumption of a meal, the body stores the ingested foods as carbohydrate (glycogen) or fat (triglycerides), with excess amounts of carbohydrate and protein being converted to fat.

When digested foodstuffs are not entering the blood stream from the small intestine, the metabolic condition of the body is referred to as the postabsorptive state (Fig. 1–17). In the postabsorptive state, blood glucose levels begin to fall, which removes the stimulus for insulin release by the pancreas. When the insulin concentration in the blood falls, glucose entry into muscle and fat cells declines. Diminished glucose entry into fat cells results in a net release of fatty acids from the adipose tissue, and the plasma fatty acid concentration rises. As mentioned previously, when fatty acids are available to muscle cells, the cells tend to metabolize fats, and glucose metabolism is retarded.

Several of the tissues in the body, particularly nerve tissue, use only glucose in their metabolism under normal conditions (although during prolonged starvation the

---

*Insulin release by the pancreas is also stimulated by the presence of glucose and amino acids in the small intestine and by elevated amino acid levels in the blood.

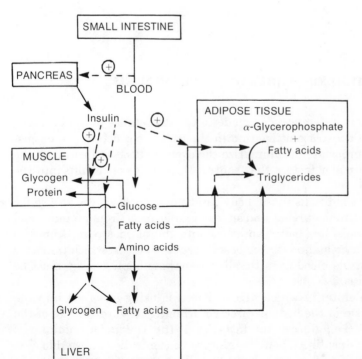

Figure 1–16. Substrate storage in the absorptive state.

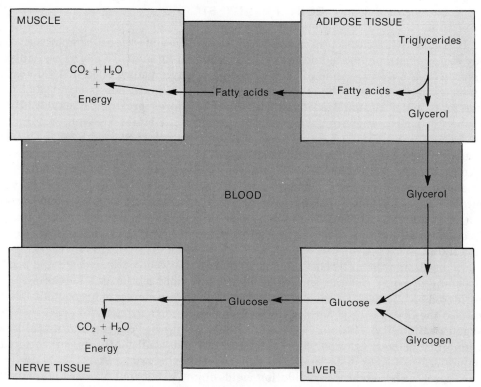

Figure 1–17. Substrate mobilization in the postabsorptive state.

brain can adapt to use other substrates). Insulin is not necessary for glucose diffusion into brain tissue. Thus, the metabolic changes that take place in the postabsorptive state are designed to insure a constant supply of glucose for these vital tissues. Under most circumstances, the blood glucose concentration does not decline much below 1 gram per liter. In the postabsorptive state, it is maintained primarily by glucose production and release from liver glycogen under normal dietary conditions (i.e., three meals per day). The liver can also use various substances, including the glycerol resulting from lipolysis in the adipose tissue, to synthesize glucose (gluconeogenesis). Lactic acid produced during muscular exercise may also be used by the liver to resynthesize glucose.

In summary, during the postabsorptive state, blood glucose is "spared" for nerve tissue because other tissues, including muscle, convert primarily to fat metabolism. As long as there is adequate blood flow to muscle to provide oxygen and fatty acids, the muscle will produce ATP primarily from energy derived from fat. However, as muscles become progressively more active, they increase their reliance on glucose.

In Chapter 9 the effects of hormones during exercise will be covered in detail. It may already be apparent, however, that the whole-body metabolism during exercise is similar to that in the postabsorptive state. During exercise, plasma insulin levels decline and the concentrations of several hormones that stimulate lipolysis are elevated. Thus, the body mobilizes fat during exercise, and the overall metabolic effect is to promote fatty acid oxidation and "spare" glucose. As the intensity of the exercise increases, however, it becomes increasingly necessary to depend upon stored glycogen when fatty acid oxidation cannot provide the required ATP to support the contractile activity.

BODY ENERGY STORES

In Table 1–4, some representative values are presented for a comparison of the body stores of carbohydrate and fat in an average 70-kg man. To put these figures in perspective, the average man of this body weight would utilize 3000 to 4000 kcal per day for normal activity. The energy cost of running a marathon is about 3000 kcal. Therefore, under normal circumstances, the fat stores provide an essentially inexhaustible source of energy, whereas the carbohydrate stores are limited.

As shown in Table 1–4, every gram of stored fat in the body contains about 9 kcal of energy that can be released during oxidation. On the other hand, one gram of glycogen contains only about 4 kcal of energy. When glucose is stored as glycogen it is associated with water, or is *hydrated,* which is not the case for fat. When the water content of glycogen is included, fat is about five times more efficient as an energy store on a per unit weight basis. Thus, for a man to store the same amount of energy in glycogen instead of fat would require an increase in body weight from 70 kg to more than 120 kg.

In discussing the differences in energy storage between carbohydrate and fat, it is important to point out the similarity in energy yield of the two substrates when considered on the basis of oxygen consumed. It has been indicated repeatedly that in exercise the factor that generally limits the muscle cell's capacity to produce ATP is oxygen availability. Therefore, given a certain amount of oxygen and an unlimited availability of both fat and glucose, which can most efficiently be metabolized to produce ATP? Reference to Table 1–5 indicates that the two substrates are similar in this respect, although glucose oxidation yields slightly more energy per liter of oxygen consumed.

Table 1–5 also includes the *respiratory quotients* (RQ) for oxidation of glucose and fat. The RQ is calculated from the ratio of CO_2 produced during metabolism to O_2 consumed:

$$RQ = \frac{CO_2 \text{ produced}}{O_2 \text{ consumed}} \tag{4}$$

For example, oxidation of glucose is given in the following equation:

$$C_6H_{12}O_6 + 6\,O_2 \longrightarrow 6\,CO_2 + 6\,H_2O \tag{5}$$

Therefore, the RQ for glucose oxidation is:

$$RQ = \frac{6\,CO_2}{6\,O_2} = 1.00 \tag{6}$$

TABLE 1–4. BODY STORES OF CARBOHYDRATE AND FAT IN AN AVERAGE 70 KG MAN

Energy Source	Energy Equivalent	Tissue Concentration	Tissue Mass	Energy Stored
Muscle glycogen	4 kcal/gm	18 gm/kg	28 kg	2,016 kcal
Liver glycogen	4 kcal/gm	70 gm/kg	2 kg	560 kcal
Blood glucose	4 kcal/gm	1 gm/l	5 liters	20 kcal
Total carbohydrate stores				2,596 kcal
Adipose tissue triglycerides	9 kcal/gm	900 gm/kg	10 kg	81,000 kcal
Muscle triglycerides	9 kcal/gm	9 gm/kg	28 kg	2,268 kcal
Liver triglycerides	9 kcal/gm	25 gm/kg	2 kg	450 kcal
Blood fatty acids and triglycerides	9 kcal/gm	1 gm/l	5 l	45 kcal
Total fat stores				83,763 kcal

TABLE 1–5.   ENERGY EQUIVALENTS OF CARBOHYDRATE AND FAT OXIDATION

| Substrate | O_2 Required to Oxidize 1 gm (liters) | Produced in Oxidation of 1 gm | | RQ | Energy Produced per Liter of O_2 Consumed (kcal) |
		CO_2 (LITERS)	ENERGY (KCAL)		
Glucose	0.829	0.829	4	1.00	4.83
Fat	2.013	1.431	9	0.71	4.47

As indicated in Table 1–5, the RQ for fat oxidation is about 0.70. Ideally, the difference in RQ for carbohydrate and fat may be utilized to determine the type of substrate the body is metabolizing, since the O_2 consumed ($\dot{V}_{O_2}$) and CO_2 produced are relatively easy to measure. When this measurement is done for the whole body, the ratio is referred to as the *respiratory exchange ratio* (RER). The problem with using RER to precisely estimate substrate utilization is that the amount of CO_2 expired is dependent upon a number of factors other than the type of substrate metabolized, including ventilation rate and body fluid pH — variables that are affected by exercise. These factors will be discussed in greater detail in Chapter 4.

SUMMARY

Muscular contraction is powered by energy released from the splitting of ATP to ADP and P_i. Since the muscle stores of ATP are small, it is necessary for the cells to be able to rapidly resynthesize ATP to support contractile activity lasting longer than several seconds. The muscle produces most of its ATP in the mitochondria through oxidative phosphorylation in the respiratory chain. This process requires oxygen; the production of ATP when oxygen is available is referred to as aerobic metabolism.

The hydrogen atoms used by the muscle cell for oxidative phosphorylation are obtained primarily from fatty acids and glucose. At rest and during low to moderate exercise, fatty acids are the major metabolic substrates in the muscle. They diffuse into the cell from the circulating blood and are broken down to produce hydrogen atoms in β-oxidation and the Krebs cycle. With increasing exercise intensities, glucose becomes more important as the hydrogen source. Glucose is obtained from the blood but may be stored as glycogen in the muscle cell for use when blood flow is impeded during intense muscular activity. Glucose is also broken down in two metabolic pathways: glycolysis and the Krebs cycle.

During periods when oxygen is limited and the cell cannot meet its energy needs aerobically, it may resynthesize ATP through several anaerobic mechanisms. Creatine phosphate donates its high-energy phosphate to ADP to resynthesize ATP, and ATP can be generated by anaerobic glycolysis with production of lactic acid. Muscle cells "attempt" to produce ATP aerobically; the anaerobic mechanisms allow the cells to go beyond their immediate aerobic potential to meet their energy needs

When fatty acids and oxygen are available to the muscle cell, fatty acids are used as a substrate in preference to glucose. This serves as a glucose-sparing device so that the limited carbohydrate stores in the body may be saved for nerve tissue, which cannot metabolize fat. Whole-body metabolism may be understood in terms of two general conditions, the absorptive state and the postabsorptive state, which are regulated primarily by the hormone insulin. During the absorptive state, nutritive substances absorbed from the digestive tract are stored as glycogen or triglycerides; during the postabsorptive state the stored substrates are mobilized for energy production in the cells.

STUDY QUESTIONS

1. What is the major energy-requiring process in muscle cells, and what constitutes the immediate energy source for the process?

2. Oxidative phosphorylation is the major means by which the muscle cell produces ATP. What is meant by the term? Where in the cell does the process occur? In your answer you should state the specific function of the respiratory chain.

3. How do NAD and FAD function in the cell?

4. What are the two major sources of hydrogen in the muscle cell for oxidative phosphorylation?

5. Describe the major pathways involved in the oxidation of fatty acids, and give the primary function(s) of each of the pathways.

6. Describe the major pathways in glucose oxidation, and give the functions of each of the pathways.

7. Explain what is meant by respiratory control. Why is this concept important in understanding the regulation of metabolism in the muscle cell?

8. What is meant by "anaerobic metabolism" and when is it important in the muscle cell?

9. Why is anaerobic ATP production less desirable than aerobic energy production in the metabolic economy of the cell?

10. What is the fate of the lactic acid formed in the muscle cell during anaerobic glycolysis?

11. Explain the relationship between aerobic and anaerobic metabolism during low-intensity and high-intensity exercise.

12. Explain what is meant by the statement "Muscles 'prefer' to use fatty acids for their energy needs." Explain how this is accomplished in the muscle cell.

13. Explain how fatty acid release from the adipose tissue is regulated, and give the effects of this control on fatty acid concentration in the blood plasma.

14. Explain the major metabolic strategies of the body during the absorptive and postabsorptive states.

15. What is the similarity in whole-body metabolism between the exercise situation and the postabsorptive state?

FURTHER READINGS

Armstrong, R. B.: Energy release in the extrafusal muscle fiber. *In* Knuttgen, H, G. (ed.): *Neuromuscular Mechanisms for Therapeutic and Conditioning Exercise.* Baltimore, University Park Press, 1976, pp. 55–77.

Gollnick, P. D., and Hermansen, L.: Biochemical adaptations to exercise: anaerobic metabolism. *In* Wilmore, J. H. (ed.): *Exercise and Sports Sciences Review,* Vol. 1. New York, Academic Press, 1973, pp. 1–43.

Holloszy, J. O.: Biochemical adaptations to exercise: aerobic metabolism. *In* Wilmore, J. H. (ed.): *Exercise and Sports Sciences Reviews,* Vol. 1. New York, Academic Press, 1973, pp. 45–71.

Lehninger, A. L.: *Biochemistry,* 2nd ed. New York, Worth Publishers, 1975.

Milvy, P. (ed.): The marathon: Physiological, medical, epidemiological, and psychological studies. Ann. N.Y. Acad. Sci. *301,* 1977.

Newsholme, E. A., and Start, C.: *Regulation in Metabolism.* London, John Wiley and Sons, 1973.

Pernow, B., and Saltin, B. (eds.): *Muscle Metabolism During Exercise.* New York, Plenum Press, 1971.

2

SKELETAL MUSCLE PHYSIOLOGY

ROBERT B. ARMSTRONG, Ph.D.

If one were asked to identify the basic body tissue in the science of physical exercise, the reply would most certainly be "muscle." Exercise physiology is the study of the acute and chronic alterations in bodily function that result from physical activity, and it is the muscular system that provides the basic ingredient of the activity — *movement*. All aspects of exercise physiology are therefore either directly or indirectly related to what the muscles are doing, and an understanding of how muscles work is essential for an appreciation of exercise physiology and sports medicine as a whole.

This chapter presents a general outline of muscle function and summarizes the structural and physiological bases that permit muscles to behave in their characteristic fashion.

WHAT MUSCLES DO

A total of about 217 pairs of skeletal muscles make up 40 to 45 per cent of the body weight in man. Although muscles display an amazing diversity of size, shape, and position in relation to the joints, they all have the same basic function: to develop contractile tension, or force, that tends to draw the ends of the muscle toward its center. Another way of stating the function of muscles is to say that they pull.

To illustrate the effects of muscle contraction, consider the calf muscle group in the leg, which is composed of the gastrocnemius and soleus muscles (Fig. 2–1). These two muscles have several individual actions at the knee and ankle joint, respectively, but one of their major group functions is to *extend* (plantar flex) the foot at the ankle. This is an essential muscular action in a wide variety of sporting events, for it provides a major portion of the thrust in the "take-off" phase of walking, running, and jumping.

The action of these muscles can be easily demonstrated by (1) standing in an upright position with the knees straight and the heels on the ground, (2) slowly rising on the toes to the highest attainable elevation, (3) maintaining that position for a few moments, then (4) slowly lowering the heels until the feet are again flat on the floor. Analysis of this relatively simple movement tells a great deal about what muscles do.

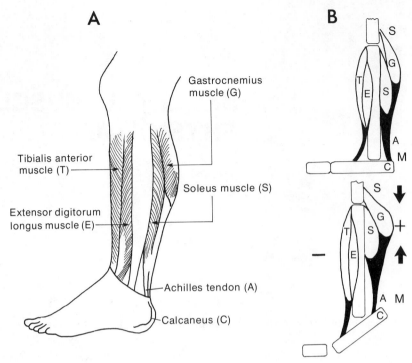

Figure 2–1. Muscles that extend the foot at the ankle.

Coordination of Muscles and Muscle Groups

It is important first to realize that although this discussion will deal only with the activity of the gastrocnemius and soleus muscles, body movements require the coordinated contraction and relaxation of large numbers of muscles and muscle groups. During the contraction of the calf muscles to elevate the heels, it is necessary for the antagonistic muscles (e.g., the tibialis anterior and extensor digitorum longus muscles) to undergo relative relaxations (Fig. 2–1). *Antagonists* are muscles that have an opposing action on the joint in question (in this case the ankle).

Simultaneously, synergistic muscles increase their contractile activity. *Synergists* are muscles that help, or have the same action on the joint. Examples of muscles synergistic to the gastrocnemius and soleus muscles in extension of the foot are the flexor hallucis longus, flexor digitorum longus, and plantaris muscles.

While the most obvious changes in muscular activity are noted in the muscles affecting the ankle when the heels are raised, it is necessary for all the body muscles involved in maintaining posture to adjust to the shift in the center of gravity that occurs during the movement; in fact, it will be noted in performing this exercise that initiation of the action includes a forward shift of the body, which requires the coordinated participation of a number of different muscles. Thus, most muscular activities require a highly coordinated effort involving a variety of muscular groups located at many joints. The muscular activity required in the spin and delivery in the discus throw is an example of the tremendous complexity this coordination may achieve.

Types of Muscular Contraction

The second thing that should be noted in the exercise described is that several different types of contraction are necessary to complete the motion. These may be referred to as (1) *shortening contractions,* (2) *isometric contractions,* and (3) *lengthening contractions.*

Shortening (Concentric) Contractions.   The first phase of the described movement involves the elevation of the heels off the floor, which results from extension of the foot at the ankle (Fig. 2–1*B*). As indicated before, this action at the ankle results from increased contractile tension in the gastrocnemius and soleus muscles, which pulls on the tendons that attach the muscles to the bones. In this example, the *origins* of the muscles (i.e., the more stable bony attachments) are located proximally* on either side of the knee. The gastrocnemius muscle attaches to the femur and the soleus muscle to the tibia and fibula. The *insertion* is the attachment to the more movable, distal† part, the heel bone (calcaneus), through the Achilles tendon (tendocalcaneus).

Points *S* and *M* in Figure 2–1B represent the respective stable and moveable attachments of the muscles. As the muscles develop increased contractile force, the more moveable of the connections (in this case the heel) is pulled toward the more stable connection.‡ As the heel is raised, the gastrocnemius and soleus muscles shorten during tension development. Hence, the contraction is called a *shortening contraction.*

Isometric (Static) Contractions.   Once the heels are elevated off the ground, a fairly stable, raised position can be maintained for a period of time. At this point, the gastrocnemius and soleus muscles develop contractile forces of magnitudes similar to those required during the shortening phase. However, the muscles are now maintaining the same lengths. Hence, the term "isometric" (*iso:* equal + *metric:* measure) is applied to this type of contraction.

Lengthening (Eccentric) Contractions.   When raising the heels off the ground, it is necessary to elevate the body's mass against the force of gravity. It might seem that simple relaxation of the calf muscles would result in a return of the body, and the heels, to the original position. Although this assumption is essentially correct, it tends to overlook the important role of lengthening contractions in muscular movement.

Perform the heel-raising exercise again. After elevating the heels, try to quickly and completely relax the muscles; the heels should "crash" to the floor. The preferred way of returning to the original position is for the calf muscles to resist the descent of the heels to the floor. This resistance is a lengthening contraction. Although the muscles generate contractile tension during this process, they are actually increasing their length. When the heels are slowly lowered to the floor, the forces developed by the gastrocnemius and soleus muscles are necessarily similar in magnitude to those generated during the shortening and isometric phases of the cycle.

In summary, shortening contractions result when the tension generated by active muscles is greater than the resistance, or load, so that the bony connections of the muscles are drawn toward one another. Isometric contractions occur when active contractile tension is equivalent to the resistance, or load, such that the distance between the bony attachments remains constant. Lengthening contractions result when the resistive load is greater than the generated contractile tension, causing the distance between the bony attachments to increase. It is important to remember that regardless of the type of contraction, the tension generated by the muscle tends to cause the muscle to shorten; hence, the muscles *pull* when they contract.

Several examples of the different types of muscle contraction used in daily activities may help in understanding their significance. As mentioned before, during the

---

*Nearer to the body.

†Farther from the body.

‡It should be pointed out that, under different conditions, the heel may serve as the more stable connection and the proximal attachments as the more movable.

take-off phase in jumping and running, the calf muscles perform an explosive shortening contraction immediately before the foot leaves the ground. This contraction provides the final phase of the muscular thrust that propels the body into the air.

Immediately before contacting the floor during the flight phase of a jump, these
same muscles undergo a shortening contraction to extend the ankle. They continue to
contract as the toes strike the floor. However, as the heels descend, the calf muscle
group generates tension while lengthening. The importance of this decelerating action
of the muscles can be appreciated by allowing oneself to land flat-footed after a fall.

The muscles function similarly during running; that is, they contract just before
the foot strikes the ground and perform a lengthening contraction after the toes touch
to decelerate the limb. In fact, during running most of the leg muscles perform both
shortening and lengthening contractions at various phases of the stride, as well as
brief isometric contractions at the end points.

HOW MUSCLES WORK

In talking about how muscles work, individual whole muscles, single muscle cells
within the muscles, contractile strands within muscle cells, and single contractile
proteins within the strands must be considered, and it is easy for the beginning
student to become somewhat confused by the spectrum of structural and functional
levels that are involved. The best way to keep one's bearings is to simply remember that
when these various levels are all put together their combined effect is to enable the
muscle to *pull*.

Like other organs in the body, muscles are composed of a number of different types
of tissue. Even an elementary comprehension of muscle physiology requires an appreciation of how these tissues interact, for their design is coordinated to contribute to the
basic contractile function of the muscle. The muscle organ possesses four basic components: (1) *muscle tissue,* composed of muscle cells; (2) *connective tissue;* (3) *nerve tissue;*
and (4) *vascular tissue,* composed of the blood vessels in the muscle.

Muscle Tissue

The major proportion (>90 per cent) of the muscle organ consists of muscle cells,
which have the specific function of producing contractile force. The other tissues in the
muscle play supportive or regulative roles. As illustrated in Figure 2–2A and B,
muscle cells are typically long, slender, multinucleated cells that lie somewhat parallel to the long axis of the muscle. Because of their geometry, muscle cells are referred
to as *muscle fibers.* Like whole muscles, when individual muscle fibers contract, the
tension developed tends to shorten the fibers, i.e., pull the ends toward the center.

Muscle Fiber Ultrastructure.   The basic structural and functional component
of the muscle fiber is the *myofibril* (Fig. 2–2C and D). This subcellular structure forms
the "contractile strand" of the cell. Each muscle fiber is packed with hundreds of
myofibrils that lie parallel to each other and to the long axis of the fiber.

The myofibrils consist of repeating individual contractile units called *sarcomeres,*
which are aligned end to end like links in a chain (Fig. 2–2D and E.). Each sarcomere
can individually develop contractile tension; when all sarcomeres within a muscle
fiber contract simultaneously, measurable pulling force is generated by the fiber as a
whole.

Skeletal muscles are sometimes called *striated muscles* because of the microscopic
light and dark banding patterns imparted to the muscle fibers by the sarcomeres (Fig.
2–2C and D). As illustrated in the electron micrograph in Figure 2–3, the sarcomeres

SKELETAL MUSCLE

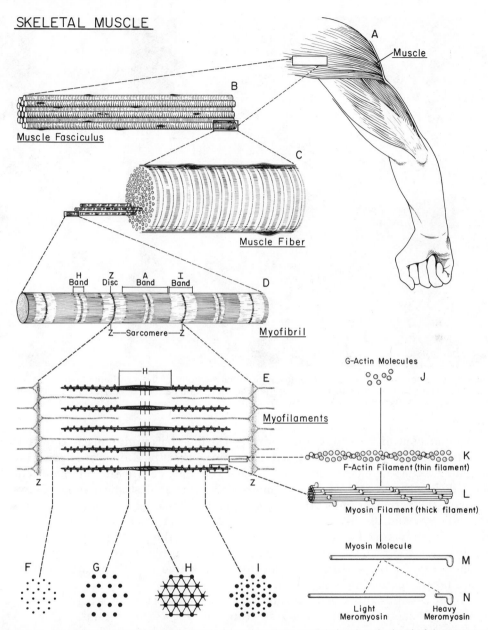

Figure 2–2. Organization of a skeletal muscle from the whole muscle level to the level of the contractile proteins. F, G, H, and I are cross sections of sarcomere taken from different levels. (From Bloom W., and Fawcett D. W.: *A Textbook of Histology.* Philadelphia, W. B. Saunders Company, 1975.)

of adjacent myofibrils are aligned so that the bands are continuous throughout the muscle fiber. The alternating dark and light bands are termed A (anisotropic) and I (isotropic) bands, respectively, and are a consequence of the different densities of the protein filaments that are present in the band regions.

Sarcomeres are delimited by the *Z lines* (Ger. *zwischen*: between). Extending toward the center of the sarcomere from each Z line are the *thin filaments* (Fig. 2–2K). These filaments form a hexagonal pattern around the *thick filaments* (Fig. 2–2L), which are situated in the center of the sarcomere (Fig. 2E, F, G, and I). It should be remembered that the myofibril and the sarcomeres within the myofibril exist in three dimensions.

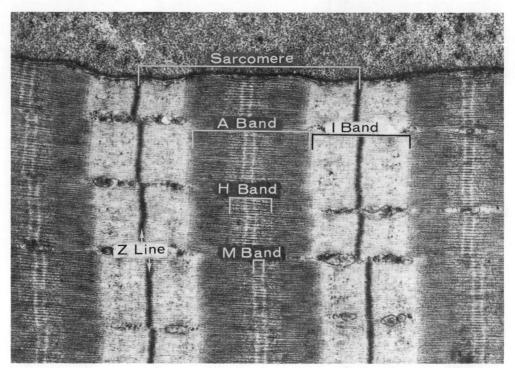

Figure 2–3. Electron micrograph showing longitudinal sections of five myofibrils labelled to indicate the various bands in relaxed skeletal muscle. (From Bloom W., and Fawcett D. W.: *A Textbook of Histology.* Philadelphia, W. B. Saunders Company, 1975.)

Mechanism of Muscle Contraction. During shortening muscle contractions, the thin filaments slide past the thick filaments so that the Z lines are drawn toward the center of the sarcomere (Fig. 2–4). Neither the thick nor the thin filaments change length during the process, so the sarcomere shortens in a telescopic manner. Conversely, during relaxation, or in lengthening contractions, the Z lines are drawn apart by an external force and the filaments slide past one another in the opposite direction. It should be reemphasized that in all types of contraction, (i.e., shortening, isometric, and lengthening), the tendency is for the Z lines to be drawn toward the center of the sarcomere, or for the sarcomere to shorten. The active force generated by the sarcomere favors shortening.

Figure 2–4 illustrates another important principle. As the three sarcomeres shorten, their diameters increase, demonstrating the *isovolumetric* relationship that is maintained by the myofibrils during shortening and lengthening. This phenomenon is obvious even at the gross muscle level. During shortening contractions, the muscle "bulges" because the same muscle volume must be maintained even though the organ has assumed a shorter length.

Protein Composition of the Thick and Thin Filaments. The exact mechanism that the sarcomere uses to generate force to pull the thin filaments past the thick filaments is not known. However, enough experimental evidence is available for muscle physiologists and biochemists to develop useful theories to explain the events. The current theories of muscle contraction take into account the properties of the molecules that form the thick and thin filaments.

The primary constituent of the thick filament is *myosin,* which is a spoon-shaped protein molecule (Fig. 2–2*M* and *N*). The "handles" (light meromyosin) of the myosin molecules form the body of the thick filament, while the "heads" (heavy meromyosin) of the molecules protrude from the filament shaft at regular intervals. These head

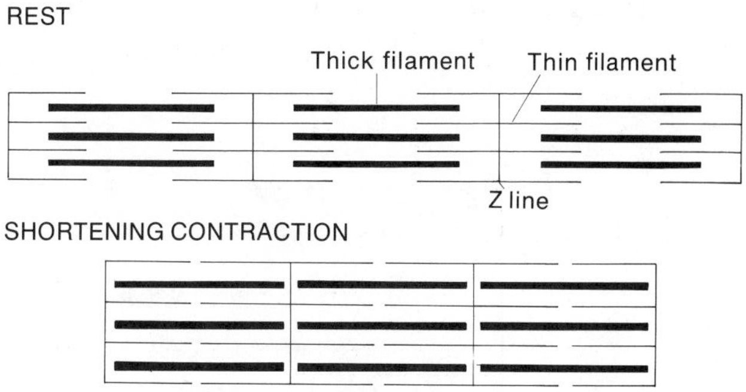

REST

Figure 2–4. Schematic illustration of three sarcomeres in a myofibril at rest and during a shortening contraction.

portions are called *cross-bridges* and possess several chemical properties that indicate that they are a basic component of the contractile system: (1) they contain an enzyme, *myosin ATPase,* that catalyzes the reaction in which ATP is hydrolyzed to ADP and P_i, releasing energy to power contraction; and (2) they have a high affinity, or attraction, for *actin,* which is the major constituent of the thin filament.

The thin filament has three major protein molecules: (1) actin, (2) *troponin,* and (3) *tropomyosin.* These exist in a numerical ratio of 7:1:1; that is, for each seven actin molecules there is one troponin and one tropomyosin molecule. Two interwoven chains of actin molecules form the backbone of the thin filament (Fig. 2–2*J* and *K* and Fig. 2–5*B*), and the other two proteins are distributed along the length of the strand (Fig. 2–5*B*).

Suggested Mechanism for Tension Development.   Actin molecules readily bind to the myosin cross-bridges under the right conditions. In resting muscle, the binding of actin and myosin is prevented by the other two major proteins in the thin filament, troponin and tropomyosin. In their resting conformational states, the troponin and tropomyosin inhibit the interaction between myosin and actin. The trigger that the muscle cell uses to remove this inhibition is *calcium ion* (Ca^{++}). When Ca^{++} binds with a troponin molecule, the actin molecules with which it is associated through tropomyosin are free to bind with myosin (Fig. 2–5*C*).

After actin and myosin bind, the ATPase enzyme — located on the myosin cross-bridge — *hydrolyzes* (splits) ATP to provide the required energy, and the cross-bridge in some way pulls on the thin filament, tending to draw it toward the center of the sarcomere (Fig. 2–5*D*). It is this process in muscle contraction that requires energy in the form of ATP, and during heavy exercise ATP must be resynthesized rapidly to support the elevated cross-bridge activity. It should be reemphasized here that the exact mechanism by which the thin filaments are pulled past the thick filaments has not been experimentally proved.

Within each sarcomere there are thousands of possible interaction sites between the myosin cross-bridges and the actin molecules of the thin filament. Although muscle contraction is initiated by increasing the concentration of Ca^{++} in the microenvironment of the myofibril, thereby releasing the inhibition on the myosin-actin interaction exerted by the troponin-tropomyosin complex, there is always some Ca^{++} present in the myofibril. Thus, even during "rest," some cross-bridges will be active, and some contractile tension will be generated by the sarcomere.

Control of Ca^{++} Concentration.   We have seen that the cellular event that triggers muscle contraction is the provision of Ca^{++} to the myofibril, which in turn removes the inhibitory influence that troponin and tropomyosin exert on the contractile process. It is obvious that the cell requires a means for regulating the Ca^{++} concentration in the microenvironment of the myofibril. This role is filled by the *sarcoplasmic reticulum* (SR).

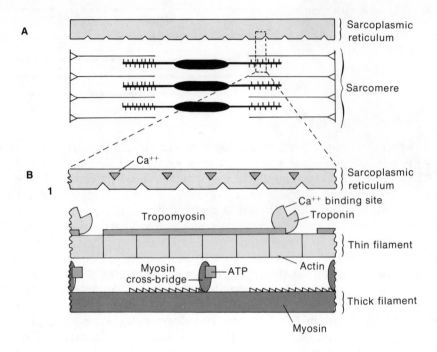

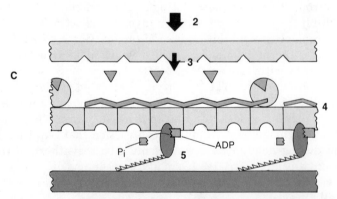

Figure 2–5. Schematic representation of the process of excitation-contraction of skeletal muscle. The summary of events in excitation-contraction is as follows.

1. *A* and *B*, During rest, the Ca^{++} is stored in the sarcoplasmic reticulum; the myosin cross-bridge is charged with ATP; and the troponin-tropomyosin system inhibits interaction between the myosin cross-bridge and the actin.

2. *C*, The action potential delivered to the muscle fiber by the alpha-motoneuron is transmitted throughout the fiber by the sarcolemma and transverse tubules.

3. *C*, The sarcoplasmic reticulum releases Ca^{++} into the microenvironment of the myofibril.

4. *C*, The Ca^{++} binds to the troponin on the thin filament, which releases the inhibition on the myosin-actin interaction imposed by troponin and tropomyosin.

5. *C*, The myosin cross-bridges bind to individual G-actin units, and ATP is split by the ATPase enzyme located on the cross-bridge.

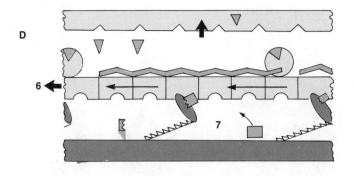

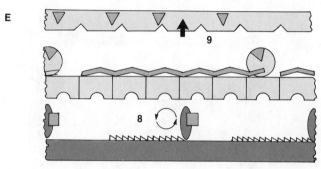

Figure 2-5 *Continued.*

6. *D,* The energy released by the hydrolysis of ATP is used to "pull" the thin filament toward the center of the sarcomere.

7. *D,* A new ATP molecule attaches to the cross-bridge, and the cross-bridge returns to its original position on the thick filament.

8. *E,* As long as Ca^{++} is bound to troponin, the cross-bridge may reattach to another actin molecule and the cycle is repeated. The cross-bridge "rows" the thin filament toward the center of the sarcomere.

9. *D* and *E,* Ca^{++} is continuously pumped back into the sarcoplasmic reticulum. Within a short time after the action potential activates contraction, the Ca^{++} concentration returns to resting levels and the inhibition of the troponin-tropomyosin system on contraction is reexerted.

Figure 2-6 illustrates the intimate relationship between the SR and the myofibril. Each sarcomere is completely enveloped by the SR, which actively accumulates Ca^{++} from the microenvironment of the myofibril and stores it. Ca^{++} is then released from the SR when the muscle fiber is stimulated to contract. The elevated Ca^{++} concentration resulting from stimulation of the SR increases the number of active cross-bridges, and the tension generated by the muscle fiber rises.

Conversely, relaxation of the muscle fiber occurs when Ca^{++} is removed from the *sarcoplasm* (cytoplasm of the muscle cell) in and around the myofibril. The membranes of the SR possess "pumps" that actively move Ca^{++} from the sarcoplasm into the SR. These pumps are continuously active, and they require a continuous supply of ATP to provide metabolic energy. After Ca^{++} has been released to initiate contraction, it is rapidly returned to the SR by the pumps, and the concentration of Ca^{++} in the sarcoplasm is lowered. The troponin and tropomyosin molecules again exert their inhibitory influence in the thin filament, and further cross-bridge interaction is prevented.

Action Potential Conduction. The final mechanisms that must be considered in the process of *excitation-contraction* are the electrochemical pathways (1) that the central nervous system uses to signal the muscle fiber to contract, and (2) that the muscle fiber uses to transmit the signal to the contractile molecules.

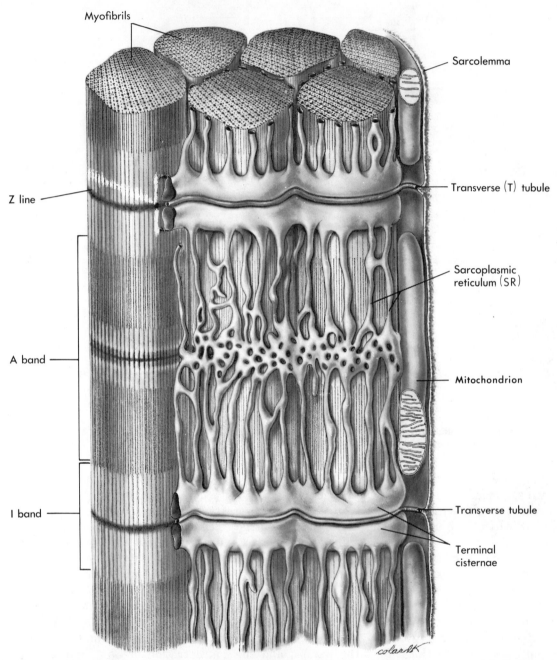

Figure 2 –6. Illustration of the distribution of the sarcoplasmic reticulum and transverse tubules around the myofibrils of frog skeletal muscle. (From Bloom W., and Fawcett D. W.: *A Textbook of Histology.* Philadelphia, W. B. Saunders Company, 1975.)

Each muscle fiber is innervated by a single *alpha-motoneuron* that arises in the ventral horn of the spinal cord (Fig. 2–7). The neural mechanisms involved in initiating an action potential (impulse) in the alpha-motoneuron and the means by which the impulse travels down the axon will be discussed in Chapter 3.

The nervous signal is passed from the alpha-motoneuron to the muscle fiber across the *neuromuscular junction* (Fig. 2–7). The arrival of the impulse at the neuron terminal results in the release of *acetylcholine* (ACh) from vesicles (sacs) located in the axonal ending. The neuronal terminal is not physically attached to the sarcolemma (muscle cell membrane) but is separated by a narrow space. The released ACh diffuses across the neuromuscular junction and complexes with specific binding sites in the *motor end plate,* which is the region of the sarcolemma located directly under the axonal ending. This interaction changes the permeability of the motor end plate to Na^+ and K^+ so that the membrane potential is lowered toward threshold. This altered potential is called the *end-plate potential* (EPP).

When the EPP reaches threshold, an action potential develops and is propagated along the sarcolemma in all directions away from the motor end plate region. This process is qualitatively similar to the propagation of action potentials on nerve cell membranes (Chapter 3).

Enzymes known as *cholinesterases* are located in the motor end plate and are responsible for destroying the ACh. It is important that the neuromuscular transmitter be rapidly inactivated; otherwise, the central nervous system would lose control of muscular contraction.

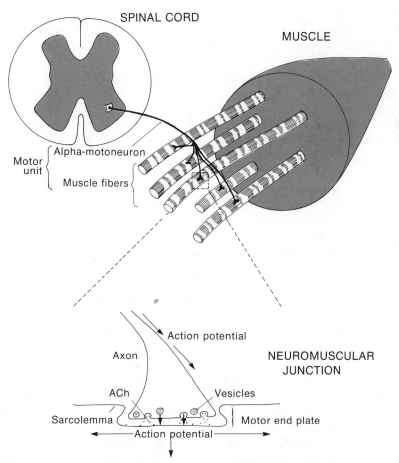

Figure 2–7. Schematic illustrations of one motor unit in a muscle and of a neuromuscular junction.

The neuromuscular junction is located near the middle of the muscle fiber. Once an action potential develops at the motor end plate, it spreads rapidly in all directions away from this point. The muscle fiber is designed in such a way that when it is stimulated, all myofibrils in the fiber, and hence all sarcomeres, contract almost simultaneously. You will recall that the muscle fiber consists of a large number of myofibrils packed together and contained within the sarcolemma. To initiate simultaneous contraction in all the myofibrils there must be a means of rapidly conducting the electrochemical impulse into the interior of the fiber. This function is fulfilled by the *transverse tubules* (T-tubules).

The relationship of the T-tubules to the SR and the myofibrils is illustrated in Figure 2–6. The T-tubules are inward extensions of the sarcolemma that run transversely through the muscle fiber. As the action potential travels down the length of the sarcolemma, it also penetrates into the interior of the cell over the T-tubules. The effect is to deliver the nervous signal to all the contractile components of the muscle almost simultaneously.

The *terminal cisternae* of the SR (Fig. 2–6) are located in close approximation to the T-tubules as they encircle the sarcomere. The passage of an action potential over the T-tubule causes the release of the Ca^{++}. However, the exact mechanism by which the SR is stimulated has not been experimentally demonstrated.

The events of the excitation-contraction process are summarized in Figure 2–5.

Metabolic Components of the Muscle Fiber.   The primary structures in the muscle fiber for ATP production are the mitochondria. These organelles are called the "powerhouses" of the cell. Their function in oxidative phosphorylation was discussed in detail in Chapter 1.

The largest accumulation of mitochondria in the muscle fiber is just under the sarcolemma (Fig. 2–6). However, they are also distributed throughout the fiber among the myofibrils.

Also distributed through the sarcoplasm between adjacent myofibrils are glycogen granules and lipid (fat) droplets (see Chapter 1). The muscle fibers thus have their own stored metabolic fuel supplies, as well as access to the blood-borne fuels (e.g., glucose and free fatty acids) from the surrounding capillaries. Most of the enzymes involved in the breakdown of glycogen and in the process of anaerobic glycolysis are associated with the glycogen granules.

Connective Tissue

Intimately associated with the muscle fibers, both structurally and functionally, is the connective tissue element of the muscle. Every muscle fiber is completely surrounded by a thin layer of loose connective tissue called *endomysium*. This tissue ultimately blends together to form the connective tissue tendons by which the muscle is attached to the bones. When the muscle fibers contract and develop tension, the force is exerted on the bony levers through this connective tissue element of the muscle. The endomysium also forms the structural matrix that contains the neurons and blood capillaries associated with the muscle fibers.

Muscle fibers are grouped into bundles of 10 to 50 fibers called *fascicles* (Fig. 2–2B). Each fascicle is surrounded by a more fibrous connective tissue sheath referred to as *perimysium*. Arteries, veins, and nerves lie in the spaces between adjacent fascicles. Every whole muscle, in turn, is covered with an *epimysium,* which is a thicker, tougher connective tissue coat.

It is important to consider the connective tissue portion of the muscle for several reasons. First, it plays an important role in muscle mechanics, which will be discussed when the elastic properties of the muscle are described later in this chapter. Second, most muscular injuries in athletics occur in the connective tissue element of the muscle. The causes and treatments for these injuries will be discussed in some detail in Chapters 12–14.

Nerve Tissue

Mixed sensory-motor nerves enter the muscle through the epimysium and course through the muscle in the interfascicular spaces. Each muscle fiber is innervated by one alpha-motoneuron, as indicated previously. However, each alpha-motoneuron innervates and controls more than one muscle fiber. Some alpha-motoneurons control as few as 10 to 20 muscle fibers, whereas others innervate more than 1000 muscle fibers. The alpha-motoneuron and the muscle fibers it innervates make up the *motor unit* (Fig. 2–7). Under normal conditions, an action potential in the alpha-motoneuron results in simultaneous contraction of all the muscle fibers in the motor unit. These concepts will be discussed in greater detail in Chapter 3. Also covered in Chapter 3 are the sensory components of the muscle, the spindles and Golgi tendon organs, which send afferent neurons back to the spinal cord through the same muscle nerves that contain the alpha-motoneurons.

Vascular Tissue

Like all bodily organs, muscle fibers receive a continuous supply of blood through one or more arteries that enter through the epimysium and run through the muscle between fascicles in a manner similar to the nerves. Small arteries enter the fascicles, and a network of capillaries branches out and surrounds each muscle fiber. From the capillaries, the blood drains into veins that leave the muscle by the same general route by which the arteries entered. Respiratory gases, nutritional molecules, and wastes pass freely between the capillaries and muscle fibers through the endomysium.

During exercise, the blood flow to the active muscles may increase by as much as 50 to 60-fold. This elevated flow is necessary to support the metabolic requirements of the muscle and results from an opening of the capillary beds that surround the muscle fibers and an increase in cardiac output.

Skeletal Muscle Mechanics

The study of muscle mechanics has allowed physiologists to measure precisely the effects of the forces generated by contracting muscles. Several of the concepts that have evolved from this type of laboratory experimentation are essential to a basic understanding of how muscles work.

Muscle Twitches. A single action potential in an alpha-motoneuron causes the stimulated fibers to produce a *twitch*. Muscle twitches may be recorded in the laboratory in two general ways: (1) isometrically or (2) isotonically.

In recording an *isometric twitch,* the muscle is fixed so that it cannot shorten. The variable that is measured is tension. Figure 2–8A shows that the tension in the fibers rises to a peak (contraction time) after a brief latent period, and then declines over a longer time interval (relaxation time).

In an *isotonic twitch,* the muscle is allowed to shorten against a constant load. The distance that the muscle shortens and the rate of shortening are measured in an

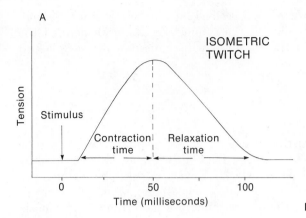

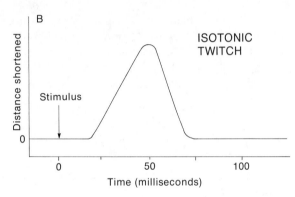

Figure 2-8. Recordings of muscle twitches.

isotonic contraction (Fig. 2–8*B*). When the muscle develops contractile tension sufficient to overcome the resistance of the load, the muscle shortens at a fairly constant rate. As active tension development ceases, the load overcomes the contractile force and the muscle returns to its original length.

Summation and Tetanus.   The contractile behavior of the motor unit is controlled by the patterns of action potentials that arrive at the motor end plates through the alpha-motoneuron. Figure 2–9 illustrates how changing the pattern of stimuli affects the isometric tension developed by the motor unit. When the alpha-motoneuron is stimulated with successively shorter intervals between impulses, the resulting twitches *summate*. Summation continues with increasingly higher stimulation frequencies until a smooth, maximal tension is produced. This smooth contraction is referred to as *tetanus*. The differences in tension among twitches, summated twitches, and tetanus are a consequence of the elastic component of the muscle.

Before external force can be exerted on a load by a contracting motor unit, the *series elastic component* must be "stretched." This principle may be illustrated by fastening a spring to a weight and slowly raising the weight by lifting the spring. The spring must stretch to the point at which the tension in the spring equals the mass of the load before the weight is raised. In this example, the person lifting the weight is analogous to the cross-bridges in the muscle, the spring is analogous to the series elastic component, and the weight corresponds to the load the muscle is pulling against. Thus, when a motor unit undergoes a twitch, a good share of the tension produced by the active cross-bridges (internal tension) is used to stretch the elastic component, and the measureable external tension is less than the tension actually generated by the contractile proteins. By stimulating the motor unit with repetitive stimuli, a greater proportion of the tension produced by the cross-bridges may be measured as external force. Once the elastic component is completely stretched, all of the contractile tension may be exerted on the load. The structural components of the series elastic element are the connective tissues in the muscle and the tendons, the Z lines, and the passive elasticity in the cross-bridges.

Neural Control of Muscle Tension

There are two general means by which the nervous system controls the contractile tension in a given muscle. The more important of the two mechanisms is *motor unit recruitment*. Muscles possess hundreds of motor units, each consisting of one alpha-motoneuron and the muscle fibers it innervates. To generate low tensions in a muscle, a small number of motor units may be activated; higher tensions can be achieved by recruiting larger numbers of motor units.

The second method the nervous system uses to control muscle tension is to vary the frequency or the pattern of stimuli, or both, to a given motor unit. As has been pointed out, increasing the frequency of action potentials to a motor unit produces elevated tensions.

Of these two general mechanisms, motor unit recruitment is more important for producing the wide range of contractile forces that muscles are called upon to produce. However, the two are never completely dissociated; normally, recruitment and frequency variation are coordinated to produce the fine control of muscle tension that the motor system provides.

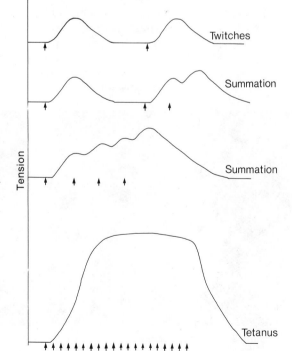

Figure 2–9. Isometrically recorded twitches, summations, and tetanus. Arrows represent action potentials (stimuli).

SPECIAL CONSIDERATIONS

Skeletal Muscle Fiber Types

To this point, general properties of skeletal muscle that are common to all muscle fibers have been discussed. It is important to realize, however, that muscles are composed of a mixture of different fiber types that are specially designed to participate in specific types of muscular activity.

In human locomotory muscles there are two distinct populations of fibers, one that will be referred to as *fast-twitch* (FT), and the other as *slow-twitch* (ST). It is possible to further subdivide the FT fibers, but this discussion will be restricted to the two basic types. All muscle fibers within a given motor unit are of the same type, and the fibers of FT and ST motor units are mixed together in the muscles so that they form a checkerboard pattern when viewed in a muscle cross section (Fig. 2–10).

Table 2–1 summarizes some of the characteristics of the two fiber types. FT motor units are capable of generating high peak forces because of the large numbers of muscle fibers innervated by each alpha-motoneuron. Stimulation of these units produces strong, rapid muscular contractions. These fibers are therefore ideally suited for generating the explosive shortening contractions needed for sprinting, jumping, and throwing. The FT fibers have relatively high anaerobic enzyme potentials, which allow them to effectively resynthesize ATP for contractile energy in the absence of oxygen for brief periods of time (see Chapter 1). This metabolic characteristic is important for these fibers because, during explosive bursts of contractile activity, the muscle is not able to obtain sufficient oxygen to aerobically produce ATP.

On the other hand, the FT fibers have fewer mitochondria and capillaries than ST fibers, resulting in a relatively low capacity to resynthesize ATP through oxidative phosphorylation. They therefore tend to fatigue relatively fast during continuous activity and are not as suitable as the ST fibers for producing tension for postural support or for prolonged endurance activities.

ST motor units contract more slowly and, because of their low innervation ratios, do not deveop the high total tensions produced by FT units.* Because of the high

---

*Specific tensions for the two fiber types are probably the same; that is, per cross-sectional area of active muscle, ST and FT fibers develop similar maximal tensions.

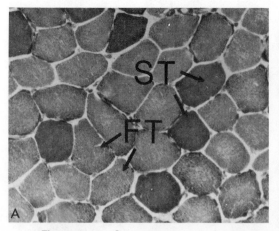 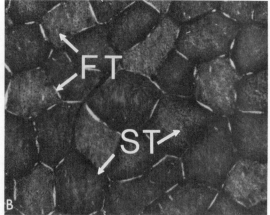

Figure 2–10. Cross sections of human muscles histochemically stained for mitochondrial enzymes (DPNH-diaphorase). The intensity of the stain indicates the density of mitochondria in the fibers. *A* is from the vastus lateralis (thigh) muscle of a sedentary adult male. *B* is from the same muscle of an active adult male (jogger). FT = fast-twitch fiber; ST = slow-twitch fiber. Both fast-twitch and slow-twitch fibers in the muscle from the jogger have a greater density of mitochondria and, thus, a larger aerobic capacity.

TABLE 2–1. CHARACTERISTICS OF THE FIBER TYPES IN HUMAN MUSCLE

Characteristic	Fiber Type	
	SLOW-TWITCH	FAST-TWITCH
Contraction time	Slow	Fast
Relaxation time	Slow	Fast
Fatigue resistance	High	Low
Mitochondrial density	High	Low
Capillary density	High	Low
Anaerobic potential	Low	High
Innervation ratio (muscle fibers/motoneuron)	Low	High

mitochondrial (Fig. 2–10) and capillary densities associated with ST fibers, they have a high capacity for oxidative phosphorylation. They are therefore more resistant to fatigue than FT fibers and are ideally suited for the contractions needed in postural support and endurance activities.

Different muscles have varying proportions of the two fiber types, depending upon their specific functions. Earlier in the chapter, the gastrocnemius and soleus muscles were used to illustrate the effects of muscle contraction. Although these muscles have similar actions on the ankle joint, the soleus muscle serves a more important postural role than the gastrocnemius muscle. Thus, as you might predict, the soleus muscle has a higher proportion of ST fibers.

Training Effects on Skeletal Muscle

Muscles display a high degree of both specificity and adaptability in the ways in which they respond to different types of training programs. Two general categories will be briefly considered: (1) adaptation to strength training, and (2) adaptation to endurance training.

Strength Training. The strength of an individual muscle, or the maximal tension it is capable of producing, is dependent upon the total cross-sectional area of its muscle fibers. It follows that the way to increase muscular strength is to increase the total fiber cross-sectional area of the muscle. This might be accomplished either by increasing the total number of fibers in the muscle (*hyperplasia*) or by increasing the diameters, or areas, of the existing fibers (*hypertrophy*).

It is generally believed that the number of fibers in a muscle is set before a child is born and that this number does not change. Although animal experiments have demonstrated that muscle enlargement resulting from severe overload conditions is accompanied by an increase in the number of fibers, it is probable that the muscle enlargement associated with strength training in humans is entirely attributable to hypertrophy of existing fibers.

The increased girth of hypertrophied muscle fibers results primarily from increases in the diameter and number of the myofibrils within the fibers, although all the other constituents of the muscle cell (mitochondria, sarcoplasmic reticulum, etc.) increase somewhat proportionally. Both FT and ST fibers hypertrophy during weight training, although the greater enlargement occurs in the FT fibers.

The stimulus that causes a muscle to enlarge is long-term heavy resistance exercise. Endurance exercise (e.g., distance running or swimming) does not result in significant hypertrophy of muscle fibers.

It should be emphasized that bodily strength is dependent upon a number of factors other than the maximal tensions attainable by individual muscles. Thus, differences in bony leverages, coordination, learning, motivation, age, and a number of other variables affect a person's applicable muscular strength.

Just as overuse tends to increase the girth of muscle fibers, underuse causes the fibers to diminish in size, or *atrophy*. This is a problem in many types of athletic injuries, for it is often necessary for the athlete to cease his training and rest the injured part. An extreme example of the process of atrophy in the muscles may be observed when it is necessary to cast a joint: while the cast is in place, the muscles that work on the joint decrease in size and hence, in strength.

The process of atrophy is essentially the reverse of that of hypertrophy; that is, there is a loss of myofibrils and the other muscle fiber constituents. However, there is a disproportionately large decrease in mitochondria in the atrophying fibers. The ST fibers atrophy to a greater extent than the FT fibers during short-term periods of muscle inactivity.

Endurance Training. The primary adaptation to long-term endurance training in the muscles that are involved in the exercise is an increased resistance to fatigue. This is accomplished by increasing the capacity of the muscle fibers to produce ATP through oxidative phosphorylation. Thus, endurance training increases (1) the blood flow to the muscle fibers through increased capillarization; (2) the myoglobin content of the fibers for enhanced intracellular oxygen transport; and (3) the density of mitochondria in the muscle fibers. It should be emphasized that these training effects occur only in the muscles that are actually used in the exercise.

Champion endurance athletes tend to have more ST fibers in their muscles than untrained individuals or athletes in nonendurance events. It is not known if these differences are simply genetic (in which case children with high proportions of ST fibers presumably would be predisposed toward success in endurance events), or if FT fibers can be transformed to ST fibers through long-term training. From the evidence available at this time, it appears doubtful that fibers change from slow twitch to fast twitch with training. However, both ST and FT fibers are able to markedly increase their oxidative capacities (Fig. 2–10) and hence their resistance to fatigue.

It should be remembered that increases in the capacities of other bodily systems, in particular the cardiovascular system, must be considered in understanding the response to endurance training. These factors will be discussed in succeeding chapters.

SUMMARY

The function of the skeletal muscles is to pull, thereby exerting tension on the bones to which they are attached. Muscles undergo shortening, isometric, and lengthening contractions, depending on the relationship between the force the muscle generates and the resistance against which it pulls.

Changes in muscle length are accomplished through the sliding filament mechanism: the thin filaments slide past the thick filaments in a telescopic fashion, allowing the muscle fiber to shorten or lengthen. The development of the pulling force involves an interaction between the major proteins in the thick and thin filaments — the myosin and actin, respectively.

The contraction of a motor unit in the muscle is controlled by the alpha-motoneuron innervating the unit. Action potentials delivered by the alpha-motoneuron stimulate Ca^{++} release from the sarcoplasmic reticulum in the muscle fiber. Ca^{++} "triggers" the actin-myosin interaction that generates muscular force by removing the inhibition imposed on the interaction by troponin and tropomyosin.

Single action potentials result in muscle twitches, whereas repetitive stimulation causes tetanus. The difference in external tension developed in twitches and tetanus is explained by the presence of the series elastic component.

Different fiber types in muscles have varying contractile and metabolic properties. Fast-twitch muscle fibers are fast contracting and better suited for explosive muscular activity of short duration. Slow-twitch units are better designed for prolonged endurance activity because of their higher aerobic capacities.

In strength training, an increase in muscle fiber cross-sectional area occurs, permitting the muscle to generate higher maximal forces. Endurance training stimulates an increase in mitochondria, myoglobin, and capillaries in the muscles.

STUDY QUESTIONS

1. What is the single basic function of all skeletal muscles?

2. Name the three different types of muscular contraction, and give examples of each of the three from your daily activities.

3. Name the four different types of tissue in a muscle, and give the basic function of each.

4. How do muscles shorten and lengthen? Describe these processes in terms of the sarcomere and the thick and thin filaments.

5. Name the two properties of the myosin cross-bridge that indicate it is involved in the generation of contractile tension.

6. What is the function of the protein molecules troponin and tropomyosin?

7. Explain how a nervous signal originating in the central nervous system is transmitted to the sarcomeres in the muscle.

8. Discuss the functional significance of the series elastic component of the muscle.

9. What is a motor unit? Why is the concept of the motor unit important in understanding how muscular tension is controlled by the nervous system?

10. What are the differences between an isometric muscle twitch and an isotonic muscle twitch?

11. Describe summation and tetanus. Why does the muscle develop maximal tension during tetanus?

12. What characteristics of the fast-twitch fibers make them suitable for rapid, powerful muscle contractions? Why are the slow-twitch fibers better suited for postural and endurance work?

13. Describe the major differences in the ways in which muscles adapt to strength training and endurance training.

FURTHER READINGS

Bloom, W., and Fawcett, D. W.: A Textbook of Histology, 10th ed. Philadelphia, W. B. Saunders Company, 1975.
Burke, R. E., and Edgerton, V. R.: Motor unit properties and selective involvement in movement. Exercise Sports Sci. Rev. 3:31–81, 1975.

Close, R. I.: Dynamic properties of mammalian skeletal muscles. Physiol. Rev. *52*:129–197, 1972.

Ebashi, S.: Excitation-contraction coupling. Ann. Rev. Physiol. *38*:293–313, 1976.

Fuchs, F.: Striated muscle. Ann. Rev. Physiol. *39*:461–502, 1974.

Goldberg, A., Etlinger, J., Goldspink, D., and Jablecki, C.: Mechanism of work-induced hypertrophy of skeletal muscle. Med. Sci. Sports 7:185–198, 1975.

Gollnick, P. D., Armstrong, R. B., Saubert, C. W., IV, Piehl, K., and Saltin, B.: Enzyme activity and fiber composition in skeletal muscle of untrained and trained men. J. Appl. Physiol. *33*:312–319, 1972.

Hill, A. V.: *First and Last Experiments in Muscle Mechanics*. Cambridge, England, Cambridge University Press, 1970.

Huxley, H. E.: The mechanism of muscular contraction. Science *164*:1356–1366, 1969.

Weber, A., and Murray, J. M.: Molecular control mechanisms in muscle contraction. Physiol. Rev. *53*:612–673, 1973.

3

THE NERVOUS SYSTEM

V. REGGIE EDGERTON, Ph.D.

There is a general tendency to overlook the importance of the nervous system in controlling movement, adapting to exercise, and resisting the fatigue caused by emotional and physical overloads. One reason for this is that it is not clearly understood how the nervous system performs such functions. However, current ideas lead to the conclusion that the nervous system has greater control of biological functions during exercise than has been generally recognized.

The functions of the nervous system during exercise are illustrated in Figure 3–1. For example, a movement may be initiated by the higher nerve centers in the outer layer (cortex) of the portion of the brain called the cerebrum, or it may begin as a result of activation of neurons (nerve cells) located in the base of the brain or even the spinal cord (Fig. 3–2). Higher nerve centers send information to the support systems at the same time that they send information to the motor (muscle) systems. That is, the heart, lungs, and the "involuntarily" controlled functions know when movement is occurring and react in a supportive manner. The muscle's role is only to be responsive to the nervous system; the neural and hormonal segments of the organism control most, if not all, related functions.

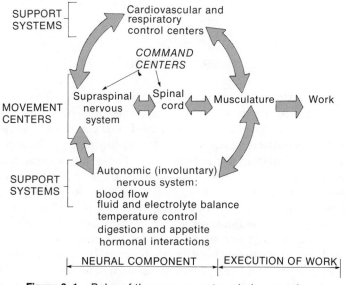

Figure 3–1. Roles of the nervous system during exercise.

49

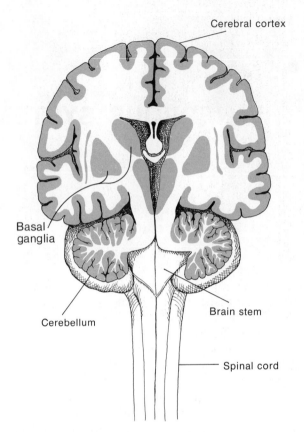

Cerebral cortex

Basal
ganglia

Cerebellum

Brain stem

Spinal cord

Figure 3–2. Anatomy of the central nervous system.

This chapter will discuss the role of the nervous system in movement and adaptation to movement as outlined in Figure 3–1. Conceptually, the neural components can be viewed as command centers or support systems. The command centers include the spinal cord and the supraspinal (above the spine) nervous system (brain and brain stem). They initiate the chain of events that leads to muscle contraction, and they also communicate, directly or indirectly, with all support systems in order to influence their functions.

SPINAL CORD

The spinal cord is the source of direct excitation of muscle. The total quantity and quality of muscular activity is directly determined by the alpha-motoneurons (α-MNs). These neurons are located in the ventral (front) portion of the spinal cord (Fig. 3–3). All skeletomotor muscle fibers are excited to contract by these α-MNs.

What is meant by skeletomotor muscle fiber? These are the long fibers of a muscle that actually cause movement (Fig. 3–3). A second kind of muscle fiber is called fusimotor, and its function is to aid in sensing the length of a muscle. This type of fiber is very small, comprising only 10 to 20 per cent of the diameter of a skeletomotor muscle fiber and less than 1 per cent of the muscle's length. Fusimotor muscle fibers usually occur in groups of three to five and are surrounded by a connective tissue sheath. Muscle spindles (Fig. 3–3) are made up of these fusimotor muscle fibers and the nerve endings that send sensory information back to the spinal cord. The nerves that send signals to the muscle spindles are called gamma-motoneurons (γ-MNs). Within the spinal cord,

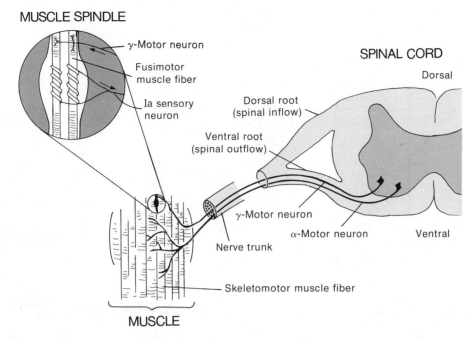

Figure 3–3. Cross section of spinal cord at lumbar region. In addition, a muscle spindle is shown enlarged.

γ-MNs that lead to a muscle are located in the same region as the α-MNs that innervate that muscle. The γ-MNs are much smaller than the α-MNs. The function of γ-MNs and fusimotor muscle fibers will be discussed more thoroughly later in this chapter.

Alpha-Motoneurons

The α-MN is often referred to as the final common pathway to muscle, because any excitation signals related to muscular efforts eventually converge on the appropriate α-MN. Within the ventral portion of the spinal cord, the α-MNs are located in groups, commonly referred to as pools. Each pool of α-MNs has a similar function: for example, one pool excites the extensors of the knee while another excites the knee flexors. Within the spinal cord these pools overlap anatomically; this makes sense because these two pools of α-MNs must communicate in order to integrate their actions so that movements are rhythmical.

The α-MN pools for the lower extremities are located in the lower back (lumbar) region. Other α-MN pools are located at the spinal level at which their axons exit from the spinal cord to innervate a particular muscle group. For example, neurons that innervate the muscles of the rib cage that are used in ventilation are located at the thoracic level of the spinal cord.

A single α-MN may innervate only a few muscle fibers or several hundred. An α-MN, along with all the muscle fibers innervated by it, is called a motor unit (Fig. 3–4). This is the basic functional unit of the neuromuscular system. An action potential (electrical impulse) (see below) initiated in the cell body (soma) of an α-MN generally reaches the neuromuscular junction of all muscle fibers of its motor unit, causing all muscle fibers of that unit to respond simultaneously. The action potential is transmitted to the muscle membrane (sarcolemma) by release of acetylcholine at the neuromuscular junction (see Figure 2–7, p. 39).

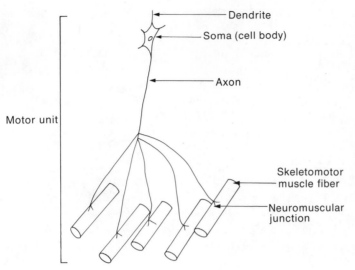

Figure 3–4. A motor unit includes the alpha-motor neuron (α-MN) and the muscle fibers that it innervates.

Dendrite

Soma (cell body)

Axon

Motor unit

Skeletomotor muscle fiber

Neuromuscular junction

ACTION POTENTIAL

An action potential is a nerve impulse. It provides one of the main ways in which neurons communicate. It is referred to as an "action" potential because the event is propagated from one point (cell body) of the neuron to another (terminal nerve endings of the axon). The event itself is simply a change in the electrical potential across the nerve cell membrane. This potential is measured in millivolts.

The resting membrane potential (when no electrical impulse is being propagated) is about 80 millivolts; that is, the difference in concentration between ions inside and outside the cell membrane is such that the inside is 80 millivolts more negative than the outside. One of the initiating events of an action potential is a change in membrane properties that allows a rush of sodium ions into the cell, thereby changing the electrical potential. Following an action potential, an outward rush of potassium ions returns the membrane to the resting state. The ions are subsequently pumped back to their original locations. The physicochemical phenomena that explain these membrane events are well understood but are not essential to the main points of this chapter.

DETERMINATION OF MUSCLE FIBER TYPE

Alpha-motoneurons not only excite the muscle fibers that they innervate but also determine the biochemical and contractile properties of muscle fibers.[1] This was demonstrated in cross-reinnervation experiments in which a nerve to a slow muscle and a nerve to a fast muscle were transected, crossed, and sutured together. That is, the nerve that originally projected into the slow muscle was made to innervate the fast muscle and vice versa. Under these circumstances, the slow muscle became fast contracting and the fast muscle became slow contracting. Therefore, one could conclude that the speed of muscle shortening is dictated by the α-MN that innervates it.[2] The α-MN also determines other properties that are related to metabolism. For example, whether a muscle fiber relies predominantly on glycolytic or oxidative metabolism is controlled by the α-MN.[1]

An obvious question is how does the motor neuron exert this control? Two hypotheses have been offered. One is that the muscle properties are determined by the pattern and/or quantity of impulses that reach the muscle. The second hypothesis is that there is (are) some chemical substance(s) produced by the α-MN that reach the muscle fibers and instruct the nuclei to synthesize a given kind and amount of protein. This second phenomenon is commonly referred to as the neurotrophic effect.

Regardless of the mechanism, the control must be accomplished by regulating the quality of protein synthesized within the muscle fibers. For example, there are two "types" of myosin protein in skeletal muscle. Fast-contracting muscle has one type that has the capacity to break down adenosine triphosphate (ATP) rapidly. Consequently, the actin and myosin filaments, with their specific regulatory proteins, can interact rapidly and produce high-velocity shortening. On the other hand, slow-muscle protein has a lower maximal rate at which it can break down ATP (lower ATPase activity)and the muscle contracts more slowly. Thus, speed of shortening seems to be determined in part by the kind of contractile protein synthesized. As described previously, this property can be reversed for any given muscle fiber by changing its source of innervation (cross innervation). Similarly, metabolic properties are dictated by the quantity and quality of enzymes synthesized. These enzymes are also determined by the type of α-MN that provides the innervation. All muscle fibers innervated by a given α-MN are homogenous; that is, they have the same biochemical and physiological properties.

Alpha-motoneurons can be categorized into at least two overlapping populations with regard to the speed of the muscle. These populations can be identified to some degree on the basis of their optimal and peak firing frequencies. For a given excitatory input, the α-MN that innervates the fast muscle fibers will respond with a higher firing frequency than one that innervates slow muscle fibers. There is some evidence that this difference may be due to a qualitative difference in cell membrane properties. The difference in frequency response is quite important because muscle speed and tension capabilities are matched well with the optimal frequency at which the α-MN tends to generate action potentials.[1]

Interneurons

A rather sophisticated network of neurons and fibers exists in the spinal cord. The α-MNs and γ-MNs are only part of the population. Many of the other neurons are collectively referred to as interneurons. These neurons functionally connect the neurons of different pathways. The interneurons that have been studied the most are the Ia inhibitory interneurons that inhibit antagonistic α-MNs and excite agonists (those having similar function) (Fig. 3–5). This is commonly referred to as reciprocal inhibition. This kind of interneuron simplifies the function of the nervous system in maintaining a normal walking or running pattern and other rhythmic efforts. For example, when a flexor contracts, it is usually efficient to relax the extensors. The Ia interneuron can provide an excitatory impulse to one muscle group and simultaneously inhibit the opposing muscle group (Fig. 3–5). The classification "Ia" is based on axon diameter. The axon diameter is critical because it determines the velocity at which an impulse is conducted.

These Ia axons are also well known for their role in the "reflex arc" involved in the knee jerk when the tendon is suddenly stretched by a tap just below the patella (knee cap). The knee jerk is caused by the excitation of the Ia nerve endings in the spindles of the muscle that is suddenly stretched. The resulting sensory impulse reaches α-MNs, which excite the skeletomotor muscle fibers of the same muscle. At the same time, the antagonist muscles are inhibited via the Ia interneurons.

Even though most interneurons are not of the Ia type, the involvement of Ia fibers in locomotion would seem to be of great importance in light of their sensitivity to muscle length and activity during movement. Another indication of their importance is the large-scale convergence of many axons from supraspinal and spinal neurons onto these specific interneurons.[3]

Neuronal Generators

It is now clear that the spinal cord has a neural network that is capable of generating remarkably normal locomotor patterns without supraspinal or peripheral input. That is, a portion of the spinal cord isolated from supraspinal and peripheral sensory inflow can be stimulated to generate rhythmic output by injecting a chemical called L-dopa (L-dihydroxyphenylalanine). This drug is used to relieve the symptoms of some motor control disabilities in humans (e.g., Parkinsonism) caused by certain neural deficits.

Isolated spinal (neuronal) generators can execute their own motor programs for the appropriate rhythmic excitation of the leg muscles, as in walking. These spinal generators are capable of receiving input and modifying the motor program in a purposeful, rather than stereotypic, manner.[4] When a "spinal" cat (spinal cord transected in the lower thoracic region) walks on a treadmill, the level of neural sophistication is such that the stepping rate increases when the belt speed increases, even to a gallop.[5] However, the spinal animal cannot maintain its balance. There is some evidence that spinal generation of movement is possible in humans. Other types of neuronal generators control ventilation, cardiovascular activity and chewing.

Glial Cells

Another component of the nervous system is the population of glial ("glue") cells. These cells perform a more sophisticated function than merely gluing neurons together and filling in spaces. Glial cells seem to interact metabolically with adjacent neurons, thereby having a metabolically supportive role. They also are responsible for synthesis of myelin, a multilayered membrane that serves to electrically insulate neurons from one another. There are several kinds of glial cells, each with its own set of functions.

The Muscle Spindle and Gamma-Motoneuron

The function of the muscle spindle (Fig. 3–5) is to sense the length of the muscle that contains it; this aids in fine control of movement. The knee jerk (patellar) reflex mentioned previously is mediated by muscle spindles. When the quadriceps (thigh) muscle is stretched slightly by tapping the tendon below the patella, the spindles are stretched. A sensitive portion within the spindle generates impulses that are transmitted to the spinal cord along a sensory neuron (Fig. 3–5). The sensory neuron synapses (connects) with an α-MN. At the synapse, a chemical transmitter is released in a manner similar to that at the neuromuscular junction. The α-MN then fires, causing its muscle fibers to twitch. This sequence is shown more clearly in Figure 3–6A.

The spindle is "in parallel" with the skeletal muscle fibers. Therefore, when the muscle contracts, one might expect tension within the spindle to decrease and the spindle to become insensitive to stretch. However, this does not normally occur because when the α-MN fires, the corresponding γ-MN also fires. The γ-MN innervates fusimotor muscle fibers within the spindle and causes them to contract, thus preventing slack (Fig. 3–6B). If the γ-MN is prevented from firing, as can be done with drugs, the spindle does indeed lose its sensitivity to muscle length (Fig. 3–6C). As a result, a dart thrower whose γ-MNs have been blocked will release the dart too soon. The nervous system seems to assume that the muscles are contracting faster than they actually are.[6]

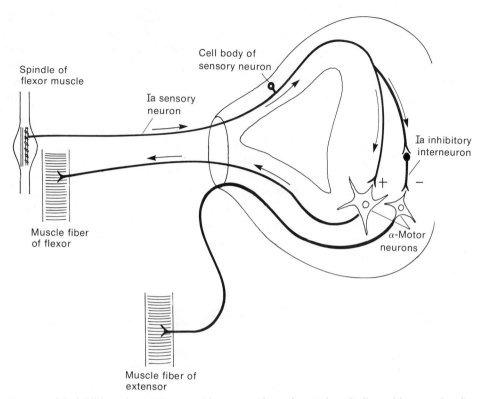

Figure 3–5. A Ia inhibitory interneuron and its connections. A muscle spindle and its stretch reflex are shown.

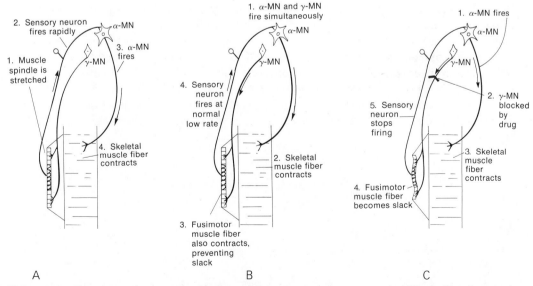

Figure 3–6. Functions of a muscle spindle and its gamma motor neuron (γ-MN). *A,* Muscle stretch reflex. *B,* Voluntary contraction of skeletal muscle with normal contraction of α-MN and γ-MN. *C,* Voluntary contraction of skeletal muscle with γ-MN blocked by drug.

SUPRASPINAL NERVOUS SYSTEM

The α-MNs located within the spinal cord excite the skeletomotor muscle fibers directly. However, the α-MNs receive their input from several neural pathways, and the input from each of these pathways can excite both skeletomotor and fusimotor muscle fibers. Supraspinal input originates from the motor cortex and basal ganglia of the brain and from the brain stem (Figs. 3–2 and 3–7). In addition, the cerebellum provides indirect input via feedback to the motor cortex, basal ganglia, and several brain stem centers.

Cerebral Motor Cortex

The motor cortex contains nerve cells called pyramidal tract neurons (PTNs), of which about 10 to 20 per cent terminate directly on the spinal α-MN and the rest terminate via another neuron (Fig. 3–7). The axons that descend from PTNs form a bundle of fibers called the corticospinal or pyramidal tract. This is the largest tract descending to α-MNs and it is relatively slow conducting.

The motor portion of the cerebral cortex also controls the spinal αMNs via other relay centers in other areas of the brain. PTNs provide direct input to the basal ganglia, which in turn send axons to other centers in the brainstem (Fig. 3–7). Each of these can relay signals indirectly or directly to spinal α-MNs at various levels of the spinal cord.[7]

The PTNs must function in relation to an almost infinite number of possible combinations of muscle forces, velocities, and directions. It appears that the PTNs act as one component of a set of neurons involved in a movement. The set varies when the movement is modified. The activity of specific PTNs seems to be related to the part or joint involved rather than to a specific muscle or muscle group. The firing rates of some PTNs are closely related to the force and, to a somewhat lesser degree, to the direction of the displacement.[8]

Trains of action potentials often occur in a PTN before a movement is made in response to visual or other cues. Some PTNs consistently fire after a specific movement is begun, demonstrating the sensory (afferent) feedback from a limb to the motor cortex. Despite the evidence accumulating to demonstrate a correlation between PTN activity and movement of a specific group of muscles, it should be recognized that these events do not necessarily indicate a cause-and-effect relationship. In general, it seems that the PTN by itself lacks tight control over many aspects of movement.

The function of the motor cortex in normal movement also is indicated to some degree by studies in which cats have been decorticated (cerebral cortex removed).

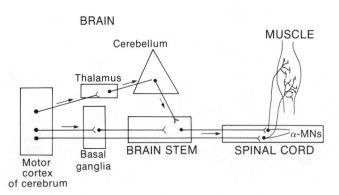

Figure 3–7. Supraspinal connections to motor neurons.

After decortication they can still walk, run, and right themselves. Decortication has more severe effects in monkeys, but they remain able to right themselves and move about, although somewhat awkwardly. This shows that, although most learning of motor patterns is thought to occur in the cerebral cortex, other areas of the brain, such as the cerebellum and brain stem area, are also intimately involved.[9]

Basal Ganglia

The functions of the basal ganglia (Figs. 3–2 and 3–7) seem to be totally motor related. They relay information from the ears, muscles, skin, and joints to the motor cortex and brain stem. It has been hypothesized that the basal ganglia are the generators for slow, smooth movements. Diseases of the basal ganglia are characterized by akinesia (a tendency to use a part of the body less than normally), increased muscle tone rigidity, and involuntary movements.[9]

Brain Stem

The brain stem (Figs. 3–2 and 3–7) receives input from the cerebral cortex, cerebellum, basal ganglia, and spinal cord. One region of the brain stem acts as a regulator for involuntary and reflex motor reactions. This region provides strong inhibitory as well as excitatory input to a large number of α-MNs. Another region can provide a selective inhibitory effect on α-MNs that innervate slow-twitch muscle fibers and an excitatory effect on α-MNs that innervate fast-twitch muscle fibers. This differential input to α-MNs provides a mechanism by which the nervous system might be capable of selectively recruiting a fast unit without, or prior to, recruiting a slow motor unit. Whether or not such selective recruitment actually occurs in normal movements is controversial.

Other brain stem neurons receive input from the inner ear, which helps in maintaining equilibrium, providing sensations of movement and spatial orientation, and adjusting input for maintenance of posture. Some of the other pathways in the brain stem assist in controlling eye position during head movements.

Cerebellum

The cerebellum (Fig. 3–2 and 3–7) is responsible at least in part for the integration of information regarding motor programs, which leads to effective and efficient movement. The cerebellum receives information from the cerebral cortex, muscle receptors, joints, tendons, skin, eyes, and auditory and vestibular receptors. This information is processed and then used to modify subsequent motor programs. The efferent (outward) pathways of the cerebellum connect to the brain stem. The connection of the cerebellum to the cerebral cortex may be very important in assisting the cortex to initiate rapid repetitive movements by informing it of the previous movement to be repeated. Thus, although information may travel from muscle to cortex too slowly to influence the next movement, the movement after that can be altered.[9]

Cerebellar lesions are characterized by deficits in muscular control that relate to rate, force, direction, and range of movement. The deficits become more apparent when motor demands increase; for example, a tremor at rest becomes worse when the person reaches for a pencil.

SUPPORT SYSTEMS

Neuromuscular activity requires a number of adjustments in order for the activity to be continued and in order to normalize basic function after activity is terminated. For example, neuromuscular activity is associated with functional alterations of the heart, blood vessels, lungs, metabolism, digestion, renal function, and body temperature. The autonomic nervous system (ANS) plays a major role in assuring that the rate at which these functions occurs is matched rather precisely with the intensity of neuromuscular activity. Figure 3–8 diagramatically illustrates the large number of critical functions that are associated with neuromuscular activity and controlled to some degree by the ANS. The ANS can be subdivided into two components — sympathetic and parasympathetic — on the basis of anatomical features (origin in the central nervous system and peripheral distribution) and physiological effects.

Sympathetic Autonomic Nervous System

The neurons of the sympathetic nervous system originate in the ventral portion of the spinal cord. They are located at levels ranging from the first thoracic vertebra to the upper lumbar portion (L-2) of the spine. These neurons are short: their axons synapse in ganglia located just outside the spinal cord. The spinal ganglia consist of a group of neurons with similar functions. Thus, neurons with their cell bodies located in the spinal cord (preganglionic neurons) send impulses to neurons within the ganglia (postganglionic neurons). This is functionally important because the preganglionic neurons release acetylcholine as the neurotransmitter (just as do α-MNs at the neuromuscular junction), but the postganglionic fibers release primarily norepinephrine. (In contrast, in the parasympathetic nervous system, acetylcholine is released from both

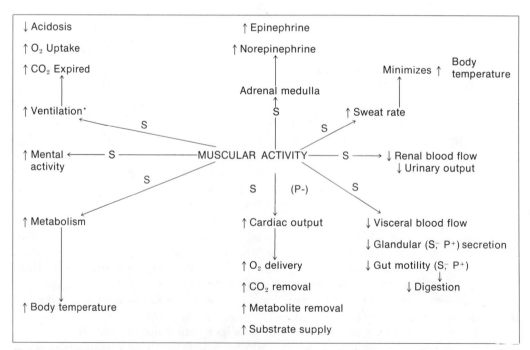

Figure 3–8. Influence of muscular activity on the autonomic nervous system. S = sympathetic; P = parasympathetic; + = excitation; − = inhibition.
  *Ventilatory neurons are not considered part of the autonomic nervous system.

pre- and postganglionic neurons.) Because two different neurotransmitters are at work, the effects of the input from both sympathetic and parasympathetic postganglionic neurons can counteract one another in the receiving organ. As indicated in Figure 3–8, several support systems are regulated by the relative strengths of the inputs from the sympathetic and parasympathetic nervous systems.

When the nervous system initiates a movement, it simultaneously informs the neurons that control cardiovascular function, ventilation, endocrine systems, secretory functions, and metabolism. Modification of cardiovascular function includes an initial elevation in blood pressure, heart rate, and cardiac output. In addition, blood redistribution is an effective means of increasing exercise tolerance because it permits a greater proportion of the elevated cardiac output to be delivered to the active muscles while proportionally less is delivered to the less active muscles, intestines, liver, and kidneys. Blood redistribution is also important in body temperature control. Control of body temperature is accomplished by regulating the amount of blood distributed to the skin as opposed to the core of the body. The greater the blood flow to the skin, the greater the rate of body heat loss.

Regulation of the amount of blood flow to the various organs is accomplished by changes in the diameters of the small arteries (arterioles) that supply the organs. Diameter is controlled by sympathetic nerve fibers that innervate the muscular wall of an artery. Sympathetic activity causes vasoconstriction, thereby increasing resistance to blood flow. During exercise there is a level of general sympathetic nervous activity in the vessels of most organs that matches the exercise intensity. However, in working muscles, this sympathetic effect is counteracted by a vasodilatory effect caused by increased metabolite concentrations. The vasodilatory effect of the metabolites is stronger than the vasoconstricting stimuli of the sympathetic nerves. The general excitation level of the sympathetic nervous system causes vasoconstriction in the liver, intestines, and kidneys. In these organs, there is no increase of metabolites to overcome the sympathetic vasoconstricting effect.

The sympathetic nervous system can regulate local or general body reactions to temperature. Localized reactions are easily observed when a small area of skin is heated or cooled. For example, the skin can become red owing to elevated blood flow or the lips may become blue (cyanotic) owing to a lowered blood flow. During prolonged exposure to cold, there may be a redistribution of blood away from the skin to the core of the body in order to preserve a critical core temperature. This will occur in spite of the damage that may be caused to the skin (frostbite).

The adrenal gland essentially is a part of the sympathetic nervous system. In fact, the medulla (core) of the adrenal gland consists of cells that release epinephrine (mainly) and norepinephrine in response to sympathetic stimulation. In effect, the cells of the adrenal medulla are postganglionic sympathetic nerve fibers. The adrenal medulla is capable of releasing large quantities of epinephrine and norepinephrine very rapidly. These hormones are released into the general systemic circulation and are effective in many ways, in practically all tissues, in preparing the body for stress. For example, release of epinephrine and norepinephrine can markedly elevate metabolic rate, increase cardiac output, activate enzymes, increase activity of some neurons and inhibit others, and induce many other reactions. This is often referred to as the "fight or flight" syndrome.

The adrenal cortex differs from the adrenal medulla. The cortex is not regulated by sympathetic nerves and it releases different hormones, as discussed in Chapter 9.

The neurons that control ventilation are not considered to be a part of the autonomic nervous system. However, their function obviously serves a major supporting role for neuromuscular activity. Although ventilation can be controlled voluntarily to some degree, voluntary activation is not essential. Rhythmic ventilation occurs even if a person is unconscious. Within the brain there are groups of neurons that interact with one another as well as with sensory input from the lungs, respiratory muscles, and blood to maintain a steady, rhythmic pattern of inspiration and expiration.

Parasympathetic Autonomic Nervous System

Neurons of the parasympathetic nervous system originate in the base of the brain, above the pituitary, in an area called the hypothalamus (see Chapter 9) and in the brain stem. In addition, some neurons originate in the sacral (tail bone) region of the spinal cord. The axons of these neurons exit the brain with cranial nerves and as sacral nerves from the spinal cord. The tenth cranial nerve, the vagus, contains about 75 per cent of the parasympathetic nerves. The vagus nerve leaves the base of the brain and travels through the neck adjacent to the jugular vein and carotid artery. Its parasympathetic nerves innervate the heart, digestive tract, liver, and pancreas. Unlike those of the sympathetic nervous system, the preganglionic nerve fibers usually extend to the wall of the organ that they innervate before synapsing with the postganglionic neurons.

The parasympathetic effect on the heart reduces the rate and decreases the strength of contraction; therefore, it reduces blood pressure and cardiac output. The bradycardial (heart slowing) effect of training may be due in part to adaptations of the parasympathetic nervous sytem. The parasympathetic influence in the liver and digestive system generally opposes the sympathetic effects; that is, digestion is enhanced by parasympathetic and depressed by sympathetic nerves.

There are other bodily functions that are controlled by the autonomic nervous system. However, since they do not involve neuromuscular activity directly, they are not discussed in this chapter. Information on such functions can be obtained from most basic physiology texts.

ADAPTATION OF THE NEURAL COMPONENT OF THE MOTOR UNIT

Can neural portions of the motor unit adapt to changes in activity level? Some parts can, but the significance of these changes is not entirely clear at this time. The soma (cell body) of the motor neuron responds to acute (single bout) and chronic (daily) exericse. Acute exhaustive exercise enlarges the soma. However, chronic daily exercise reduces soma size, below control levels if the exercise program is intense enough.

The α-MN can adopt biochemically as well. Nuclear material and nucleoproteins in the soma are reduced by acute exhaustive exercise. However, if animals are subjected to moderate chronic daily overload the soma will develop significantly greater levels of nucleoprotein (general protein synthesizing activity), acetylcholinesterase activity (related to neurotransmission), and glucose-6-phosphate dehydrogenase activity (important metabolically for synthesizing ATP).[10]

The axon of the α-MN probably does not adapt morphologically to overload and disuse; the neuromuscular junction, on the other hand, does seem to adapt.[11] Its area and enzymatic activity increase when the muscle fiber increases in size (hypertrophy) and decrease with decreased fiber size (atrophy).

SUMMARY

One of many roles of the nervous system is to execute and regulate complex movement patterns. This control occurs via the α-MNs (alpha-motoneurons) that synapse directly with muscle fibers. The α-MNs, with the muscle fibers that they innervate, form at least two types of motor units. The α-MNs control not only the activity of the muscle fibers but also biochemical and contractile properties of those fibers. This control may be due to the activity of the motor unit or to a neurotrophic influence on the muscle fibers.

The α-MNs function synergistically with smaller γ-MNs that maintain tension in small muscle fibers within spindles so that the spindles remain sensitive to muscle length during active muscle shortening. Both the α-MNs and γ-MNs are interconnected to spinal cord interneurons, which seem to play a major role in coordinating flexion and extension. Input from stretch receptors of the muscle spindle also converges on the interneurons.

The spinal cord has a remarkable autonomy with respect to its ability to execute locomotor patterns without specific supraspinal or peripheral sensory input. Direct supraspinal input to the spinal cord originates from the sensorimotor cortex of the cerebrum and from the brain stem. The brain stem, motor cortex, cerebellum, and basal ganglia are motor control centers that interact in order to synthesize the appropriate motor program for a given moment.

The autonomic nervous system controls most functions that support neuromuscular activity. It consists of the sympathetic and parasympathetic nervous systems. The sympathetic nervous system releases epinephrine and norepinephrine, which excite the cardiovascular system and inhibit functions related to digestion. Metabolic rate is elevated by the sympathetic nervous system. The parasympathetic system generally opposes these effects.

STUDY QUESTIONS

1. Neurons associated with the initiation of movement are found in what portions of the nervous system?

2. One's response to environmental stress is controlled by what part of the nervous system?

3. How does the autonomic nervous system act to support prolonged exercise?

4. How does an alpha-motoneuron differ from a gamma-motoneuron?

5. What is a fusimotor muscle fiber?

6. What is a skeletomotor muscle fiber?

7. What part of the adrenal gland can be considered to be a postganglionic sympathetic ganglion?

8. What are the major neurotransmitters released from sympathetic postganglionic neurons?

9. Which neurotransmitter is released from postganglionic parasympathetic nerve fibers?

10. What evidence is there that motoneurons control the properties of muscle fiber types?

11. What is meant by a spinal (neuronal) generator?

12. Can alpha-motoneurons adapt to chronic exercise?

FURTHER READINGS

Creed, R. S., Denny-Brown, D., Eccles, J. C., Linddell, E. G. T., and Sherrington, C. S.: *Reflex Activity of the Spinal Cord.* Oxford, Oxford University Press, 1972.

Edington, D. W., and Edgerton, V. R.: *The Biology of Physical Activity.* Boston, Houghton-Mifflin, 1976.

Ginzel, K. H.: Interaction of somatic and autonomic functions in muscular exericse. *In* Keogh, J., and Hutton R. (eds.): *Exercise and Sports Sciences Reviews.* Santa Barbara, Journal Publishing Affiliates, 1977.

Granit, R.: *Mechanisms Regulating the Discharges of Motoneurons.* Springfield, Ill., Charles C Thomas, 1972.

REFERENCES

1. Burke, R. E., and Edgerton, V. R.: Motor unit properties and selective involvement in movement. *In* Keogh, J., and Hutton, R. (eds.): *Exercise and Sports Sciences Reviews,* Vol. 3. New York, Academic Press, 1975, pp. 31–81.

2. Buller, A. J., Eccles, J. C., and Eccles, R. M.: Interaction between motoneurons and muscles in respect of the characteristic speeds of their responses. J. Physiol. (Lond.) *150*:417–439, 1960.

3. Hultborn, H. Illert, M., and Santini, M.: Convergence on interneurons mediating the reciprocal Ia inhibition of motoneurons. I. Disynaptic Ia inhibition of Ia inhibitory interneurons. Acta Physiol. Scand. *96*:193–201, 1976

4. Edgerton, V. R., Grillner, S., Sjostrom, A., and Zangger, P.: Central generation of locomotion in vertebrates. *In* Herman, R., Grillner, S., Stein, P. S. G., and Stuart, D. G. (eds.): *Neural Control of Locomotion.* New York, Plenum Publishing Corporation, 1976, pp. 439–464.

5. Orlovsky, G. N., and Shitz, M. L.: Control of locomotion: A neurophysiological analysis of the cat locomotor system. *In* Porter, R. (ed.): *Neurophysiology II,* Vol. 10. Baltimore, University Park Press, 1976, pp. 281–317.

6. Smith, J. L.: Fusimotor loop properties and involvement during voluntary movement. *In* Keogh, H. and Hutton, R. (eds.): *Exercise and Sports Sciences Reviews.* Santa Barbara, Journal Publishing Affiliates, 1977, pp. 297–334.

7. Henneman, E.: Motor functions of the cerebral cortex. *In* Mountcastle, V. B. (ed.): *Medical Physiology,* 13th ed. St. Louis, the C. V. Mosby Company, 1974, p. 772.

8. Evarts, E. V.: Sensorimotor cortex activity associated with movement triggered by visual as compared to somesthetic inputs. *In* Evarts, E. v. (ed.): *Central Processing of Sensory Input Leading to Motor Output.* Cambridge, Mass., The MIT Press, 1975, pp. 327–337.

9. Kornhuber, H. H.: Cerebral cortex, cerebellum, and basal ganglia: An introduction to their motor functions. *In* Evarts, E. V. (ed.): *Central Processing of Sensory Input Leading to Motor Output.* Cambridge, Mass., The MIT Press, 1975, pp. 267–280.

10. Gerchman, L., Edgerton, V. R., and Carrow, R.: Effects of physical training on the histochemistry and morphology of ventral motor neurons. Exp. Neurol. *49*:790–801, 1975.

11. Crockett, J. L., Edgerton, V. R., Max, S. R., and Barnard, R. J.: The neuromuscular junction in response to endurance training. Exp. Neurol. *51*:207–215, 1976.

4

THE RESPIRATORY SYSTEM

RICHARD H. STRAUSS, M.D.

Animal cells respire: they consume oxygen and produce carbon dioxide. Single-celled animals, such as the amoeba, support their respiration simply by allowing oxygen to diffuse into the cell from the surrounding liquid and carbon dioxide, the waste product, to diffuse out. Diffusion of gases through water and tissues is slow, but because the distances involved are small (less than 1 millimeter), amoebae function effectively.

Humans, being larger, require tubes and plumbing to transport gases between the outside environment and the cell surface. The respiratory system and the circulatory system transfer gases at a rate that is determined by the needs of the cells. For example, ventilation in the human can vary from about 6 liters of air per minute at rest to 180 liters of air per minute at maximum exercise. This chapter discusses how air gets into and out of the lungs (ventilation); how gases diffuse between air and blood in the lungs; how blood transports gases to and from tissue; and what changes in respiration take place during exercise.

MECHANICS OF VENTILATION

In order for air to be pumped into and out of the lungs, the muscles of respiration exert forces that result in pressure changes within the lung. These pressure changes cause air to flow, but not entirely freely, because resistance develops as air passes through various structures.

Resistance to Airflow

Any gas or liquid that flows smoothly through a tube (laminar flow) resists movement because of friction among its molecules and between them and the tube wall. This resistance is highly dependent on the radius of the tube: the smaller the tube, the greater the resistance.* The energy that is required to overcome resistance is provided by a drop in gas pressure between the two ends of the tube.

---

*Resistance is inversely proportional to the fourth power of the radius.

During exercise, the pressure difference between the environment and the inside of the lungs must increase in order to increase gas flow (velocity). In addition, as gas velocity increases, flow tends to become increasingly turbulent (swirling), which causes more resistance than does smooth flow.

Airways

Airways are the structures that conduct air from the outside environment to the *alveoli,* the tiny sacs of the lung where gases diffuse between air and blood. It is in the upper airways (Fig. 4–1), which include the nose, mouth, and pharynx, that incoming air is generally warmed, humidified, and cleansed of large particles. These functions are performed most efficiently when air is breathed through the nose, rather than the mouth, because the nasal passages provide a larger surface area of mucous membranes for the air to come in contact with. The irregular bony turbinates of the nose help to increase surface area. During the high ventilations of strenuous exercise, people find that it is necessary to breathe through the mouth because it offers less resistance to air flow than does the nose.

The lower airways (from the larynx downward) include the trachea, bronchi, and bronchioles (Fig. 4–1). These tubes branch repeatedly, becoming smaller and more numerous until reaching every alveolus. As the airways branch, their *total* cross-sectional area actually increases, and resistance to airflow lessens. Consequently, in normal individuals, most airflow resistance occurs in the large and medium-size airways.

Most portions of the lower airways are lined by cells that produce mucus in which particles are trapped. Thus, air is almost sterile by the time it reaches the alveoli. Cleansing of the airways is normally accomplished by the rhythmic motion of the cilia (Fig. 4–2), which sweep mucus up the airways to the pharynx where it is swallowed unconsciously. Coughing helps to eliminate excess secretions and foreign material from the lower airways.

The walls of most of the lower airways contain cartilage and smooth muscle. Cartilage adds rigidity and helps to prevent airway collapse during expiration. During exercise, the smooth muscle relaxes and allows airways to dilate slightly, which in turn permits air to flow more easily. Contraction of the smooth muscle causes increased resistance to airflow and is one of the mechanisms that make breathing difficult during an asthma attack.

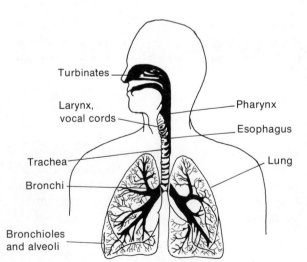

Turbinates

Larynx,
vocal cords

Pharynx

Esophagus

Trachea

Lung

Bronchi

Bronchioles
and alveoli

Figure 4–1. Airways of the respiratory system. (Redrawn from Guyton, A. C.: *Textbook of Medical Physiology.* 5th ed. Philadelphia, W. B. Saunders Company, 1976, p. 526.)

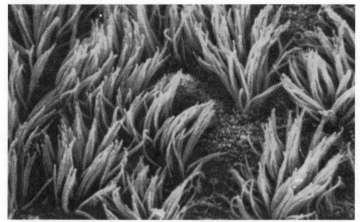

Figure 4–2. Cilia line lower airways and beat in a coordinated manner to move mucus toward the larynx and out of the respiratory system. (Hamster trachea is shown.) (From Comroe, J. H.: *Physiology of Respiration,* 2nd ed. Chicago, Year Book Medical Publishers Inc., 1974, p. 223.)

Muscles of Respiration

The lungs are passive. They expand and contract only because the thoracic (chest) cavity changes in volume. During inspiration at rest, the thoracic cavity enlarges as the diaphragm contracts and moves downward (Fig. 4–3A). This contraction also tends to pull the ribs upward by using the abdominal contents as a fulcrum. When the ribs move upward they pivot forward, enlarging the rib cage (Fig. 4–3B and C). The external intercostal muscles (between the ribs) also help to pull the ribs upward during ventilations of greater intensity than those at rest. During heavy exercise, other muscles assist in enlarging the thoracic volume. Such muscles are called accessory muscles of respiration and include neck and back muscles which can be seen working in persons who have just finished a hard race.

In contrast to inspiration, expiration at rest is passive; that is, it occurs without the aid of contracting muscles. The chest wall and lungs are stretched during inspiration and therefore get smaller when the respiratory muscles relax. During exercise, air

Figure 4–3. *A,* Changes in dimensions of chest and abdomen during breathing. Positions in expiration are shown by solid lines; positions in inspiration, by dashed lines. *B* and *C,* During inspiration, the ribs pivot upward and forward, increasing the diameter of the rib cage. (*B* and *C* from Goss, C. M. (ed.): *Gray's Anatomy of the Human Body,* 28th ed. Philadelphia, Lea & Febiger, 1966, p. 317.)

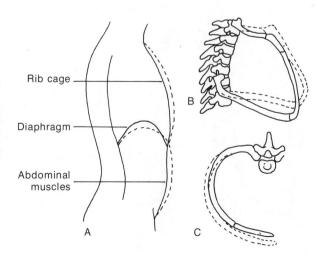

Rib cage

Diaphragm

Abdominal
muscles

can be forced out more rapidly by the contraction of the abdominal muscles (Fig. 4–3A). These muscles push the abdominal contents against the diaphragm, forcing it upward. At the same time, internal intercostal muscles contract to pull the ribs downward and make the rib cage smaller.

Work of Breathing

The muscles of respiration use a portion of the oxygen respired, varying from about 1 per cent at rest to 10 per cent during heavy exercise. The largest portion of the work done by these muscles is used to overcome airflow resistance. In addition, energy is also required to overcome elastic forces during expansion of the lungs and chest wall. Part of the force opposing expansion of the lungs comes from the surface tension of the thin film of water and other material that lines the alveoli. Because water molecules are attracted to each other, they tend to decrease the water-gas surface area and oppose expansion. This attraction is reduced by a surface active agent (surfactant) that is produced by the lung and that floats on the water's surface.

Intrapleural Pressure

Because the lungs are elastic, they will collapse like deflated balloons if removed from the chest. The lungs remain inflated within the chest because the pressure surrounding them is less than the pressure within them. Normally, there is no air surrounding the lungs. The inside of the chest wall and the outside of the lungs are lined by smooth transparent membranes called *pleurae* (Fig. 4–4). These surfaces rub against each other during breathing and are lubricated by a thin film of fluid. The space between the pleural surfaces is called the pleural space or cavity, even though there is normally no true space there.

The pressure within the pleural space is called the *intrapleural pressure*. At the end of quiet expiration it is about -5 cm H_2O; that is, a little less than the pressure surrounding the body. During inspiration, the intrapleural pressure becomes more negative and the lungs expand. Pressure within the alveoli falls and air flows inward.

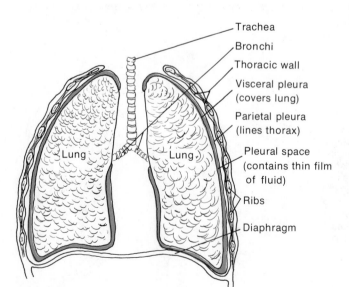

Trachea
Bronchi
Thoracic wall
Visceral pleura (covers lung)
Parietal pleura (lines thorax)
Pleural space (contains thin film of fluid)
Ribs
Diaphragm
Lung
Lung

Figure 4–4. The pleural space. (Redrawn from Mathews, D. K., and Fox, E. L.: *The Physiological Basis of Physical Education and Athletics.* Philadelphia, W. B. Saunders Company, 1976, p. 180.)

During forced expiration, the intrapleural pressure becomes positive, although this does not occur during quiet breathing. Very high pressures (about 200 cm H_2O) can be generated within the chest by trying to exhale forcefully against the glottis (vocal cords), which is closed so that air cannot escape. Sometimes this is done (inadvisably) in weight lifting. If a high intrapleural pressure is maintained for several seconds, it can prevent return of venous blood to the heart from the rest of the body. The heart then has little blood to pump and the decreased flow of blood to the brain can cause loss of consciousness (blackout).

When air gets into the pleural space the condition is termed a *pneumothorax*. The lung then collapses partly or entirely, depending on how much air has leaked in. One cause of a pneumothorax is a stab wound of the chest which allows air to enter the pleural space either through the chest wall or through a wound in the lung. Blood may also enter the pleural space.

A more common cause of collapsed lung is a *spontaneous pneumothorax* (Fig. 4–5) in which a weak area on the surface of the lung ruptures for no apparent reason, causing an air leak. Because the pleural spaces of the left and right sides of the chest

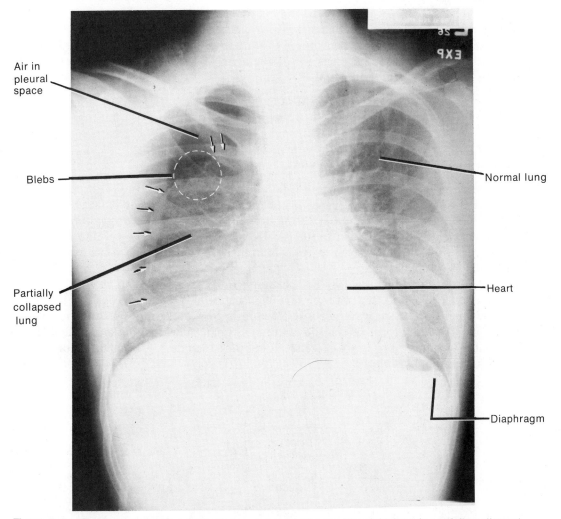

Figure 4–5. Chest x-ray showing a spontaneous pneumothorax. The right lung is partially collapsed (arrows) because a moderate amount of air has leaked into the pleural space from a ruptured bleb on the surface of the lung. Several unruptured blebs are visible (circled). (Courtesy of Peter Bent Brigham Hospital Boston.)

are separated, only one lung collapses. Spontaneous pneumothorax occurs most commonly in young men of about college age, either at rest or during exercise. In a small pneumothorax, in which the leak seals almost immediately, the air is absorbed spontaneously by the body over a few days. A large pneumothorax may require specific treatment (see Chapter 16).

Respiratory Volumes

During respiration the volume of the lungs changes and the volume of gas inspired or expired can be measured. That volume of gas that is inspired or expired during a single normal respiratory cycle is called the *tidal volume* (Fig. 4–6). Tidal volume can increase from about 0.5 liter at rest to about 3.0 liters during severe exercise. *Vital capacity* is a measurement of the maximum amount of air that can be expired — from one's deepest inhalation to maximum exhalation. Vital capacity is generally larger in larger people and is abnormally small in persons with diseases that restrict the movement of the lungs or chest wall. Even at the end of a maximum exhalation the lungs are not empty. The remaining volume of air is called the *residual volume*. The *total lung capacity* is the volume of gas in the lungs at maximum inspiration — that is, the vital capacity plus the residual volume.

The amount of gas breathed in one minute is called the *minute volume* (MV). It can be calculated from the *respiratory frequency* (f) — the number of breaths per minute — and the tidal volume (V_T):

$$MV = (f) (V_T)$$

For example, at rest:

$$MV = (12 \text{ breaths/min}) (0.5 \text{ liter/breath})$$
$$= 6 \text{ liters/min}$$

During exercise, both frequency and tidal volume increase.

Not all the air breathed reaches the alveoli. Some — about one-third of it at rest — remains in the airways at the end of inspiration and is unavailable for gas exchange with the blood. This volume is called the *dead space*. The volume of gas that reaches the alveoli in a period of time is known as the alveolar ventilation and is available for gas exchange.

The ability to ventilate does not normally limit exercise. Even though a runner may feel that he can go no faster or farther because he is "out of breath," he usually can still ventilate more if he wishes. The limits to exercise are not known but are believed to reside within the cardiovascular system. However, abnormalities of the respiratory system may limit exercise. Examples include the removal of one lung, asthma, and emphysema.

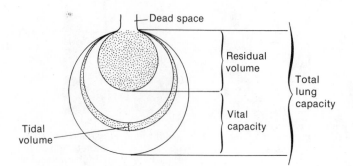

Figure 4–6. Lung volumes and capacities. (Redrawn from Comroe, J. H.: *Physiology of Respiration,* 2nd ed. Chicago, Year Book Medical Publishers, Inc., 1974, p. 15.)

GAS EXCHANGE

Venous blood from the body passes through the lungs where it gains oxygen and loses carbon dioxide. The exchange of gases between air and blood takes place through the thin alveolocapillary membrane, which presents little barrier to diffusion of gases under normal conditions (Fig. 4–7). Gas exchange must take place rapidly, especially in exercise, when up to 30 liters of blood per minute pass through the lungs. Blood remains in the pulmonary (lung) capillaries for less than one second. Rapid equilibration of blood and air can take place because of the large surface area of the 300 million alveoli (Fig. 4–8). The blood in the capillaries of the lung is spread out so that each alveolus is in effect surrounded by a thin sheet of blood. It is as though one glassful of blood were spread over half a tennis court.

A gas diffuses down its partial pressure gradient — from a location of higher to lower partial pressure.* The partial pressure of oxygen (P_{O_2}) decreases in transit from inspired air to tissue cells (Fig. 4–9). In dry air at sea level, $P_{O_2} = 160$ mm Hg. When air is humidified in the airways, $P_{O_2} = 150$ mm Hg because air is diluted by water vapor. In the alveoli, P_{O_2} drops to about 100 mm Hg because the air is further diluted with carbon dioxide and some of the oxygen is used up. Blood leaving most of the pulmonary capillaries has the same P_{O_2} as the alveoli (100 mm Hg), but in the arteries the P_{O_2} is slightly lower because a small amount of blood gets through the lungs without being fully oxygenated. This occurs mainly because ventilation and perfusion (blood flow) are not precisely matched in some parts of the lung. As arterial blood passes through the capillaries of the body, it loses some of its oxygen by diffusion to the cells of the tissues and becomes venous blood. Mixed venous blood, from throughout the body, has a P_{O_2} of about 40 mm Hg at rest. During strenuous exercise, the mixed venous P_{O_2} may drop below 20 mm Hg, with the venous blood from working muscles having an even lower value.

During exercise, arterial blood remains fully oxygenated. Thus, transfer of oxygen to blood by the lungs does not normally limit exercise. The blood is well oxygenated because (1) more lung capillaries are open during exercise than at rest; and (2) although blood spends less time in lung capillaries (about 0.3 sec), that time is still sufficient for complete equilibration of gases between blood and alveoli.

---

*Partial pressure is that gas pressure contributed by a single gas in a mixture of gases or in solution.

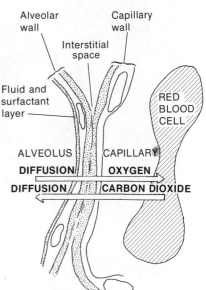

Figure 4–7. Diffusion of gases through the alveolo-capillary membrane. (Redrawn from Guyton, A. C.: *Textbook of Medical Physiology,* 5th ed. Philadelphia, W. B. Saunders Company, 1976, p. 539.)

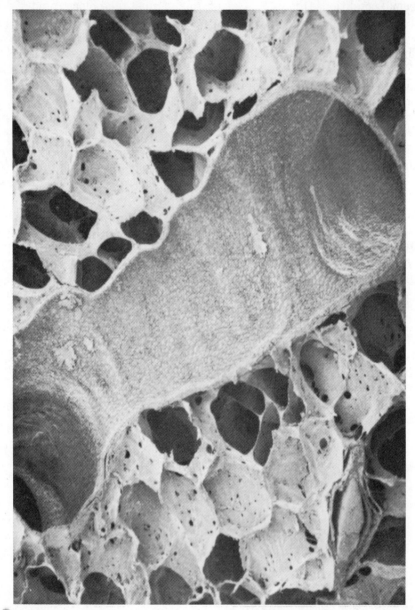

Figure 4–8. Section of lung showing many alveoli and a small bronchiole. The pulmonary capillaries run in the walls of the alveoli. The holes in the alveolar walls are the pores of Kohn. (Scanning electron micrograph by J. A. Nowell and W. S. Tyler.) (From West, J. B.: *Respiratory Physiology.* Baltimore, The Williams and Wilkins Company, 1974, p. 4.)

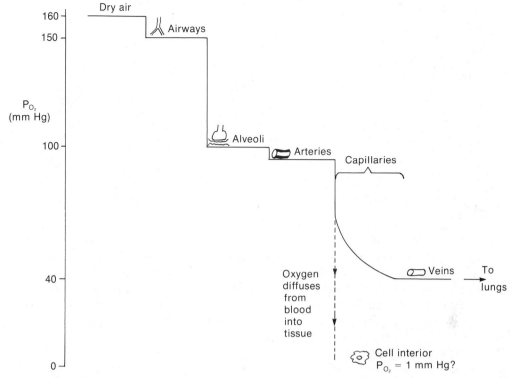

Figure 4–9. Oxygen pressure falls in transit from external air to the cell.

TRANSPORT OF OXYGEN AND CARBON DIOXIDE BY BLOOD

Oxygen

Oxygen is not very soluble in water; thus, little oxygen is carried dissolved in the plasma of blood. Most is transported bound to hemoglobin, which is contained in red cells and is responsible for the red color of blood. The hemoglobin molecule consists of a protein portion and four heme groups to which oxygen is attracted (Fig. 4–10). One oxygen molecule can combine with each heme group because it is moderately attracted to the iron in heme. The oxygen-hemoglobin bond is readily broken — that is, oxygen can leave the hemoglobin molecule easily when it reaches tissue and encounters a lower oxygen pressure.

As blood passes through the capillaries of the lung, the partial pressure of oxygen rises and oxygen molecules combine with the available hemoglobin until it becomes saturated (Fig. 4–11). As blood passes through the capillaries of the body it loses oxygen. The P_{O_2} falls from about 100 mm Hg in arterial blood to an average of 40 mm Hg in mixed venous blood during rest. Under such conditions, hemoglobin saturation falls from about 100 per cent to 75 per cent. Blood passing through working muscle loses more oxygen and leaves with a lower P_{O_2}. In addition, several conditions found within exercising muscle cause a decrease in the attraction between oxygen and hemoglobin and thus promote the unloading of oxygen in the tissue capillaries. These local factors are (1) increased partial pressure of carbon dioxide; (2) increased acidity as a result of carbon dioxide and lactic acid production; and (3) increased temperature (Fig. 4–11).

Myoglobin is a compound similar to hemoglobin, but it is located within muscle cells. It acts as a storage depot for a small amount of oxygen, which probably can be

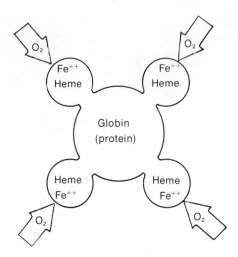

Figure 4–10. The hemoglobin molecule is composed of a protein called globin and four iron-containing groups called heme. Oxygen is carried by the heme groups. (Redrawn from Mathews, D. K., and Fox, E. L.: *The Physiological Basis of Physical Education and Athletics.* Philadelphia, W. B. Saunders Company, 1976, p. 194.)

used by the muscle cell during contraction when blood is unable to flow through the muscle. Between contractions the myoglobin is recharged with oxygen.

Abnormalities and Poisons. Hemoglobin that is saturated with oxygen appears bright red. A significant loss of oxygen (desaturation) results in the darker red color of venous blood. The presence of desaturated blood in the skin causes the skin to look blue. This blue coloration is called *cyanosis.* Exposure to a cold environment may cause the skin and lips to turn blue because cold can greatly reduce the flow of blood to skin, which results in unusually great desaturation of that blood that remains in the skin. A decrease in blood flow to the skin, and thus cyanosis, may also be found in cardiac arrest or circulatory shock. Breathing a gas that contains too little oxygen can also cause cyanosis.

Cyanide poisoning interferes with the function of the cytochrome system (see Chapter 1) and stops respiration within the cells. It does not decrease hemoglobin saturation and does not cause cyanosis. Carbon monoxide poisoning occurs primarily because the carbon monoxide molecule is attracted to hemoglobin about 210 times more strongly than is oxygen. Hemoglobin with carbon monoxide attached is unavailable for transport of oxygen to tissues. Such hemoglobin is even brighter red in color than hemoglobin that is saturated with oxygen, so the skin of people dying of carbon monoxide poisoning has a healthy pink color.

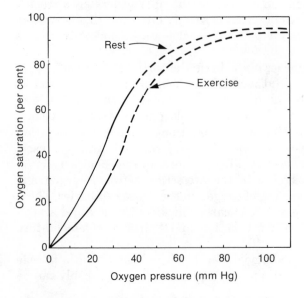

Figure 4–11. Saturation of hemoglobin by oxygen. Broken lines indicate the loading and unloading of oxygen as it normally occurs in the body. During exercise there is greater unloading of oxygen because oxygen pressure is lower in the working muscle. In addition, exercise shifts the entire curve to the right because oxygen is further driven off by increases in acidity, P_{CO_2}, and temperature, which occur in the working muscle. (Redrawn from Chapman, C. B., and Mitchell, J. H.: The physiology of exercise. Scientific American, May 1965, p. 94. Copyright © 1965 by Scientific American, Inc. All rights reserved.)

Carbon Dioxide

In contrast to oxygen, carbon dioxide is very soluble in water and does not require a special molecule to carry it. Carbon dioxide produced by tissue diffuses into capillary blood where it reacts with water to form acid and bicarbonate:

$$CO_2 + H_2O \underset{\text{anhydrase}}{\overset{\text{carbonic}}{\rightleftharpoons}} H_2CO_3 \rightleftharpoons H^+ + HCO_3^-$$

This reaction, if unaided, would proceed so slowly that it could not keep up with metabolic requirements. However, the reaction is catalyzed (speeded up) by carbonic anhydrase, which is located primarily within red cells.

Although most carbon dioxide is transported as bicarbonate, a small amount is transported attached to the protein portion of the hemoglobin molecule and a little remains in physical solution in water.

In the lung capillaries, the processes that occur in blood in the body tissues are essentially reversed, so that carbon dioxide is lost from blood and oxygen is gained.

CONTROL OF VENTILATION

As the cells of the body increase their metabolism during exercise, ventilation increases to meet the demand for gas exchange. How this is accomplished is not completely understood, but parts of the control system have been analyzed. Signals are transmitted from working muscles as neural impulses or as chemical changes in the blood stream.

Neural Control

The rhythmic pattern of breathing is generated by the *central respiratory neurons* that form a network within the brain stem (Fig. 4–12). This network acts as a type of pacemaker and transmits impulses to the respiratory muscles. (The phrenic nerve goes to the diaphragm, and intercostal nerves run to the intercostal muscles.) It is through the central respiratory neurons that stimuli act to influence respiration. For example, the cerebral cortex of the brain can affect ventilation, as is seen in breath-holding, speaking, and playing a wind instrument. Similarly, excitement before a race often causes breathing that is deeper and faster than necessary (*hyperventilation**). Neural reflexes from many parts of the body, such as moving limbs and the lungs themselves, can also modify ventilation.

Chemical Control

There are specialized areas within the body that contain nerve endings capable of sensing certain chemicals in their immediate environment. These are called chemoreceptors. An important one is the *central chemoreceptor* that is located at the base of the brain stem in the medulla (Fig. 4–12). The job of the central chemoreceptor is to "taste" the acidity of cerebrospinal fluid that surrounds the brain. Cells of the body function

---

*Hyperventilation is ventilation in excess of that required by metabolism. Symptoms and treatment of the hyperventilation syndrome are discussed in Chapter 16.

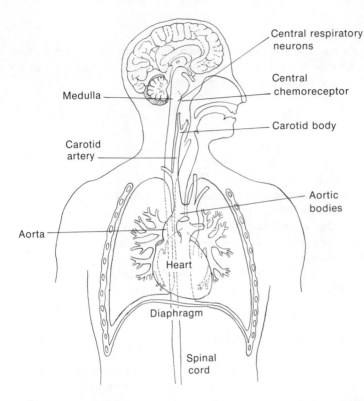

Medulla

Carotid
artery

Aorta

Heart

Diaphragm

Spinal
cord

Central respiratory
neurons

Central
chemoreceptor

Carotid body

Aortic
bodies

Figure 4–12. Location of chemoreceptors and central respiratory neurons. (Modified from Comroe, J. H.: The lung. Scientific American, February 1966, p. 62. Copyright © 1966 by Scientific American, Inc. All rights reserved.)

well only if the acidity of their environment is carefully controlled, so clearly this is an important function. The central chemoreceptor can sense changes in acidity caused by a change in the partial pressure of carbon dioxide. If acidity becomes too high, the central chemoreceptor signals the central respiratory neurons to increase ventilation. The increased ventilation causes more carbon dioxide to be "washed out" of the body, which lowers not only P_{CO_2} but also the acidity of arterial blood and cerebrospinal fluid. Conversely, if acidity becomes lower than normal, ventilation decreases. Experimentally, breathing air that contains carbon dioxide causes increased ventilation, as does adding acid, such as lactic acid, to the blood stream.

The *peripheral chemoreceptors* consist of the carotid bodies, which are located on the carotid arteries in the neck, and the aortic bodies, on the arch of the aorta, the main artery coming from the heart (Fig. 4–12). These chemoreceptors (primarily the carotid bodies) are moderately sensitive to changes in arterial P_{CO_2} and acidity and, in addition, are the only important monitors of oxygen in arterial blood. A low arterial P_{O_2} can cause a small increase in ventilation. However, low P_{O_2} is a weak stimulus for ventilation and causes little conscious desire to increase breathing. Elevated arterial P_{CO_2} is a stronger respiratory stimulus. For example, an individual who hyperventilates immediately before making a breath-hold dive may become unconscious underwater without warning owing to low arterial oxygen. The hyperventilation causes an abnormal loss of carbon dioxide from the body, and the stimulus to breathe that carbon dioxide causes is thereby decreased. Hyperventilation does not significantly increase the body's stores of oxygen (see Chapter 23).

Ventilation During Exercise

An example of the way in which ventilation increases during exercise is shown in Figure 4–13. When exercise begins, there is a sudden, moderate increase in ventilation possibly due to neural signals from the brain and the moving joints and muscles. Over

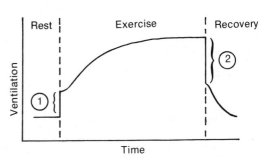

Figure 4–13. Schematic representation of changes in ventilation during exercise, showing (1) the abrupt increase at the onset and (2) the abrupt, larger decrease at the end of exercise. (Redrawn from Dejours, P. *In* Fenn, W. O., and Rahn, H. (eds.): *Handbook of Physiology.* Washington, D.C., American Physiological Society, 1964, Sec. 3, vol. 1.)

the next few minutes there is a gradual increase in ventilation, which tends to plateau. This increase may be due to chemical stimuli but the mechanism is not understood. Working muscles give off more carbon dioxide and lactic acid and use more oxygen, but arterial P_{CO_2} and P_{O_2} remain constant except during very strenuous exercise. Increased arterial acidity alone cannot account for the ventilation. When exercise stops there is a sharp fall in ventilation, followed by a more gradual return to the resting level as metabolism returns to normal and lactic acid is consumed.

Physical training can increase both the maximum oxygen uptake and the ventilation that accompanies it.

Second Wind. Second wind is a subjective phenomenon that is difficult to study. Not everyone believes that it exists. After a few minutes of reasonably hard exercise, some people experience an easing of their initial sensation of difficult breathing (dyspnea). Among the many suggested causes are the various adjustments in the respiratory and cardiovascular systems that take place during the early part of exercise. For example, initially elevated levels of lactic acid in muscle and blood may decrease.

CIGARETTE SMOKING

It is generally felt that cigarette smoking causes a decrease in endurance. The reasons for this are not entirely clear, but cigarette smoke is known to increase airway resistance and the amount of carbon monoxide combined with hemoglobin. In addition, the nicotine in cigarette smoke causes constriction of blood vessels and an increase in resting heart rate.

College students who smoke were found to have more cough, mucus production, and shortness of breath than nonsmokers. Smoking over a period of years is known to damage health in several ways. The epidemic of lung cancer in many Western countries is almost wholly due to cigarette smoking. Chronic bronchitis and emphysema are caused in large part by smoking, which also contributes significantly to heart disease and peptic ulcer disease.

SUMMARY

The function of the respiratory system, in conjunction with the circulatory system, is to transfer oxygen to the cells of the body and to remove carbon dioxide. The airways not only conduct air but also clean, warm (or cool), and humidify it before it reaches the alveoli. The forces that pump air in and out of the lungs are generated by muscles and transmitted through the intrapleural space to the lungs. Energy is used mainly in overcoming resistance to airflow. The work of breathing is much greater during high ventilations of exercise than at rest. Gases diffuse readily between air and blood through the walls of the alveoli. Hemoglobin carries most of the oxygen, which is poorly soluble in plasma. Carbon dioxide, in contrast, is transported mainly as bicarbonate dissolved in plasma. During heavy exercise, many respiratory and circulatory mechanisms work at rates that are near their maxima. The respiratory system, however, does not normally determine the upper limit to exercise. The cause of increased ventilation during exercise is not known.

STUDY QUESTIONS

1. Where in the airways does most of the resistance to airflow occur?

2. What is the primary muscle (or groups of muscles) used in resting ventilation?

3. What is the function of the cilia that line the airways?

4. What effect does surfactant have on lung expansion?

5. Why does the lung collapse in the event of a pneumothorax?

6. Calculate the approximate *alveolar* ventilation in a resting individual with a tidal volume of 0.6 liter per breath and a respiratory frequency of 10 breaths per minute. Do not ignore dead space.

7. Does ventilation normally limit exercise?

8. Why, even at high blood flows, does blood leave the lungs well oxygenated?

9. Why is iron necessary for oxygen transport?

10. (a) Give a chemical reaction that relates carbonic anhydrase to the transport of carbon dioxide by blood.

    (b) Where is carbonic anhydrase found in high concentrations?

11. (a) What is the main reason that oxygen dissociates (unloads) from hemoglobin in muscle capillaries?

    (b) What are three additional factors found in exercising muscle that promote this dissociation?

12. Why do people sometimes appear blue when cold?

13. Which is a stronger stimulus to ventilation, decreased inspired P_{O_2} or increased inspired P_{CO_2}?

14. Plot the time course of ventilation before, during, and after a period of exercise.

15. What happens to arterial P_{O_2} and P_{CO_2} in moderate exercise?

16. Give three detrimental effects of smoking.

FURTHER READINGS

Åstrand, P.-O. and Rodahl, K.: *Textbook of Work Physiology*. New York, McGraw-Hill Book Company, 1977.

Comroe, J. H.: *Physiology of Respiration*. Chicago, Year Book Medical Publishers, 1974.

Guyton, A. C.: *Textbook of Medical Physiology*. Philadelphia, W. B. Saunders Company, 1976.

Ruch, T. C., and Patton, H. D. (eds.): *Physiology and Biophysics*. Philadelphia, W. B. Saunders Company, 1973.

West, J. B.: *Respiratory Physiology — The Essentials*. Baltimore, The Williams & Wilkins Company, 1974.

5

THE CIRCULATORY SYSTEM

MICHAEL M. DEHN, M.S.
and JERE H. MITCHELL, M.D.

The primary function of the circulation is to supply fuel to tissues of the body and to remove metabolic waste products. The blood and the components of the cardiovascular system (i.e., the heart and blood vessels) are responsible for carrying out this task. Changes in metabolic activity necessitate that the circulatory system be dynamic. Continuous feedback with respect to the specific needs of the organs and tissues results in an appropriate response for the most effective distribution of blood flow and maintenance of mean arterial blood pressure. The regulation of blood flow often involves complex mechanisms, some of which are not totally understood. This chapter examines the basic structure and function of the cardiovascular system's components and discusses principles relating to the acute and chronic responses of the cardiovascular system to dynamic and static exercise.

THE HEART

The heart is simply a muscle that acts as the pump for the circulatory system. Actually, the heart consists of two pumps, as shown in Figure 5–1. The right heart (right side of the heart) receives oxygen-desaturated blood from the body and delivers it to the lungs (pulmonary circulation). The left heart accepts the now oxygen-saturated blood from the lungs and pumps it to the organs and tissues of the body (systemic circulation). Each side of the heart consists of an upper chamber (atrium) and a lower chamber (ventricle). The atria are primarily reservoirs, but they also serve some "booster pump" functions, although the thicker-walled ventricles do most of the pumping.

The direction of the blood flow within the heart is controlled by valves. The tricuspid and mitral (atrioventricular) valves (Fig. 5–1) prevent blood from regurgitating back into the atria during the contractions of the ventricles. The pulmonic and aortic valves prevent blood from flowing back into the ventricles from the pulmonary artery and aorta. The difference in pressures between chambers and major vessels causes these one-way valves to open and close. The fibrous connections (chordae tendinae) between the ventricular wall and the atrioventricular valves prevent these valves from becoming everted but do not actively participate in their opening or closing.

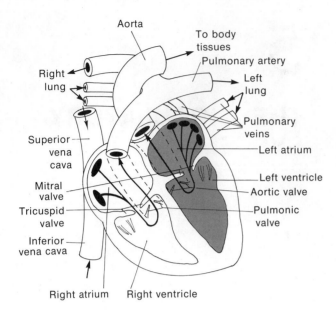

Figure 5–1. Diagram of the heart. The arrows indicate the direction of blood flow. (Redrawn from Vander, A. J., et al.: *Human Physiology: The Mechanisms of Body Function,* 2nd ed. Copyright © 1975 by McGraw-Hill, Inc. Used by permission of McGraw-Hill Book Company.)

Cardiac Muscle

The heart is made up largely of cardiac muscle cells having scme properties similar to those of skeletal muscle and some properties similar to those of smooth muscle. Similarities to skeletal muscle include a striated ultrastructure having myofibrils that utilize a sliding filament type of contraction. Like smooth muscle, cardiac cells are autorhythmic and are thus able to spontaneously generate their own rhythmic excitation impulses. The presence of gap junctions between adjacent cells allows propagation of electrical impulses (action potentials) from cell to cell as in smooth muscle. Furthermore, neural control of cardiac muscle is maintained primarily by the autonomic nervous system.

Electrical Activity

Contraction of the heart is stimulated by depolarization of the cardiac muscle membrane. The impulse spreads through the heart via special conduction fibers and unique junctions between adjacent cells that allow action potentials to be transmitted from cell to cell. The coordinated conduction of the electrical impulse produces effective cardiac contraction that could not be accomplished by random cellular depolarization.

The action potential originates in the sinoatrial (SA) node, the primary pacemaker of the heart. It spreads through the atria and along special conduction fibers to the atrioventricular (AV) node. Conduction through the AV node is relatively slow, which permits optimal filling of the ventricles before their contraction. Depolarization spreads from the AV node through conductive tissues called the bundle of His and the bundle branches, which are located in the wall between the ventricles and extend into most regions of the ventricles. Conduction continues to be transmitted from cell to cell until depolarization of the heart is complete.

The electrical current generated by the impulse conducted through the heart can be detected by a galvanometer when electrodes are placed on the body. This is essentially the mechanism by which the electrocardiogram (ECG) is produced. A typical

ECG is shown in Figure 5–2. The graph shows, as a function of time, the variations in voltage created by the depolarization and repolarization of cardiac cells. The depolarization of the atria results in a small deflection called the P wave. The QRS complex follows about 0.15 seconds after the P wave and reflects ventricular depolarization. Repolarization of the ventricles creates the T wave. The atrial repolarization wave is of low amplitude and is partially hidden in the QRS complex.

The clinical ECG usually displays twelve different projections of the heart's electrical activity. Each projection produces deflections that describe the magnitude and direction of the electrical impulse with respect to a set of electrodes (one positive and one negative) placed in standardized positions on the body. When the impulse is directed toward the positive electrode, the deflection is positive (upward). Impulses traveling toward the negative electrode produce negative (downward) deflections. Variations from standard patterns reflect underlying anatomical or physiological disorders. The ECG is thus a very useful clinical tool in the diagnosis of heart conditions.

Mechanical Activity (Cardiac Cycle)

The mechanical sequence in the cardiac cycle begins when the electrical depolarization of the heart muscle (myocardium) initiates a period of contraction, first of the atria and then of the ventricles. The atria are in their period of contraction (systole) when the ventricles are in their period of relaxation (diastole). However, the terms systole and diastole are generally used to denote ventricular systole and diastole since the ventricle is the primary pump on each side of the circulation. A diagram of the cardiac cycle on the left side of the heart is shown in Figure 5–3. For the purpose of simplicity, only the left side will be described since the events on the right side are similar.

Ventricular contraction rapidly increases the pressure in the ventricle during the initial fractions of a second before the aortic valve opens. This phase, called isovolumic (constant volume) contraction, involves an isometric-like contraction of cardiac fibers with tremendous tension producing very little shortening in fiber length. As ventricular pressure exceeds aortic pressure, the aortic valve opens and ventricular ejection

Figure 5–2. Typical electrocardiogram. P wave — depolarization of atria. QRS complex — depolarization of ventricles. T wave — repolarization of ventricles. (From Vander, A. J., et al.: *Human Physiology: The Mechanisms of Body Function,* 2nd ed. Copyright © 1975 by McGraw-Hill, Inc. Used by permission of McGraw-Hill Book Company.)

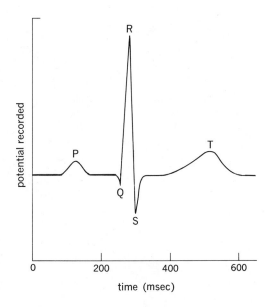

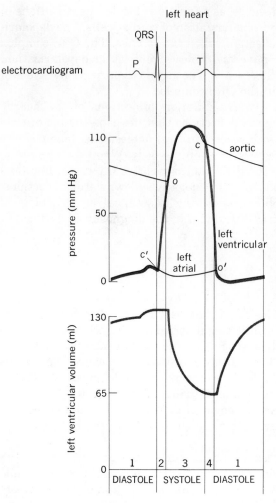

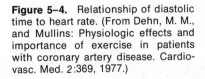

Figure 5–3. Events of the cardiac cycle on the left side of the heart. 1, Filling of the ventricle. 2, Isovolumic contraction of the ventricle. 3, Ejection of blood from the ventricle. 4, Isovolumic relaxation of the ventricle. C', Mitral valve closes. O, aortic valve opens. C, aortic valve closes. O', mitral valve opens. (From Vander, A. J., et al.: *Human Physiology: The Mechanisms of Body Function,* 2nd ed. Copyright © 1975 by McGraw-Hill, Inc. Used by permission of McGraw-Hill Book Company.)

Figure 5–4. Relationship of diastolic time to heart rate. (From Dehn, M. M., and Mullins: Physiologic effects and importance of exercise in patients with coronary artery disease. Cardiovasc. Med. 2:369, 1977.)

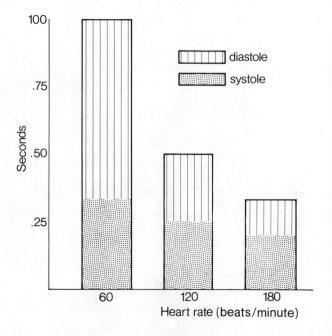

occurs. The ventricles normally eject only about 50 to 75 per cent of the blood in their chambers. Blood surging through the vascular system increases arterial and venous pressures and actually enhances atrial filling at the other end of the circulation. As ventricular pressure diminishes below aortic pressure at the conclusion of systole, the aortic valve closes and ejection ceases.

During the initial stage of ventricular relaxation, the ventricular pressure remains greater than that in the atrium, preventing the AV valves from opening. This brief period of isovolumic relaxation is followed by a precipitous fall in ventricular pressure, the opening of the AV valves, and a phase of rapid ventricular filling. Since most ventricular filling is accomplished during the initial third of diastole, the disproportionate shortening of diastole with increasing heart rates (Fig. 5–4) does not significantly diminish the amount of blood in the ventricle at the end of diastole (end-diastolic volume) at heart rates below 200 beats per minute. By the time the atrium begins to contract during the last phase of diastole, more than 75 per cent of the ventricular filling has already occurred. The fall in atrial pressure after the atrium ejects a small volume of blood into the ventricle causes the AV valves to close and concludes the diastolic period. By this time, the aortic pressure has fallen as blood has passed on through the vascular system.

THE VASCULAR SYSTEM

Systemic Circulation

This vascular system consists of a complex network of conduits for the blood. Arteries take blood away from the heart and veins return blood to the heart. The arteries branch into progressively smaller vessels, called arterioles. These vessels play the primary role in controlling total peripheral resistance (TPR) and regional blood flow by means of expansion (vasodilatation) and reduction (vasoconstriction) of vessel diameter. Arterioles are sometimes referred to as resistance vessels. Arterioles branch into capillaries where the exchange of oxygen, nutrients, and metabolic waste products takes place. The greater percentage of the 70,000 miles of blood vessels in the body are capillaries. They could hold the entire blood supply of the body, but only a fraction are open at any instant. Blood flow through these small vessels (less than 1/1000 inch in diameter) is very slow (5 feet per hour, versus 40 miles per hour in the arteries). This allows maximal exchange of oxygen, fuel, and metabolic waste products to take place.

The smallest branches of the veins, called venules, accept the oxygen-desaturated blood from the capillaries and deposit it in the larger systemic veins. These veins serve as blood reservoirs with the capability of constricting during hemorrhage or exercise to maintain effective blood volume elsewhere in the circulatory system. The systemic veins contain nearly 50 per cent of the body's blood volume (more than three times the volume of the arterial system) and are commonly referred to as capacitance vessels. The veins empty into the venae cavae (Fig. 5–1), the great veins through which all blood returns to the heart. As one can easily see, the blood vessels play an active role in the circulatory system and are not static plumbing.

The heart, being a muscle, requires its own blood supply since it receives no oxygen from the blood that passes through its chambers. The coronary arteries provide the heart muscle (myocardium) with its blood supply. These arteries are the first branches originating from the aorta, which is the largest artery in the body and which receives the blood pumped from the left ventricle. The left coronary artery branches into the anterior descending and the circumflex arteries, which supply most of the front and lateral portions of the left ventricle. The right coronary artery usually supplies the right ventricle and the back wall of the left ventricle.

The heart muscle is very efficient in its utilization of the oxygen provided by the coronary arteries, extracting about 70 per cent of that present in the blood at rest. (Skeletal muscle normally extracts 20 to 25 per cent at rest.) However, this means that any increase in oxygen demand by the heart muscle (usually due to increased heart rate and/or blood pressure) must be met by increased oxygen delivery, primarily from augmented blood flow, since oxygen extraction is almost maximally taxed at rest. This is why the coronary circulation is particularly vulnerable to any obstruction to blood flow, such as is present in coronary artery disease.

The oxygen supply to skeletal muscle must also undergo great change according to its state of activity. This is accomplished both by an increase in blood flow and by an increase in extraction of oxygen from the blood. The diameter of the resistance vessels in skeletal muscle is controlled by sympathetic nerve activity and by local metabolites released during muscular activity. During activity, local factors are much more important than sympathetic nerve activity.

Pulmonary Circulation

The blood returning from the body to the right side of the heart is pumped through the pulmonary circulation to the lungs and back to the left heart. Although the volume of blood passing through the pulmonary circulation normally equals the volume being pumped by the left heart to the body through the systemic circulation, there are distinct differences in these circuits. The blood in the pulmonary artery is low in oxygen content compared to that in the systemic arteries. The pressure in the pulmonary artery (20 mm Hg/5 mm Hg) is significantly lower than that in the systemic arteries (120 mm Hg/80 mm Hg). This lower pressure in spite of similar flow is due to a lower vascular resistance in the pulmonary vessels. The right ventricle is thinner walled than the left because it performs less work.

REGULATION OF CIRCULATION

Blood flow requirements of the body demand that the circulation be able to adjust almost instantaneously to a wide range of needs. The regulation of how much blood is pumped by the heart and its regional distribution within the body involves the integration of various control mechanisms.

Two predominant factors are critical to the regulation of the circulation: satisfaction of the body's metabolic needs, and maintenance of arterial blood pressure. The body's metabolic needs must be met by the volume of blood pumped around the circulatory system per minute, which is called the cardiac output. The determinants of cardiac output are shown in Figure 5–5. Cardiac output is the product of the heart rate (number of strokes by the ventricle per minute) and the stroke volume (amount of blood ejected with each stroke). The stroke volume is the difference between the amount of blood in the heart when it is filled (end-diastolic volume) and the amount after ejection is completed (end-systolic volume). The end-diastolic volume is dependent upon the filling pressure, which is in turn determined by the amount of blood returned by the veins. The end-systolic volume is dependent upon the level of sympathetic nerve activity to the heart and the resistance to ejection by the peripheral circulation.

Blood pressure is the driving force of the circulation and involves the coordinated

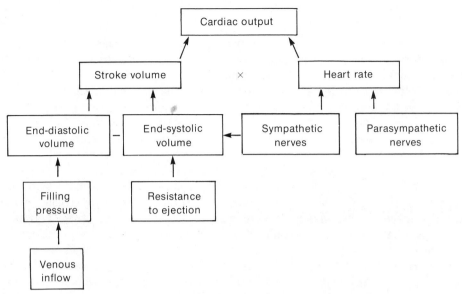

Figure 5–5. Major factors that determine the cardiac output.

interplay of cardiac output and peripheral resistance, as illustrated in Figure 5–6. This means there must be pressure sensors within the body that monitor blood pressure and provide feedback to the heart and autonomic nervous system. These pressure-sensitive areas are called baroreceptors. The primary ones are located in the carotid arteries of the neck and in the aortic arch. The baroreceptors have nerve endings that are stimulated by stretch within the arterial wall, reflecting a change in pressure. The appropriate autonomic response is triggered, and cardiac output and peripheral resistance are altered to maintain arterial pressure.

Measurement of Blood Pressure. Arterial blood pressure is normally measured at the upper arm with an inflatable cuff and pressure gauge (sphygmomanometer). One listens with a stethoscope at the point where a large artery (brachial) emerges from under the cuff. A cuff pressure greater than systolic blood pressure prevents any blood flow and there is no sound. As the cuff is deflated, interrupted flow occurs. A sharp "pulse" sound first appears when the cuff pressure drops below the peak pressure, thus indicating systolic pressure. When cuff pressure falls below the lowest arterial pressure, flow becomes constant and the "pulse" sounds disappear. The point of disappearance indicates diastolic pressure.

Although the classic "normal" for systolic blood pressure is 120 mm Hg and for diastolic pressure 80 mm Hg (reported 120/80 mm Hg), this is by no means the most desirable blood pressure. Studies have indicated that, within reasonable limits, the lower the blood pressure the lower the risk of heart attack and stroke.

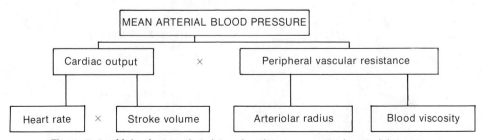

Figure 5–6. Major factors that determine the mean systemic arterial pressure.

Heart

In very simple terms, intrinsic control of the heart (without influence by the nervous system) involves properties of cardiac muscle that affect the force of ventricular contraction and, therefore, the amount of blood ejected with each beat (stroke volume). Cardiac muscle is like skeletal muscle in the sense that the strength of its contraction will increase when it is stretched. Therefore, the greater the volume of blood in the heart at the end of its filling phase, the greater the cardiac fiber length and consequently the greater the force of contraction (Fig. 5–7). This relationship is called Starling's law of the heart.

Starling's law cannot totally account for all the changes in performance that take place in the heart. Increases in the force and velocity of the heart's contraction can and do occur in the absence of changes in end-diastolic volume. These take place by means of extrinsic mechanisms, primarily sympathetic nerve stimulation and circulating hormones from the adrenal medulla. The effect of sympathetic stimulation on the performance of the ventricle is shown in Figure 5–8. With the increased force of contraction caused by the sympathetic stimulation, the ventricle can eject a larger stroke volume from any given end-diastolic volume. This occurs because the ventricle is able to eject down to a smaller end-systolic volume.

Sympathetic discharge not only increases the force and velocity of contraction but also increases heart rate via direct stimulation of the SA node, as shown in Figure 5–9. Epinephrine released into the blood by the adrenal medulla increases heart rate as well as contractility.

Sympathetic nerve activity also affects ventricular filling by causing constriction of the veins and improved function of the atrium. Respiration, the skeletal muscle "pump" (exercise), and blood volume also contribute to venous pressure and venous return with their ultimate influence on stroke volume and cardiac output.

Parasympathetic nerves affect heart rate via the vagus nerve. Vagal stimulation diminishes heart rate by means of its direct effect on the SA node. Atrial contractility is depressed by vagal stimulation, and ventricular contractility may also be diminished slightly. Parasympathetic activity, therefore, produces effects opposite to sympathetic stimulation: decreased cardiac output through decreases in myocardial force, velocity, and frequency of contraction.

Peripheral Circulation

Distribution of cardiac output to various regions within the body is regulated primarily by the arterioles. Variation in sympathetic nerve activity can cause vasoconstriction (from more activity) and vasodilation (from less activity) to dramatically shift blood flow from one region of the body to another and maintain an appropriate

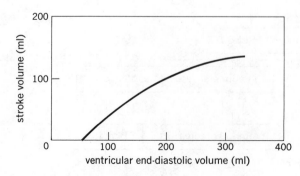

Figure 5–7. Relationship between stroke volume and ventricular end-diastolic volume (Starling's law of the heart). (From Vander, A. J., et al.: *Human Physiology: The Mechanisms of Body Function*, 2nd ed. Copyright © 1975 by McGraw-Hill, Inc. Used by permission of McGraw-Hill Book Company.)

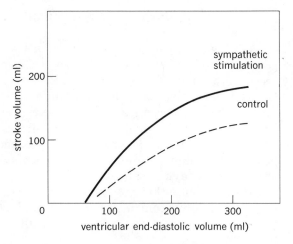

Figure 5–8. Effect of stimulation of the sympathetic nerves to the heart. (From Vander, A. J., et al.: *Human Physiology: The Mechanisms of Body Function,* 2nd ed. Copyright © 1975 by McGraw-Hill, Inc. Used by permission of McGraw-Hill Book Company.)

arterial blood pressure at all times. Again, plasma epinephrine contributes to the control of arteriolar radius in the same way that sympathetic stimulation does. The final factors affecting regional distribution of cardiac output are the local metabolic needs (hypoxia), blood levels of potassium and carbon dioxide, blood acidity, and concentrations of histamine and various metabolites.

Although each of the *individual* intrinsic and extrinsic mechanisms described responds in a relatively simple fashion, the combined effect of their simultaneous responses involves complex integration to regulate the circulation with the precision necessary for optimal function. In adjusting to changing body needs, the autonomic nervous system is capable of finely graded differential responses controlling cardiac output and its distribution. The primary centers for control of the cardiovascular response reside within the brain, particularly in the medulla. These centers regulate the neural output to the sympathetic and parasympathetic fibers of the autonomic nervous system for control of heart rate, myocardial contractile state, and vascular resistance and capacitance.

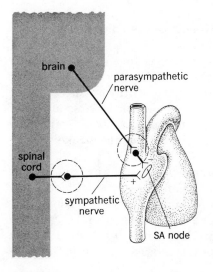

Figure 5–9. Control of heart rate by the effect of autonomic nerves on the SA node. (From Vander, A. J., et al.: *Human Physiology: The Mechanisms of Body Function.* Copyright © 1970 by McGraw-Hill. Used by permission of McGraw-Hill Book Company.)

RESPONSES TO DYNAMIC AND STATIC EXERCISE

During the performance of muscular exercise, the cardiovascular system undergoes important adaptive changes. The exact nature of these changes depends on the specific type of exertion undertaken. Broadly speaking, there are two types of muscular activity — dynamic and static. Muscular exercise in which the contraction causes principally a change in length with little change in tension is termed dynamic or isotonic. Exercise in which the contraction causes principally a change in tension with little change in length is termed static or isometric. Most muscular exercise is neither purely dynamic nor purely static, but a mixture of both types. Activities that are predominantly dynamic include running, swimming, bicycling, rowing, and rhythmic calisthenics; those that are predominantly static include lifting, carrying, or pushing heavy weights and contracting muscles against fixed objects. The physiologic response to these two forms of muscular activity differs greatly on both an acute and chronic basis.

During dynamic exercise involving a large mass of skeletal muscle, there is great demand for oxygen to supply the increased metabolic needs of the contracting muscles. This type of activity results in large increases in cardiac output, heart rate, and stroke volume with relatively little change in mean arterial pressure. Systolic pressure increases, but diastolic pressure remains unchanged or falls. In contrast, during the static contractions of even a small mass of muscle, there is a marked increase in mean arterial pressure with relatively small increases in heart rate and cardiac output. Both systolic and diastolic pressures are increased. Thus, dynamic exercise may be thought of as causing primarily a *volume load* on the heart, whereas static exercise produces primarily a *pressure load*.

Dynamic Exercise

ACUTE EFFECTS

The capacity of an individual to perform dynamic exercise is determined primarily by the ability to transport oxygen to the working muscles. The oxygen requirement of working muscle must be satisfied by a commensurate oxygen uptake, or fatigue quickly ensues. Oxygen uptake is the product of the cardiac output times the amount of oxygen extracted by the tissues of the body per unit of blood (called the arteriovenous oxygen difference):

$$\text{oxygen uptake} = (\text{cardiac output}) \times (\text{arteriovenous oxygen difference})$$

The typical effects that occur in the circulatory system when one goes from rest to heavy exercise are shown in Figure 5–10 and Table 5–1. Cardiac output during standing rest is approximately 6 liters per minute and represents the product of heart rate (90 beats per minute) and stroke volume (66 ml per beat). During maximal exercise, cardiac output increases fourfold (to 24 liters per minute) as a result of an approximate doubling of both heart rate (to 190 beats per minute) and stroke volume (to 126 ml per beat).

The arteriovenous oxygen difference is the difference between the oxygen content of the blood leaving the left ventricle (approximately 20 ml O_2 per 100 ml blood) and that returning to the right atrium from the body (approximately 14.4 ml O_2 per 100 ml blood during standing rest). This arteriovenous oxygen difference of 5.6 ml O_2 per 100 ml blood at rest is widened to approximately 15.8 ml O_2 per 100 ml blood during maximal exercise. Although the arterial oxygen content is relatively uniform through-

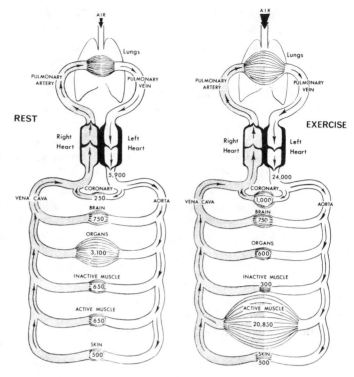

Figure 5–10. Schematic representation of the cardiopulmonary system of a sedentary man during standing rest and during exercise at the maximal oxygen uptake. Organs include kidneys, liver, gastrointestinal tract, spleen, and others. Blood flow is indicated in milliliters per minute. (Reprinted, by permission, from The New England Journal of Medicine, 284: 1020, 1971.)

out the body, the venous oxygen content of blood leaving the various tissues varies. The relatively high blood flow to the visceral organs (e.g., kidney, liver) in comparison to their oxygen needs is reflected in their higher venous oxygen content and lower arteriovenous oxygen difference (4 ml O_2 per 100 ml blood) in comparison to the body as a whole. In heart muscle, however, the arteriovenous oxygen difference is very high at rest (approximately 14 ml O_2 per 100 ml blood). Although this provides the heart with a "cheaper" source of oxygen under resting conditions, very little additional oxygen extraction can occur, and any increased oxygen demand during exercise must be met by increased coronary blood flow. The heart is, therefore, vulnerable to any condition that impairs coronary blood flow, such as coronary artery disease.

TABLE 5–1. CARDIOVASCULAR RESPONSES OF A NORMAL MAN TO EXERCISE AT MAXIMAL OXYGEN UPTAKE*

Conditions of Study	Oxygen Uptake (liters/min)	Oxygen Uptake (ml/kg/min)	Cardiac Output (liters/min)	Heart Rate (beats/min)	Stroke Volume (ml)	Arteriovenous Oxygen Difference (ml of oxygen/100 ml of blood)	Blood Pressure (mm hg)		
							SYSTOLIC	DIASTOLIC	MEAN
Standing rest	0.3	4	5.9	90	66	5.6	130	80	106
Maximal exercise	3.8	48	24.0	190	126	15.8	185	86	115

*Calculated for 25-year-old man weighing 80 kg. Table adapted from Mitchell, J. H., and Blomqvist, G.: Maximal oxygen uptake. N. Engl. J. Med. 284:1018–1022, 1971.

Arteriovenous oxygen difference is widened during exercise via greater oxygen extraction by the exercising muscle coupled with redistribution of cardiac output to areas of greatest demand. This shift in regional blood flow is accomplished by profound vasodilation in the working muscle concomitant with vasoconstriction in the viscera and nonworking muscle.

At rest, the muscles receive only about 20 per cent of the cardiac output, or approximately 1.2 liters per minute. At maximal exercise, however, nearly 90 per cent of the 24 liters per minute cardiac output (approximately 21 liters per minute) is redirected to the muscles — almost a 20-fold increase. Because of the high metabolic needs of the skeletal muscle cells during maximal exercise, the regional oxygen extraction is almost 100 per cent.

The vasoconstriction in the kidney, liver, gastrointestinal tract, and other visceral organs allows a greater percentage of the cardiac output to be "shunted" to the working muscles. As blood flow in these organs diminishes, oxygen supply is maintained by widening the arteriovenous oxygen difference. Redistribution of cardiac output is proportional to the intensity of work (per cent of one's maximal capacity). Very light workloads require minimal shifts in regional blood flow, whereas heavy workloads require significant redistribution.

During maximal exercise, the coronary blood flow increases four times, but the arteriovenous oxygen difference for the heart is only slightly greater than at rest. Individuals with arteriosclerotic obstructions in their coronary arteries often are limited by chest pain at low levels of exercise because the retarded oxygen supply cannot keep up with increased requirements. Cerebral blood flow remains the same during maximal exercise and at rest, with essentially no change in the arteriovenous oxygen difference.

Maximal Oxygen Uptake.   Oxygen consumption at a maximal work, or maximal oxygen uptake ($\dot{V}_{O_2 max}$), represents the maximal circulatory transport of oxygen from the lungs to the metabolically active tissues. It is physiologically defined as the product of maximal cardiac output and maximal arteriovenous oxygen difference. Maximal oxygen uptake is proportional to body weight (particularly lean body mass) and diminishes with advancing age. The effect of age on maximal oxygen uptake is shown in Figure 5–11. A peak in maximal oxygen uptake between 15 and 20 years of age and a gradual decline with advancing age was found in this group of males. The average maximal oxygen uptake of a 60-year-old man is two thirds the mean value at age 20.

Ample evidence exists that the habitual level of physical activity is an important factor in determining maximal oxygen uptake. A decrease in activity causes a prompt fall in maximal oxygen uptake. With bed rest, a 20 to 25 per cent drop below control values occurs after three to six weeks in young normal subjects. The data plotted in Figure 5–11 demonstrate results from two studies on the effect of physical training. Three sedentary college students increased their maximal oxygen uptake by 33 per cent after a two-month period of intensive physical training. A group of nine extremely sedentary middle-aged blind men were subjected to less intensive training over a longer period and showed an increase of almost 20 per cent after 15 weeks. Similar results have been reported by many investigators.

Because the circulatory transport of oxygen is achieved both by cardiac output and by peripheral extraction, $\dot{V}_{O_2 max}$ is the best physiological reference for functional capacity of the circulation and is a standard measure of cardiovascular fitness. The maintenance of arterial oxygen tension during heavy exercise demonstrates that pulmonary factors, ventilatory or diffusive, do not limit oxygen transport in normal subjects.

Maximal oxygen uptake is measured in the laboratory by analysis of expired gas

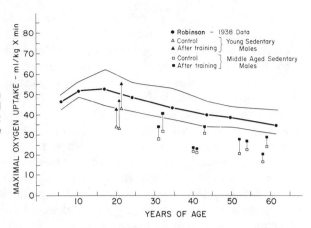

Figure 5–11. Effect of age and training on maximal oxygen uptake in males. (Adapted from Robinson, S.: Arbeitsphysiologie *10*: 251–323, 1938, with the permission of the publishers).

during maximal exercise, usually on a treadmill or bicycle ergometer. This is illustrated in Figure 5–12. Oxygen uptake is determined at progressively increasing workloads until a workload is reached at which oxygen uptake fails to increase significantly over that of the previous workload. This highest level of oxygen uptake represents maximal oxygen uptake and is associated with a high concentration of blood lactate.

CHRONIC EFFECTS

Probably the most significant physiological change induced by a well-designed program of dynamic exercise is an increase in maximal oxygen uptake. This results in improved functional capacity and allows a conditioned individual to perform at higher workloads for longer periods of time before being limited by fatigue, dyspnea, or chest pain. Increases in maximal oxygen uptake of up to 33 per cent have followed physical conditioning. The magnitude of the increase is determined by several factors, including the intensity, duration, and frequency of training and the initial level of maximal oxygen uptake.

Average maximal oxygen uptake in any population of moderately active, healthy 20-year-old men is probably about 45 ml per kilogram per minute. Virtually all Olympic champions in endurance events have a maximal oxygen uptake between 75

Figure 5–12. Determination of maximal oxygen uptake on a treadmill. (Reprinted, with permission, from The New England Journal of Medicine, *284*:1018, 1971.)

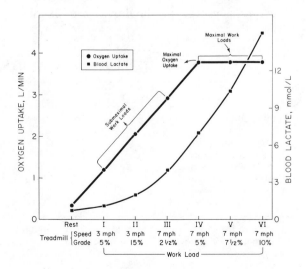

and 80 ml per kilogram per minute. Values above 55 ml per kilogram are rarely recorded among subjects who do not train regularly. These data suggest that it takes an exceptional genetic background plus hard physical training to produce a gold-medal winner in an Olympic endurance event.

In most individuals, maximal cardiac output increases after physical conditioning, mainly as a result of increased maximal stroke volume, with very little, if any, change in maximal heart rate. During submaximal work, cardiac output remains unchanged for a given level of oxygen uptake. Heart rate during submaximal work, however, decreases in direct proportion to the increase in stroke volume.

The changes in maximal arteriovenous oxygen difference after training contribute less to increases in maximal oxygen uptake than does enhanced cardiac output. Increased oxidative enzymes, size and number of mitochondria, and more efficient distribution of cardiac output after physical conditioning contribute to increased arteriovenous oxygen difference.

Static Exercise

ACUTE EFFECTS

In the cardiovascular laboratory, static exercise is studied by having a subject perform graded degrees of handgrip contractions. A strong static contraction of the forearm muscles of one arm causes a marked increase in mean arterial blood pressure (50 to 70 mm Hg), a slight increase in cardiac output (1 to 2 liters/min), and a moderate increase in heart rate (30 to 40 beats/min). Stroke volume remains relatively constant. Thus, as was stated earlier, static exercise produces primarily a pressure load on the heart, whereas dynamic exercise produces primarily a volume load on the heart. A comparison of acute responses to static and dynamic exercise is presented in Table 5–2. Such changes usually present little problem to a young, healthy individual but could trigger dangerous irregularities in heart rhythm or other hazardous responses in a patient with heart disease.

The rise in heart rate and blood pressure during static exercise is directly proportional to the *relative* tension, that is, the percentage of that tension developed during a maximal voluntary contraction (MVC) of the muscle group involved. Thus, the response to a 50 per cent MVC would be greater than that of a 25 per cent MVC. Sustained contractions exceeding 15 to 20 per cent MVC compromise blood flow into the working muscle sufficiently to require a shift to anaerobic energy supply, thus precipitously limiting the duration of exercise.

TABLE 5–2. ACUTE RESPONSES TO DYNAMIC AND STATIC EXERCISE*

	Dynamic	Static
Cardiac output	+ + + +	+
Heart rate	+ +	+
Stroke volume	+ +	0
Peripheral resistance	– – –	+ + +
Systolic blood pressure	+ + +	+ + + +
Diastolic blood pressure	0 or –	+ + + +
Mean arterial blood pressure	0 or +	+ + + +
Left ventricular work	Volume load	Pressure load

*From Dehn, M. M., Panesgrau, D. G., and Mitchell, J. H.: Exercise training after acute myocardial infarction. *In* Brest, A. N. (ed.): *Cardiovascular Clinics: Exercise and the Heart.* Philadelphia, F. A. Davis Company, 1978, pp. 117–132.

CHRONIC EFFECTS

Static exercise has been shown to increase significantly muscle strength and mass; thus, it certainly has a place in competitive athletics and orthopedic rehabilitation. Static training also has benefits for persons engaged in occupations or recreational pursuits that require lifting, carrying, or pushing heavy objects.

Intense and prolonged programs of static exercise lead to no significant increase in maximal oxygen uptake. Although endurance athletes have consistently high maximal oxygen uptakes, wrestlers and weight lifters usually measure just above the average for untrained subjects.

Athletes participating in dynamic exercise training have larger hearts and larger maximal oxygen pulses (amount of oxygen delivered each heart beat) than do athletes participating in static exercise training. Although it is possible that champion athletes choose their events because of genetic predisposition, a study of one set of identical twins has shown that this is probably not the case. One of the twins trained for several years in weight lifting and the other in endurance running. The weight lifter was 16 kg heavier than the runner, but both his maximal oxygen uptake (1.8 liter/min) and heart volume (560 ml) were less than those of the runner, whose maximal oxygen uptake was 2.5 liters/min and heart volume was 710 ml.

From a cardiological viewpoint, training with isometric exercise is relatively useless and should not be substituted for dynamic exercise, which has possible prophylactic and therapeutic value in certain types of cardiac disease. In fact, it is possible that intense static exertion should be avoided by some cardiac patients.

SUMMARY

Blood from the veins of the body drains into the right side of the heart. It is then pumped through the lungs where it is oxygenated, returned to the left side of the heart, and then pumped to all parts of the body. Contraction of the heart is triggered by its pacemaker, the SA node. The electrical activity of the heart can be recorded on the surface of the body by means of an electrocardiogram. Contraction of the ventricles (systole) pumps blood out of the heart. During relaxation (diastole), the ventricles refill with blood. The valves of the heart cause blood flow to be one way.

Blood can be sent where it is particularly needed (e.g., exercising muscle) because the small arterioles can change diameter, thus altering resistance. Beyond the arterioles, capillaries permit exchange of oxygen, fuel, and metabolic wastes between blood and tissues. Small veins (venules) act as reservoirs for blood and can contract if necessary (e.g., following blood loss) to put more blood into the rest of the circulatory system.

Exercising skeletal muscle receives increased oxygen by extracting more oxygen from blood than it does at rest and by increasing its blood flow. In contrast, the heart muscle extracts 70 per cent of the oxygen from blood even at rest and thus is especially sensitive to obstruction of blood flow, as in coronary artery disease.

Blood pressure must be maintained in order to drive blood. Changes in blood pressure are sensed by baroreceptors. The autonomic nervous system then alters the amount of blood pumped and the peripheral resistance to keep pressure stable.

Increasing quantities of blood that reach the heart stretch the muscle more and cause it to contract with more force. The force from any given stretch, as well as heart rate, is increased by sympathetic nerve stimulation and by epinephrine and norepinephrine from the adrenal gland. Flow of blood through a particular region of the body is controlled mainly by local metabolic factors, but also by sympathetic nerves and circulating epinephrine and norepinephrine.

Dynamic exercise causes a large increase in cardiac output but little change in mean arterial blood pressure. In contrast, static exercise causes a small increase in cardiac output but a relatively large increase in blood pressure — which may be unhealthy for some cardiac patients. During dynamic exercise, blood is shunted largely to the working muscles, away from the kidney, digestive system, and other visceral organs. Blood flow to the heart increases during exercise but that to the brain remains unchanged.

Maximal oxygen uptake indicates the upper limit of oxygen transport by the circulation. Maximal uptake in a 60-year-old man is about two thirds that in a 20-year-old man. Maximal oxygen uptake can increase or decrease as dynamic physical training is altered.

STUDY QUESTIONS

1. Name the properties of cardiac muscle that are similar to those of skeletal muscle and those that are similar to those of smooth muscle.

2. What major differences exist between the systemic circulation and the pulmonary circulation?

3. What major differences exist between the oxygen supply to the myocardium and to skeletal muscle at rest and during exercise?

4. In what ways would the stimulation of sympathetic and of parasympathetic nerves differ in effect on ventricular function and peripheral circulation?

5. Contrast dynamic and static exercise with respect to the nature of muscular contraction, specific types of activity, and cardiovascular responses.

6. Describe the changes in oxygen uptake, cardiac output, stroke volume, heart rate, and arteriovenous oxygen difference in a subject going from rest to maximal dynamic exercise.

7. Explain what adaptations take place to increase blood flow to working muscles.

8. What are the two primary factors that affect arterial blood pressure? How is blood pressure regulated?

9. What is the significance of maximal oxygen uptake and how is it related to cardiac output and arteriovenous oxygen difference?

10. What physiological adaptations would be expected in a regular dynamic exercise program?

11. What adaptations would be expected as a result of static exercise training and under what conditions would such changes be most beneficial?

12. Why are the arterioles and the systemic veins sometimes referred to as the resistance and capacitance vessels, respectively?

FURTHER READINGS

Astrand, P. O., and Rodahl, K.: *Textbook of Work Physiology*. New York, McGraw-Hill Book Company, 1977.
Chapman, C. B., and Mitchell, J. H.: The physiology of exercise. Sci. Am. *212*:88–96, 1965.

Dehn, M. M., Panesgrau, D. G., and Mitchell, J. H.: Exercise training after acute myocardial infarction. *In* Brest, A. N. (ed.): *Cardiovascular Clinics: Exercise and the Heart.* Philadelphia, F. A. Davis Company, 1978, pp. 117–132.

Keul, J.: The relationship between circulation and metabolism during exercise. Med. Sci. Sports 5:209–219, 1973.

Langley, L. L., Telford, I. R., and Christensen, J. B.: *Dynamic Anatomy and Physiology,* 4th ed., New York, McGraw-Hill Book Company, 1974.

Mathews, D. K. and Fox, E. L.: *The Physiological Basis of Physical Education and Athletics,* 2nd ed. Philadelphia, W. B. Saunders Company, 1976.

Mitchell, J. H., and Blomqvist, G.: Maximal oxygen uptake. New Engl. J. Med. *284*:1018–1022, 1971.

Mitchell, J. H., and Wildenthal, K.: Static (isometric) exercise and the heart: Physiological and clinical considerations. Ann. Rev. Med. *25*:369, 1974.

Vander, A. J., Sherman, J. H., and Luciano, D. S. *Human Physiology: The Mechanisms of Body Function,* 2nd ed. New York, McGraw-Hill Book Company, 1975.

6

PHYSICAL CONDITIONING AND LIMITS TO PERFORMANCE

HOWARD G. KNUTTGEN, Ph.D.

Limits to maximal efforts in running, jumping, lifting, and throwing are imposed by the skeletal muscle cells available for the effort, the skeleton upon which the muscles act, and the various systems that control and serve the muscles. Muscles respond only to stimuli received from the nervous system; therefore, the performance of the musculoskeletal system is determined by the quality of the coordinated commands received via the efferent (motor) neurons. A circulatory system that cannot deliver oxygen to the muscles involved in the repeated contractions required by the endurance athlete will cause the athlete to lessen the pace or terminate the performance. The athlete who cannot lose excess heat when necessary or whose endocrine system does not respond to the competitive situation will perform with lessened effectiveness.

Virtually all the tissues and systems of the human body have been shown to be responsive to programs of exercise. Physical conditioning does indeed result in improved performance. Because various types of performance place different demands upon the different organs and organ systems of the body, conditioning activities and conditioning programs must be highly specific to the sports involved. The purpose of this chapter is to explore the various limits to physical performance and the types of conditioning programs that can be employed to improve performance in different activities.

MUSCULAR CONTRACTIONS AND POWER

When a muscle cell is stimulated, the cell attempts to develop force and shorten itself along the longitudinal axis. When cells of a particular muscle are activated, the muscle attempts to shorten itself. The degree to which a muscle makes such an attempt depends upon the number of cells activated and the length of time each cell is stimulated repetitively by its neuron.

The success of an active muscle in shortening itself depends upon the external resistance provided through the skeletal system. The external resistance may consist

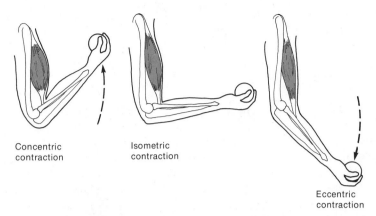

Figure 6–1. Types of muscle contraction: *concentric* — active muscle shortens; *isometric* — active muscle remains at same length; *eccentric* — active muscle is forcibly stretched.

of the athlete's own body parts (and gravity); or external objects (a ball, a weight, a discus); or other athletes (as in contact sports). If the active muscle is successful in overcoming the resistance, a shortening (*concentric contraction*) occurs and the athlete moves certain body parts, casts a ball, or moves an opponent (Fig. 6–1). If the resistance to movement is equal to the force generated by the active muscle, no movement results (*isometric contraction*) and body parts are maintained in a set posture or an opponent is held in position. If the external resistance overcomes the active muscles, a forcible lengthening of the athlete's muscles occurs (*eccentric contraction*) and the body is lowered, a ball is stopped in its flight, or an opponent's movement is retarded. Muscle contraction must, therefore, be defined as an "attempt" by the muscle to shorten. All three types of contraction require the release of energy in the active muscle cells. The type of contraction most often considered in exercise physiology and athletic performance is the shortening, or concentric, type.

Another term employed to describe skeletal movement and muscle contraction is *isokinetic*. The term refers to the maintenance of a constant velocity during a dynamic concentric or eccentric contraction. Such movement is best obtained by exercising against a motor-driven ergometer that establishes the velocity. A person may then exert any level of voluntary effort against the ergometer throughout the range of motion, including maximal voluntary effort.

Most sports activities can be characterized as an interrelationship of the coordinated movement of the body parts and the expression of power. Energy is utilized so that muscles can exert force, resulting in desired movements. *Energy* is the capacity for doing work. The release of energy is necessary for work to be accomplished, but energy is also expended in other ways, such as in the production of heat. In a concentric contraction, muscular *force* × *distance* through which the force is exerted = *work. Work* performed *per unit of time = power.*

SPORTS PERFORMANCE

Runners competing in 100-meter, 1500-meter, and 10,000-meter events must use vastly different percentages of maximal running power. Baseball pitchers vary the speed, and thus the power, of pitches. Tennis players do not hit each ball with the same force (actually power) investment. Basketball players shoot with various percentages of maximal power as appropriate to the distance from the basket. However, jumpers, shot putters, and javelin throwers attempt to attain maximal power with each attempt. The movements of a soccer player on a field or a basketball player around a court involve wide and frequent variations in the power involved in locomotion.

Aerobic and Anaerobic Power

The utilization of aerobic power in athletics requires the availability of muscle cells capable of high oxidative energy release as well as the adequate delivery of oxygen from the lungs to the muscles by the circulatory system. Metabolically, the chain of events involves ATP (adenosine triphosphate) cleavage to form ADP (adenosine diphosphate) and inorganic phosphate. The energy released is utilized for force development by the muscle cells. ATP is resynthesized when fat and carbohydrate enter the tricarboxylic acid (Krebs) cycle and respiratory chain. Oxygen must be available as an electron acceptor for the respiratory chain in order for the aerobic mechanism to function. Oxygen is taken into the lungs, diffuses from alveoli to pulmonary capillary blood, is delivered to the capillaries of the active muscle cells, and diffuses into the cells and their mitochondria.

Events lasting three to four minutes depend upon aerobic and anaerobic mechanisms in nearly equal shares (Fig. 6–2). Events lasting longer than four minutes depend more on aerobic than anaerobic energy release. The longer the duration of the event, the greater the involvement of the oxidative mechanisms. A run of 42,195 meters (a marathon) requires that more than 99 per cent of the energy come from aerobic (oxidative) energy release.

Events lasting less than three minutes depend more on anaerobic energy release. The higher the intensity of the exercise — and, therefore, the shorter the possible

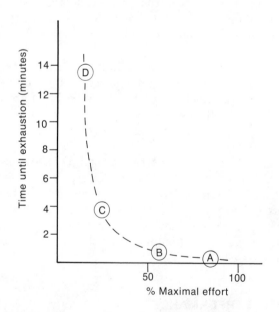

Figure 6–2. Relation of time until exhaustion (endurance time) to continuous exercise performed at various levels. The table provides relative contributions of aerobic and anaerobic processes for four sample running events.

Key to graph	Running Distance	Time	% Aerobic	% Anaerobic
A	100 m	10 sec	10	90
B	400 m	45 sec	25	75
C	1,500 m	3 min, 35 sec	55	45
D	5,000 m	13 min, 30 sec	85	15

duration (Fig. 6–2)—the greater the involvement of anaerobic mechanisms. In the shortest and most explosive efforts (weight lifting, pitching, high jumping), the energy release during the action is obtained entirely from high energy phosphates. ATP cleavage is involved directly in the contraction process, and creatine phosphate cleavage is involved in the rapid resynthesis of ATP. Oxidative mechanisms must account for eventual energy replenishment, but because this occurs during the resting or intervening recovery periods, the direct supply of energy is termed anaerobic.

If the intensity of the effort is somewhat less than maximal and the duration is for more than a few seconds, the provision of energy can still be accomplished without the involvement of oxygen because a limited amount of ATP can be resynthesized by means of anaerobic glycolysis. The end product of this process is lactic acid. The greater the duration of such activity, the greater the accumulation of lactic acid in the active muscle tissue.

Strength, Speed, and Endurance

Strength can be defined as the maximal force or power of which the involved muscles are capable. Therefore, it is better to characterize each person as having a set of different strengths. Each movement of the trunk and limbs involves a different combination of muscles, and each movement has its own maximum strength of power generation. Maximal force generation by each muscle depends upon the number of muscle cells that can be recruited and the collective size (cross section) of the active cells. It is, therefore, not surprising to see a strong relationship between muscle bulk and strength.

Considerable evidence exists to show that the prime responsibility for the development of great force resides with the fast-twitch fibers. The greater the percentage of fast-twitch muscle fibers in a muscle or muscle group, the greater is the capacity for strength. Approaching the question from the opposite direction, persons successful in strength events are found to have greater percentages of fast-twitch fibers in the involved muscles. A strength movement is by necessity a movement of short duration. Such a movement is most probably dependent on ATP cleavage alone for the provision of the energy required during the brief activity.

Speed of movement is a property that is not well understood physiologically. To a certain extent, muscle strength is necessary to move the body or its parts at high velocity. The relationship of quickness of movement to both muscle bulk and percentage of fast-twitch fibers is not as strong as might be expected. Factors other than muscle bulk and maximal force are involved but, as yet, not identified.

Endurance implies repetition of, or continuation of, effort. Adequate supplies of energy-yielding compounds must be contained in, or made readily available to, the active muscle cells. Endurance in very high intensity performances (such as 50-meter swim, 100-meter dash, a single play in football, running the bases in baseball) depends upon the capacity of the anaerobic mechanisms to provide and sustain great power generation. When performance requires energy release for several minutes to an hour or more, aerobic mechanisms are challenged. Fat and carbohydrate must be available to the active muscle cells, oxidative enzyme systems must be sufficiently developed, and the circulatory system must be capable of delivering oxygen in sufficient quantity. Endurance refers to the ability to continue an activity or sustain a particular power level. It may depend almost exclusively on anaerobic mechanisms (e.g., exhaustion in one minute); almost exclusively on aerobic mechanisms (e.g., activity maintained for one hour); or on some combination of the two mechanisms.

Specificity of Physical Fitness

Each sports activity places a different set of physiological demands on the human organism. Activities can consist of relatively constant levels of exertion (as in running and swimming); widely varying levels (as in basketball and soccer); or brief bursts (shot putting, pitching, a five-second football play). The demands for power by individual muscles and certain body parts, as well as the total energy demands for the entire body, are subject to great variation. Some sports require great strength, whereas success can be enjoyed in others without muscle bulk and capacity for great power. Different systems and different body parts are challenged in vastly different ways. Therefore, there is no single state of general fitness that would provide an athlete with the potential for championship performance in a number of sports.

Because each sports activity demands a different set of physiological capacities, conditioning programs must be highly specific to the activity in question. Sprinters and football players do not emphasize distance running in their respective conditioning programs. A marathon runner does not practice weight lifting. A high jumper does not devote time to the development of arm strength. Very often, the best conditioning programs emphasize repeated practice of the sports activities themselves. Examples include repeated runs at the competitive distance, scrimmaging in team sports, and rallying in tennis. If functional capacities are to be developed beyond levels brought about by repeated practice of specialized activities, a total program of conditioning must be planned. Such a program allows adequate time for the special activities, practice of skills, practice of strategy, and, in certain sports, teamwork.

Evaluation of Performance Capacities

In most cases, the best test of the physiological capacities necessary for top-level performance is the competition itself. While skills and motivation play important roles, a person either does or does not demonstrate the necessary capacities for power generation or maintenance. However, laboratory assessments often can give us valuable insights concerning the physiological factors underlying athletic performance and information about specific body parts and movements. A particular movement can be isolated and the strength (maximal force or power) of the movement can be measured by a mechanical or electronic dynamometer (strength gauge). The maximal aerobic power (maximum oxygen uptake) of an athlete can be assessed for a particular activity (running, skiing, swimming, cycling, rowing) by means of tests that include measurements of the expiratory exchange of the lungs during exhaustive efforts.

Samples (biopsies) of selected muscles can yield valuable information concerning such factors as muscle cell population, glycogen storage, and the capacities of enzyme systems. Many other laboratory measurements provide valuable information for physiologists, coaches, and physicians: cardiac output, limb blood flow, blood composition, body density and fat content, body proportions (anthropometry), and body fluid content, among others.

LIMITING FACTORS IN EXERCISE PERFORMANCE

Muscle Mass and Strength

The single most important factor in maximal power generation (strength) is the size of the muscles or muscle groups involved in the movement. Size, in this case, is synonymous with bulk or cross section. The greater the cross-sectional area of muscle cells that can be recruited, the greater the number of actin-myosin cross-bridges that can be involved, the greater the energy release, and the greater the force that can be generated.

The recruitment of muscle cells brings in two additional considerations: the voluntary activation of muscle cells by the neurons coming from the spinal cord; and the types of cells found in the muscles involved in the action. As regards activation, it is generally held that no voluntary (self-willed) muscle contraction ever involves the recruitment of all the contractile cells in a muscle. In fact, various inhibitory mechanisms function to insure that far less than total recruitment occurs during what is described as a "maximal voluntary contraction." For one thing, the integrity of the muscle itself, as well as its attachments, could be endangered if total recruitment and total power were allowed to develop. Part of strength training and training for an explosive effort involves the learning of release from inhibitory mechanisms to the greatest extent possible.

The types of cells found in a muscle — often referred to as muscle fiber population — has a direct bearing on strength expression. Fast-twitch fibers have greater abilities for powerful, as well as fast, contractions. The percentage of fast-twitch fibers in a muscle and the diameter of the individual fibers (i.e., the total cross-sectional area represented by these fibers) are important factors in the ability of the muscle to generate force and bring about powerful movements. The total mass of a muscle is not as important as the mass represented by fast-twitch fibers.

Anaerobic Power

The energy release of a single maximal effort, as in a strength movement, depends on energy obtained from the splitting of the high-energy phosphate compounds, ATP and creatine phosphate. No molecular oxygen is involved in these metabolic processes: they are anaerobic. However, the term anaerobic power in sports performance is more often used to describe high-intensity activity that lasts approximately five seconds to one minute. This is the range in which the capacity of the high-energy phosphate compounds dominates.

Anaerobic glycolysis (lactate formation) becomes more important as work intensity decreases and performance time increases. Fast-twitch muscle fibers have a greater capacity for glycolysis than slow-twitch fibers. Thus, the percentage of fast-twitch fibers is important for anaerobic performance. Also, the glycolytic capacities of the individual fast-twitch fibers are very responsive to conditioning.

Aerobic Power

The ability of an athlete to sustain activity by means of the oxidative release of energy is dependent on oxygen utilization and oxygen delivery. Just as fast-twitch muscle fibers are important to anaerobic activity, slow-twitch fibers are essential to aerobic activity. Slow-twitch fibers are characterized by a higher content of myoglobin (a compound similar to hemoglobin, the oxygen-carrying compound of the red blood cells) and by greater capacities of the enzyme systems involved in oxidative energy release. Therefore, muscles with a higher population of slow-twitch fibers are better able to sustain long-lasting aerobic activity. If the aerobic mechanisms of the individual cells have been enhanced by appropriate conditioning techniques, the muscles will have even greater capacities for such exercise. Appropriate increases in capillarization accompany increases in slow-twitch fibers.

Muscle cells utilizing large amounts of oxygen require adequate oxygen delivery, a responsibility of the circulatory system. Therefore, a variety of factors related to oxygen transport from the lungs to the active muscle cells become important: the ability of the heart to eject a volume of blood with each contraction or beat (stroke volume); the oxygen-carrying capacity per unit of blood; and the total volume of blood available.

Blood volume is a factor that increases only with long-term physical conditioning programs that emphasize aerobic activities of long duration — and, apparently, only in younger persons. The oxygen-carrying capacity of blood does not change with conditioning in healthy persons, although various types of anemia can reduce this capacity. Cardiac stroke volume does increase as the result of aerobic activity conditioning in persons of all ages, and markedly so in persons 25 years old and younger.

It is generally held that pulmonary ventilation (breathing) does not constitute a limiting factor for exercise tolerance. For a healthy person involved in a wide range of activities, this is probably true. In the range of exercise intensities in which exhaustion occurs in three to ten minutes, pulmonary ventilation approximates the endurance limits of the muscles of ventilation and in some athletes could limit performance.

Substrate Availability

Aerobic activity requires fat and carbohydrate as substrates for energy release. Fat is stored in individual muscle cells and at various locations in the body, such as under the skin. Fat can be transported by the blood from body depots to active muscles in the form of free fatty acids.

Carbohydrate is stored in the liver and in muscle cells as glycogen. When mobilized from the liver, it is carried by the blood as glucose (blood sugar) to active muscle cells. The total body storage of carbohydrate in a healthy, well-conditioned adult is somewhat variable but would approximate 2000 kcal (kilocalories), with 1300 kcal as muscle glycogen. The energy equivalent of fat stored in the same individual could easily exceed 50,000 kcal without the person's being obese.

At rest and during low-intensity exercise, the body depends mostly on fat as a substrate, but as soon as exercise reaches a moderately intense level, an obvious preference of the muscles for carbohydrate is observed. The closer the level of oxygen uptake is to its maximum, the greater the dependence of the muscles on carbohydrate. A certain amount of the carbohydrate metabolized by muscle comes from blood glucose.

At moderate to heavy exercise intensities, the major portion of energy derived from carbohydrate comes from the active muscle cells' own glycogen stores. The higher the intensity of exercise, the greater is the utilization. At the highest intensities of aerobic exercise, the glycogen content of the active muscles can be depleted within one to two hours. When this occurs, the person must either lower the exercise intensity drastically or cease the activity altogether. The body fat stores could sustain high-intensity activity for tremendously long periods, but a combination of factors prevents muscle from extensively utilizing fat. For one thing, fatty acids circulating with the blood do not gain easy entrance to the active muscle cells.

Environmental Factors

In spite of the optimum development of appropriate physical conditioning, skills, and motivation, an athlete's performance can be affected adversely or limited by environmental factors. The two most important factors are lowered availability of oxygen at high altitude and high environmental temperatures.

Under sea-level conditions, blood leaves the lungs of the resting or moderately active athlete with all the oxygen it can carry (fully saturated). Even during exhausting exercise, the blood reaching muscle is fully saturated with oxygen in most people. As one ascends in altitude, however, atmospheric pressure decreases, resulting in a lowered partial pressure of oxygen in the inspired air. A newcomer to an altitude of 1500 meters (5000 feet) may feel certain adverse effects from this form of hypoxia even at rest. An athlete involved in an event stressing aerobic energy release will feel increased stress during exertion. The greater the altitude, the less the oxygen availability and the greater the limitation on aerobic performance.

In ascending to altitude, the partial pressure of oxygen in the alveoli of the lungs may become too low to permit the blood to pick up all the oxygen it can carry. As a result, less oxygen is presented to the active muscle cells, and the athlete must either lessen the intensity of the exertion (slow the pace) or resort to a certain amount of anaerobic metabolism. The latter can easily result in early fatigue during competition.

The only way in which an athlete could prevent the decrease of blood oxygen saturation would be to breathe a gas having a higher percentage of oxygen than air (20.9 per cent at all altitudes). The higher percentage of oxygen (e.g., 50 to 100 per cent) would result in a higher partial pressure and complete saturation of the blood. Even if such a practice were permitted, the added weight of portable gas containers would make it impractical for the athlete.

The question of the value of training at altitude has not been completely resolved. It has been suggested that the physiological adaptations to living and training at altitude would enhance an athlete's ability to perform at sea level (i.e., result in a higher level of aerobic power capacity than would be possible with sea-level training). However, the intensity of a training program followed at sea-level cannot be maintained by a sea-level resident who goes to altitude. The net result of training at altitude for an extended period appears to be that the loss of conditioning, as a result of a lower intensity training program, is greater than any beneficial effects of living and training at altitude.

Inability to lose body heat during competition can result in detrimentally high body temperature and in dehydration. Excessive body temperature, dehydration, or both, can cause marked deteriorations in performance or even cessation of activity. In its most extreme form, hyperthermia can result in a loss of consciousness and heat stroke.

Any form of extended exertion results in production of heat that an athlete must lose. Excessively high temperature of the surrounding air will curtail or reverse heat loss. In addition, heat received as radiation by the athlete from the sun or a hot playing surface can contribute to the total thermal load on the body.

The most important heat loss mechanism available to humans is the evaporation of sweat. If high humidity results in diminished evaporation, the athlete faces an increased threat to body temperature regulation. Excessive fluid loss during extended competition, without adequate fluid replacement, can result in diminished sweat production and curtailed heat loss.

Aging

At some time between the ages of 25 and 35 years, the capacities of certain body processes begin to diminish. This can result in a deterioration of athletic performance and a lessened ability to respond to physical conditioning programs. For example, reaction time slows, vision becomes less acute, strength diminishes, and oxygen transport capacity is reduced. The tissues and organ systems of the body demonstrate a lessened ability to meet the challenges of physical exercise as well as to respond to a program of exercise.

The individual factors are quite easily identified and measured; the total syndrome is labeled aging. Limitations to athletic performance become apparent as an athlete grows olders. The order in which various types of performances appear to be adversely affected is as follows: speed events (early 20's); strength and skill events (late 20's and early 30's); and aerobic endurance events (mid to late 30's).

Skill, Strategy, and Motivation

In any discussion of limiting factors, mental (cognitive) and psychological factors must be given appropriate consideration. The most highly developed human organism in terms of musculature, circulatory system, ventilatory system, and other physical factors is still subject to the control of its nervous system. Skills represent chiefly a learning process of the central nervous system (the brain and spinal cord) from which all control signals (nervous impulses) originate. If the movements of an athlete are not finely controlled, coordinated, and made efficient in terms of energy expended, performance will suffer. Anything less than optimum skill will serve as a limiting factor.

In addition to top-level skills, an athlete must be a master of the strategies of a sport in order to be most effective as a competitor. A high jumper must know at which height to begin competition and when it would be advantageous to waive a height. A tennis player must know where and when to make certain shots. A middle-distance runner must know how to respond to different paces and when to take the lead. A team-sport player must master predetermined team offenses and defenses as well as be capable of independent initiative and response to the actions of opponents.

Motivation constitutes an additional dimension. How desirous is the athlete of performing well? In the case of events in which physical discomfort is common, how willing is the athlete to tolerate discomfort and, indeed, pain? For the best competitive results, the athlete must have all physiological and psychological variables operating at optimal levels.

PHYSICAL CONDITIONING

Virtually all the body tissues, organs, and systems are responsive to programs of conditioning and can adapt by increasing their individual characteristics and capacities. Certain adaptations diminish or become negligible as an adult advances in age; however, regardless of the sports activity involved, the average person can improve performance by initiating an appropriate physical conditioning program. The program must be appropriate in terms of duration, intensity, duration and frequency of workouts, and, above all, specificity of the conditioning activities to the physiological demands of the particular sport.

Strength Training

The most important factor in developing strength (maximal power) in a muscle group is the resistance employed in individual workouts. A person must employ maximal or near-maximal resistances for each movement. The lower the resistance employed, the slower will be the rate of increase and the less the eventual increment. If resistances much lower than 50 per cent of maximal force are used, virtually no increase in strength will occur.

The precise number of contractions for an optimal workout has not been determined, but the following can be set forth as a general guideline: six to ten repetitions of a movement performed in three sets with intervening recovery periods. Working out every other day appears to be the most effective frequency.

When weights are used as the resistance for concentric contractions, relatively slow contraction speeds should be employed in both testing sessions and actual workouts. The constant resistance of a weight is most effective at the "weakest" point in the movement; thus, the muscle produces maximum force only through a small portion of the range of motion. Isometric contractions can be performed against fixed objects and appear to be very effective for strength development. However, under normal conditions, they offer no advantage over shortening or lengthening contractions. Isokinetic devices control the speed of concentric contraction while providing a resistance equal to the force generated by the muscles throughout the entire range of a movement. They have the potential for providing maximum voluntary resistance throughout the range of motion.

Exercises in which eccentric contractions are employed require an external resistance that can overcome the forces generated by the muscles. This has the disadvantage of requiring a special device, usually motor driven. However, much greater forces can be generated with eccentric contractions than with either concentric or isometric contractions. Certain evidence exists that eccentric exercise is somewhat more effective for strength development.

Most studies of strength development have found that strength increases relatively slowly and that large increases take many months. The starting point for an individual is important. Has the person been engaging in high-resistance exercise for the movements being studied? How does the initial strength level compare with the person's genetically determined maximum?

An additional consideration in evaluating either strength studies or the progress of an individual is that the expression of strength is a voluntary process. A person produces a maximal force that is determined by motivation, tolerance of discomfort, and release from unconscious inhibitions. An increase in motivation (e.g., through either threat or promise of reward) or a decrease in inhibition brought about by practice can result in strength gains without any apparent changes in the physiology of the muscle.

Anaerobic Power

The ability to engage in levels of exertion that require energy release above that which can be provided by aerobic metabolism can be greatly enhanced by high-intensity training programs. However, the physiological changes resulting in the improved performance are not well understood. The metabolic mechanisms include high-energy phosphate splitting as well as anaerobic glycolysis leading to rapid formation of lactic acid in the muscle cells. There is some evidence that a program of intense anaerobic activity results in increased capacity of the glycolytic pathway in the muscle cells, especially in the fast-twitch fibers.

The training activities must approximate and even exceed the intensity and energy demand of the actual event. The high-intensity activity should be repeated, with appropriate intervals of rest. For example, sprints of 100 to 400 meters interspersed with 100 meters of jogging can be repeated six to ten times. Following a rest period, the entire set can be run again.

Aerobic Power

The development of aerobic power capacity for a sport depends upon (1) the development of the capacities of the individual muscle cells for oxidative phosphorylation, and (2) the development of a circulatory system capable of delivering larger quantities of oxygen. The specific muscle cells that are most active in long-lasting activity belong to the groups called slow twitch. While they do not show marked increases in size with conditioning, the capacities of the enzyme systems for oxidative metabolism are greatly increased.

In persons of all ages, capacity for cardiac output increases markedly with this type of conditioning. The maximal amount of blood that can be ejected from the heart with each contraction (cardiac stroke volume), and therefore the maximal amount of blood that can be pumped per minute (cardiac minute volume), are increased. The amount of blood pumped out by the heart is the exact amount of blood that passes through the lungs; this quantity is then available for distribution to the exercising muscles. The greater the amount pumped, the greater the capacity for oxygen delivery.

In younger persons, blood volume and total red blood cells increase with extended aerobic conditioning (i.e., six to twelve months or more). Very young people (i.e., nine to fourteen years old) can also show increases in lung volumes that remain through adulthood.

Physical inactivity can result in a marked lowering of aerobic power capacity. Vivid evidence of the effects of inactivity, followed by intensive aerobic conditioning, was presented in a study by Saltin and colleagues[1] (Fig. 6–3). Five healthy young adults underwent a three-week period of complete bedrest before beginning a two-

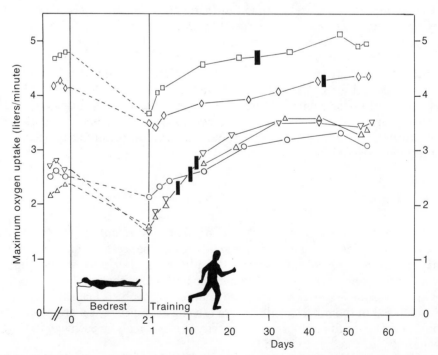

Figure 6–3. Patterns of maximal oxygen uptake for five individuals before bedrest, after three weeks of bedrest, and during the ensuing period of intensive physical training. Solid bars indicate the time in training at which prebedrest values had been reattained. (Adapted from Saltin, et al.: Response to exercise after bedrest and after training. American Heart Association, Monograph No. 23, 1968, p. VII–II. Used by permission of The American Heart Association, Inc.).

month conditioning program. Aerobic power capacity (maximum oxygen uptake) fell markedly in the subjects during the period of inactivity but improved rapidly following initiation of physical conditioning. Three subjects attained pre-bedrest values within two weeks, and all reached or exceeded pre-bedrest values by the end of the two-month program.

Additional studies have shown that an individual's aerobic power capacity follows very closely his level of physical activity. If the stimuli provided by an aerobic conditioning program are removed at any point in time, aerobic power capacity deteriorates.

Glycogen Loading

Glycogen content of muscle is important to athletes engaged in long-lasting events in which the demand for aerobic energy release is consistently high. An athlete can easily double the amount of stored glycogen over that which the average resting individual has available by following certain rules concerning the diet and exercise regimen.

An increase in carbohydrate intake by itself can cause an increase in muscle glycogen storage. Also, when glycogen levels in muscle are depleted, there is a tendency toward supercompensation — the muscle cells store more glycogen during the following days of recovery than was available prior to depletion.

The greatest supercompensation occurs when the following steps are taken: The athlete engages in the activity in question (e.g., running, walking, cross-country skiing) at a higher aerobic intensity for between one and two hours (actually, for however long it takes to deplete the glycogen in the exercising muscles). For the following three days, the athlete avoids consuming carbohydrate. Then the athlete goes on a diet rich in carbohydrate for a three-day period. Physical activity is restricted, especially during the three-day period of glycogen loading.

Whether an athlete needs to follow such a routine and, indeed, whether it is practical to follow such a regimen during a competitive season are questions the athlete must answer. Athletes engaging in training programs for long-lasting events have consistently high resting values for muscle glycogen. However, such athletes should normally have a high carbohydrate intake during their training and competitive seasons. Extensive activity should be avoided for three to four days prior to competition and the carbohydrate content of meals during this period should be increased.

It should be remembered that aerobic energy release also involves the metabolism of lipids. Experimental evidence is beginning to emerge that the mobilization of fat (e.g., by caffeine ingestion prior to performance) may have a sparing effect on glycogen stores. This would mean that if an event was long enough in duration, the athlete could lessen carbohydrate utilization during the early stages of an event and postpone the point at which muscle glycogen concentrations approached critically low levels.

Acclimatization

The process of acclimatization in athletics refers to an adaptation of physiological mechanisms for competitive performance in an unusual environment. The two most obvious environmental factors are high altitude and high ambient temperature.

As discussed previously, no special advantage has been found in having a sea-level resident train under the hypoxic conditions of altitude. For such individuals, although an increase in both red blood cells and total blood volume occurs after some months at altitude, the diminished training program that must be followed because of the decrease in aerobic power capacity overrides any beneficial effects of adaptation to hypoxia.

Athletes who will be competing for a number of days at high altitude should move to the competition location some four to seven days before the first event. This should bring the athlete through the period of general acclimatization during which symptoms such as headache, mouth dryness, and nausea may be experienced.

Acclimatization to high environmental temperature and humidity is of great importance to athletes, especially those participating in football and distance running. In addition to improving performance, such adaptations are necessary to protect the athlete's health. Repeated exposure to high heat and humidity during active training results in an increased ability of the body to lose its own metabolically produced heat and maintain satisfactory body temperature. The body is better able to direct blood flow to the skin, and sweat production is enhanced. A few days of practice under such conditions is beneficial, but some weeks are necessary to develop optimal response. Practice sessions can take place outdoors or under artificially produced conditions such as in a heated field house or in a climate chamber.

Ingestion of appropriate fluids prior to and during rigorous physical activity for extended periods at high temperatures is essential for the protection of the athlete from heat injuries. Every athlete should possess both a knowledge of proper practices in this regard as well as have the ability to recognize the early warning symptoms that precede heat injury[2] (see Chapter 21).

When athletes must wear protective padding and uniforms, as in football, everything possible must be done to expose the body surface to air circulation. When breaks in action are possible, they should be taken. Ingestion of water or commercially prepared electrolyte solutions both before and during competition should be encouraged.

Designing a Conditioning Program

The first consideration in designing a conditioning program is specifying the physiological functional capacities required for the activity or objectives in question. Does the activity require or does the person desire strength, anaerobic power, or aerobic power? In the case of strength, what movements are to be involved? For persons who are interested in conditioning for its own sake, the next question becomes how to integrate a weekly program of exercise into the normal schedule of work, study, and activities of daily living. For the athlete in an individual sport, the assignment of time for skill and strategy training as well as for conditioning must be considered. Team sports add the component of offensive and defensive team play to the practice schedule. There are, however, certain general principles that may be applied in all these situations.

Strength training should occur two or three times a week; it seems beneficial to have a day of rest between workouts. Three sets of six to ten repetitions of each movement seem to suffice. Single sets of each of the different movements can be taken in order and then the entire routine can be repeated two times. The total length of time of a workout will depend on the number of movements to be included. If the person proceeds directly from exercise set to exercise set, the total time demand will be quite small.

For anaerobic power, there is reason to believe that daily workouts are best. A slightly lower intensity of muscular contraction is used as compared to strength training. However, because the activity must be carried out for longer periods (e.g., 10 to 200 seconds) and often to exhaustion, each bout is highly stressful. Adequate time for recovery should be allowed between bouts and relatively large numbers of repetitions should be performed.

Conditioning for aerobic power requires workouts of from 30 minutes to 2 hours with exercise intensities at a high percentage of aerobic power capacity. Both the oxygen transport system and the oxidative processes of the muscle cells must be challenged. Training at 60 per cent of aerobic power capacity (equivalent to a heart rate of 140 to 150 beats per minute) results in minimal improvement; training at lower intensities can be expected to produce little or no improvement. If the amount of time per workout is kept constant, the higher the intensity employed, the greater the improvement. Three sessions per week would appear to be the minimal recommended routine, with additional sessions resulting in definite increased benefit.

The higher the intensity of aerobic exercise, the more difficult it is to maintain the intensity for an extended period. Therefore, recovery periods during which running, swimming, rowing, cross-country skiing, or other activity is done at a reduced pace can be interspersed with the intensive portions of a workout. Interval training of very high bursts of power, which the person can maintain for periods of 30 to 60 seconds, with equal periods of recovery, makes impressive contributions to aerobic power development.

Healthy young adults who begin an exercise program of stressful aerobic conditioning (three to five times a week for 30 to 60 minutes a day) can expect, on the average, a 20 per cent improvement in oxygen delivery and utilization within two months. Some members of the group might experience in excess of a 40 per cent improvement and others less than 10 per cent. These differences will be due largely to variations in the initial level of fitness as well as the genetic endowment of each individual.

Designing a conditioning program is a highly individualized operation but one that can be properly done by anyone who follows the basic principles. The fewer the objectives, the simpler the process, and vice versa. The decathlon, a group of events that challenge strength, anaerobic power, and aerobic power in a variety of configurations, represents the supreme challenge to both the versatility of an athlete and the design of a conditioning program.

SPECIAL CONSIDERATIONS

Ergogenic Aids

The term ergogenic means work-producing. An ergogenic aid is a compound that, when ingested, injected, or perhaps rubbed onto the skin, is designed to increase an athlete's capacities for or performance in competition. It has been found, however, that optimal performance in competitive sports is brought about by diligent adherence to a conditioning program, appropriate diet, maximal development of skills, mastery of the strategies of the event, and high motivation. There are no miracle potions that an athlete is allowed to use that can make a champion out of an average athlete or, indeed, enhance the performance of athletes at any level of competition.

Adding commercial vitamins or high-protein products to a normal, well-balanced diet will not increase a person's strength or enable him to run faster or shoot baskets with more accuracy. Such exotic products as the honey the worker bees manufacture for the queen bee offer no advantage over any carbohydrate, expensive or cheap.

The use of anabolic steroids in an attempt to enhance muscle growth is discouraged by physicians because of certain pathological dangers.[3] Research on the effects of these drugs on males has been inconclusive. Female athletes employing hormone treatment can expect the accompanying development of male characteristics including coarse skin, deep voice, and facial hair growth.

Amphetamines alter nervous system function but have no proven effects on muscle metabolic capacity. Because they can result in distorted judgment, they are detrimental to activities in which selection of pace and strategic decisions become important.

Laboratory tests have shown that a person's aerobic power capacity can be enhanced if the person breathes from a supply of pure oxygen or a gas mixture having a high percentage of oxygen during high-intensity exercise. This suggests that breathing pure oxygen during competition would be beneficial to the athlete engaged in an event in which aerobic energy release is important. However, the encumbrance of carrying around an oxygen supply negates the benefits of such a practice. As an aid to recovery from vigorous events, there is little chance that oxygen could benefit the athlete at sea level because the blood normally carries virtually all the oxygen it can. At altitude, a contribution can be made to the athlete who must continue high-intensity aerobic activity.

Blood Donation

The donation of 500 ml or 1 pint of blood by an athlete engaged in sports activities emphasizing aerobic power can result in a slight deterioration of performance that can last up to three or four weeks. Until the body is able to replace the lost red blood cells, the oxygen transport capacity of the circulatory system is somewhat diminished. Athletes in events not depending on oxidative energy release would notice no difference in performance.

Blood Doping

Evidence is contradictory concerning the effectiveness of reinfusing red blood cells previously removed from an athlete's circulatory system, following the natural restitution that occurs with time and conditioning. Certain studies indicate an increase in oxygen transport resulting in an increase in aerobic power capacity. The ethics and competitive legality of such a practice are important considerations for athletes and sports authorities.

Warmup

The procedure of engaging in calisthenics, running, or the sports activity in question prior to actual competition has been followed for many years and is termed warmup. It is believed that warming up will enhance competitive performance and aid in injury prevention.

Little or no data exist on injury prevention through warmup, but athletes and coaches have great faith in its effectiveness. Certain data support the effectiveness of warmup for enhancing performance of a predominantly anaerobic nature. If the temperature of the muscles is appropriately elevated prior to competition, the person can perform high intensity activity (such as sprinting) more rapidly.

Second Wind

Some athletes report that after some minutes of high-intensity aerobic activity a feeling of relief occurs as though certain body processes had become more effective. The phenomenon has not been documented with physiological evidence.

Stitch (Pain in Side)

During stressful exercise, athletes can experience a very sharp pain in the side in the upper abdominal or lower thoracic region. Hypotheses exist that such a "stitch" is caused by muscular spasm of a portion of the diaphragm, spasm of the deep intercostal musculature, or even intestinal gas. Such pain disappears with cessation of activity. Certain distance runners report that very deep breathing can relieve the discomfort while they continue to run.

SUMMARY

The physiological and environmental factors that limit physical performance are highly specific to the particular physical activity. Therefore, a conditioning program for a specific sport must be designed with an appreciation of the physiological bases for performance and a knowledge of the factors that can be improved by appropriate exercise activity. Artificial aids to performance have proven generally ineffective and will never constitute substitutes for intensive exercise and adequate nutrition.

Performances in different sports impose a wide variety of demands on the musculoskeletal system of the body as well as on the support systems. Because of the variety of physiological factors that may limit physical performance in different sports activities, as related to the unique sets of physiological demands imposed, conditioning programs must be planned with specificity as the foremost consideration.

An inverse relationship exists between the intensity of the physical activity and the duration of time a person can endure the activity. Short bursts of extremely high-intensity activity rely primarily on the quantity of muscle available. Activities demanding high levels of energy release for 5 to 50 seconds depend primarily on anaerobic energy release. Activities lasting four minutes or longer depend primarily on aerobic energy release and, therefore, on the delivery and utilization of oxygen. Long-lasting activities depend not only on the oxidative energy release mechanisms but also on the availability of carbohydrate and lipid substrate. Environmental factors, such as temperature and the hypoxia of altitude, can also affect activities of long duration.

Conditioning programs for strength activities are designed around extremely high resistance exercises, while conditioning programs for anaerobic and aerobic performance correspond in intensity to the levels of actual performance. Aerobic activities that are dependent on substrate storage require a conditioning program carefully coordinated with a prescribed food intake.

STUDY QUESTIONS

1. Discuss the physiological limits to performance in a wide variety of activities, such as archery, bowling, pole vaulting, soccer, and 1500-meter swim.

2. What are the differences among concentric, isometric, and eccentric muscle contractions?

3. Which body systems and physiological mechanisms are involved in oxidative energy release and aerobic performance?

4. Performance would suffer in which sports events at an altitude that causes a lowered saturation of blood with oxygen in the lungs?

5. What sports events can be effected adversely by performance at high temperature and high relative humidity? What steps can be taken to avoid a decrement in performance and to safeguard against heat injury?

6. What relationships might exist between muscle fiber populations for individual athletes and potential for performance in various sports events?

7. At what approximate age would an athlete be expected to achieve peak performance in each of the following: 100-meter run, volleyball, baseball, shot put, marathon?

8. What fitness objectives might be appropriate for a 30-year old not engaged in sport as a profession but interested in the health benefits of maintaining an adequate level of physiological functional capacity for physical exercise?

9. Which of the following have proven to be beneficial as ergogenic aids for specific sport activities without having potentially harmful side effects: sugar, amphetamines, anabolic steroids, spaghetti, gelatine, beefstock, bread?

FURTHER READINGS

Astrand, P.-O., and Rodahl, K.: *Textbook of Work Physiology*. New York, McGraw-Hill Book Company, 1977.

Dempsey, J. A., and Reed, C. E. (eds.): *Muscular Exercise and the Lung*. Madison, University of Wisconsin Press, 1977.

Edington, D. W., and Edgerton, V. R.: *The Biology of Physical Activity*. Boston, Houghton-Mifflin Company, 1976.

Knuttgen, H. G. (ed.): *Neuromuscular Mechanisms for Therapeutic and Conditioning Exercise*. Baltimore, University Park Press, 1976.

Medicine and Science in Sports. (The research journal of the American College of Sports Medicine.) Madison, Wis.

Nadel, E. R. (ed.): *Problems With Temperature Regulation During Exercise*. New York, Academic Press, 1977.

Shepro, D., and Knuttgen, H. G.: *Complete Conditioning*. Reading, Mass., Addison-Wesley Publishing Company, 1975.

REFERENCES

1. Saltin, B., Blomqvist, G., Mitchell, J. H., Johnson, R. L., Wildenthal, K., and Chapman, C. B.: Response to submaximal and maximal exercise after bed rest and training. Circulation *38*(Suppl. 7): 1–78, 1968.

2. American College of Sports Medicine; *Prevention of Heat Injuries During Distance Running*. Madison, Wis. (See Apprendix B of this book.)

3. American College of Sports Medicine; *The Use and Abuse of Anabolic-Androgenic Steroids in Sports*. Madison, Wis. (See Appendix B of this book.)

ADVANCED TOPICS IN EXERCISE PHYSIOLOGY AND IN MEDICINE

This section contains topics that, because of their complex natures, often are not included in books on exercise physiology. Such material is included here for those readers who desire a more complete view of sports physiology.

7

THE BIOMECHANICS OF MOVEMENT

PETER R. CAVANAGH, Ph.D.
and DON W. GRIEVE, M.Sc., Ph.D.

When muscle cells respond to stimuli and produce force, the focus must shift from biochemistry to biomechanics if the next link in the chain of human movement is to be understood. Biomechanics is the application of mechanical principles to the study of the living body. The application of mechanics allows us to make deductions about what is happening inside the body as it moves or adopts a posture. This approach is distinct from that of physiologists, who are better equipped to determine the energy cost and economy of an activity that is continued for any extended period of time. The biomechanist's main concern is with the analysis of postures and movements that may exist for only brief periods of time.

The aim of biomechanical analysis is to deduce the implications of movement for the bones, joints, and muscles; to make statements about individual regions of the body; and to recognize potentially hazardous activities. In sports, for example, complex movements occur in very brief periods of time — usually faster than the eye can comprehend. Special techniques have been developed to record the details of these movements, the forces exerted, and the muscle actions as they occur. As the subject develops, these data can be more precisely analyzed in terms of efficiency, safety, and quality of performance. This knowledge has immediate implications for participation in athletic activity and can have an important influence on coaching and performance.

The techniques developed in biomechanics are also used in the evaluation of sports equipment, training techniques, and rehabilitation procedures. For example, biomechanics research has determined the desirable characteristics for football helmets, running shoes, tennis racquets, weight training equipment, and exercise prescriptions. These achievements were based upon a biomechanical understanding of the body.

Every human movement and posture is the result of forces imposed on the body and developed within it. It is, therefore, important to understand how these forces are developed, how they lead to movement, and what effect they have on the structure of the body.

FORCE TRANSMISSION WITHIN THE LIMB

If a person weighing 700 Newtons* stands on the ball of the right foot, the foot would be acted upon by the forces shown in Figure 7–1, which is known as a *free body diagram*. In this type of presentation the object of interest, in this case the foot, is isolated from its contact with all other objects. A force is drawn acting at each point of contact, allowing the problem to be treated with the techniques of mechanics. The reaction force due to the weight of the body shown in Figure 7–1 acts through the ball of the foot. To maintain equilibrium, the Achilles tendon must pull upward on the heel bone with a tension that can be calculated from the lever ratios about the ankle. The tendon pulls at a mechanical disadvantage because it is closer to the joint than is the reaction at the ground. The actual tension required is ($^{12}/_5$) × 700 Newtons = 1680 Newtons.

The muscles of the calf (soleus and gastrocnemius muscles) are responsible for this tension. These muscles collectively contain about 2400 motor units, each of which can develop a maximum tension of approximately 1.5 Newtons when the 2000 individual fibers in each unit are working at full capacity. In the example given, only about half this capacity is being utilized.† At full capacity, this musculature could probably support the load if an even heavier person were carried on the shoulders of the subject. However, for some people this would be a dangerous exercise since direct tests of human Achilles tendons indicate that the point at which the ligaments rupture — the ultimate tensile strength — may be as small as 2000 Newtons. Under the conditions shown in Figure 7–1, the tendons of the calf muscles may have stretched as much as 1 cm.

---

*A Newton (N) is the unit of force in the International System of Units.

† $\dfrac{1680 \text{ N}}{2400 \text{ motor units} \times 1.5 \text{ N/motor unit}} = 0.47$

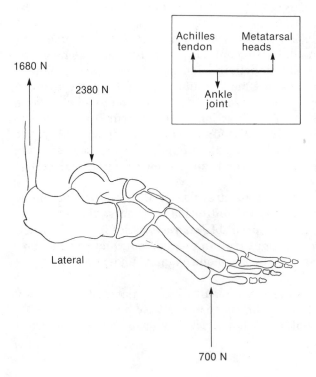

Figure 7–1. A *free body diagram* of the foot in which all points of contact of the foot with other structures have been replaced by forces. Since the subject is standing on the ball of the right foot, the body weight of 700 N acts at this point. The tension in the Achilles tendon must be 1680 N, since the lever ratio is approximately 5/12. The force acting through the ankle joint is 2380 N, the sum of the other forces but in the opposite direction. (The weight of the foot is assumed to be negligible in these calculations.)

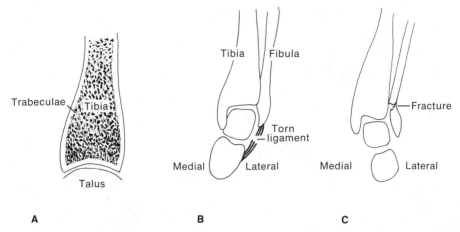

Figure 7–2. *A,* Section of tibia at ankle showing trabecular structure. *B,* Sprain (tear) of ankle ligament. *C,* Fracture of fibula near ankle.

At the same time that the collagen fibers of the tendon are elongating under stress, the skeleton in the ankle region is under severe compressive stress and it too becomes deformed. Turning back to the figure, it can be seen that a compressive force must exist at the ankle equal to 2380 Newtons (700N + 1680N). The end of the tibia is adapted to meet this stress, as can be seen in the radiating system of trabeculae that lead to the surface of the joint (Fig. 7–2A). Unlike tendon, bone is not well adapted to resist tensile (stretching) forces, and the body sometimes resorts to muscular and ligamentous arrangements that serve to relieve or avoid tension in bone. In Figure 7–1, the ligaments of the plantar (bottom) surface of the foot are under tension while the tarsal (foot) bones are in compression.

Ligaments generally play a major role in stabilizing the skeleton. At the ankle joint, strong medial and lateral collateral ligaments exist that maintain the joint surfaces in close proximity. These ligaments are designed to permit the normal movements of dorsiflexion and plantar flexion but to prevent unwanted movement in other planes. The joints may be stressed to their limits in sports, as, for example, when a player changes direction at high speed. Ligament sprains (Fig. 7–2B) and fractures of bones near joints (Fig. 7–2C) are common sports injuries.

At some joints, muscles help to relieve the tension in bone. In the forearm (Fig. 7–3), the biceps brachii muscle is necessary for supporting a weight in the hand. However, this muscle would place the upper surfaces of the forearm bones under tension if it acted alone. Fortunately, the brachioradialis muscle is suitably located to reduce this undesirable stress in the bone. Another example is found in the thigh (Fig. 7–4), where the lateral surface of the femur would come under tension if weight were placed on the limb. The iliotibial band, pulled upon by gluteus maximus and tensor fascia lata muscles, substantially reduces the tensile stress.

Bone does not articulate directly with bone. It is unusual for the opposing surfaces to have matching contours. The joint surfaces are lined with deformable articular cartilage, which is impregnated with synovial (joint) fluid and has a very smooth surface. A thin film of synovial fluid must always be present to prevent the two surfaces from coming into contact under the diverse conditions of loading and movement. Even in an extensive structure such as the hip joint, only a small part of the surface is bearing a load at any one time. When movement occurs, wedges of fluid under pressure form and serve to force the surfaces safely apart (Fig. 7–5).

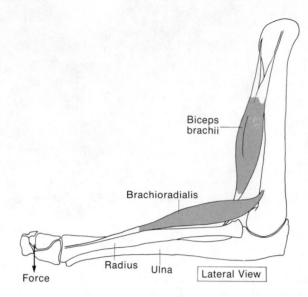

Figure 7–3. If the biceps brachii muscle acted alone to support a weight in the hand, there would be considerable tension stress on the upper surfaces of the radius and ulna. The brachioradialis muscle is in a position to reduce this undesirable stress.

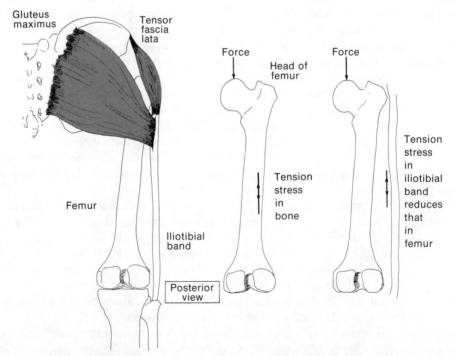

Figure 7–4. When forces act on the head of the femur, tension stress appears on the lateral surface of the femur. The iliotibial band, into which the muscles gluteus maximus and tensor fascia lata insert, helps reduce the stress.

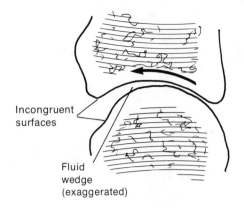

Figure 7–5. In a joint, the contours of opposing surfaces do not match perfectly. A wedge of fluid under pressure builds up during movement and drives the surfaces safely apart.

Incongruent surfaces

Fluid wedge (exaggerated)

MUSCLE ACTION

Figure 7–1 shows the ankle joint in one position. If the joint is moved to a new position, the effectiveness of the calf muscles alters. One reason is that the line of pull of the tendon changes its position relative to the center of the joint. Although this is not a particularly large change at the ankle joint, the effects at other joints, such as the elbow, knee, and hip, may be considerable (Fig. 7–6).

The other major reason for change in the competence of the calf muscles is the tension-length characteristics of the muscle fibers. Although the approximate distances between the bony attachments of the soleus and gastrocnemius muscles are 30 and 40 cm, respectively, 90 per cent of these distances are occupied by tendon. When the joint moves, the muscle fibers, in particular, accommodate the length change, as shown in Figure 7–7A and B.

The combined effects of changes in both leverage and muscle length are seen in Figure 7–7C. These data were collected from an experiment in which the foot was strapped to a lever centered on the ankle joint. The maximum torques that subjects could exert were measured with the ankle and knee joints in different positions. Changes of ankle joint angle affected both soleus and gastrocnemius muscles, whereas changes of knee angle affected only the gastrocnemius muscle.

It can be seen that with a fully extended knee and a fully dorsiflexed ankle (forefoot raised as far as possible) torque output is almost five times greater than in the least effective position: a flexed knee and plantar-flexed ankle (toes pointed as far as

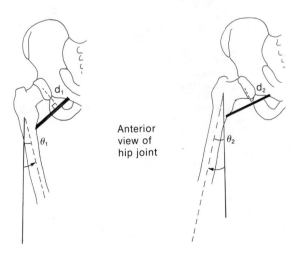

Figure 7–6. The line of action of the pectineus muscle moves closer to the center of the hip joint as the hip is moved outward from 20 degrees of adduction (θ_1) to 20 degrees of abduction (θ_2). The lever arms (d_1 and d_2) are obtained by finding the perpendicular between the center of the joint and the muscle line of action; d_2 is shorter than d_1.

Anterior view of hip joint

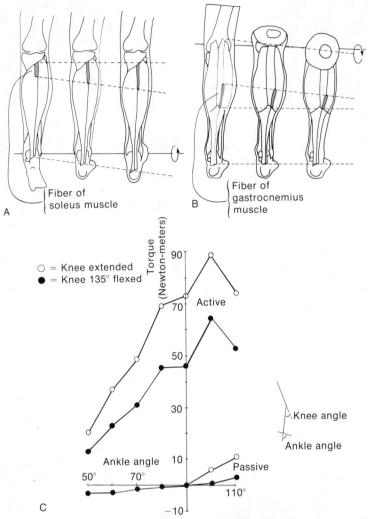

Figure 7–7. *A,* A single muscle fiber in the soleus muscle is depicted in three postures of the ankle joint. Although the fractional change of length of soleus between its attachments is modest, the effect upon the shorter muscle fibers within it is dramatic.

    B, Gastrocnemius muscle acts across the knee as well as the ankle, and therefore the length of its muscle fiber is affected by both knee and ankle posture. Here the knee is shown bent progressively; the muscle fiber shortens.

    C, The active plantar-flexor torques that can be exerted at the ankle diminish rapidly as the ankle is plantar-flexed below 90°. Flexion of the knee leads to further weakness at the ankle. Passive torques exist partly because the connective tissue in the gastrocnemius and soleus muscles tightens when stretched. Only one-joint muscles act across the front of the ankle joint, and passive torques during plantar flexion are not affected by knee posture.

possible). Because of these dramatic differences in effectiveness, the postures adopted in athletic performance greatly affect the external forces that can be developed. Tensions can also be exerted by resting muscles when they are stretched because of the connective tissue framework. These effects are an order of magnitude smaller than active tensions. Such forces are not, however, negligible and can limit the range of joint motion as, for example, in those persons who cannot touch their toes.

SIGNALS FROM MUSCLES

With the aid of a sensitive amplifier (an electromyograph), the small voltage changes produced by an active muscle can be detected between electrodes placed on the skin surface. These signals indicate that the muscle fibers are being activated by the nervous system. Muscle tension and useful output do not occur instantaneously; the elastic structures, such as tendon, joint surfaces, and skin, must first be tightened.

The muscle begins to develop tension within a few hundredths of a second after being stimulated, but it may be almost a tenth of a second before full output is obtained (Fig. 7–8). When this delay is added to reaction time, which ranges from .01 to .03 sec depending upon the complexity of the task, the importance of anticipation in sports activities becomes apparent.

If several channels are used simultaneously, electromyography shows how the coordinated use of the muscles leads to body movement. Figure 7–9 shows the activity of four lower extremity muscle groups in a man running uphill on a treadmill, together with tracings from a cine film of the action. It can be seen that each muscle group is used in bursts for a few tenths of a second. The quadriceps muscles are activated just before foot strike and remain active while they first cushion the initial impact and then drive the knee into extension. The forward thrust also requires hip extension, and the hamstring muscles are recruited for this purpose. It is interesting to recall that the hamstring and the quadriceps muscles have opposing actions at the knee and that they are both active simultaneously as knee extension occurs. In this

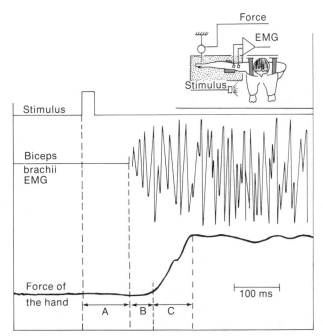

Figure 7–8. The electromyogram (EMG) from the biceps brachii is shown together with force output at the hand during a maximum effort of elbow flexion.

Activation of EMG begins approximately 100 milliseconds (ms) after the stimulus because of reaction time (delay A).

Force output does not begin for a further 50 milliseconds (delay B) owing to tensing of compliant structures.

Finally, maximum force output is achieved after a further delay of 100 milliseconds (delay C), making a total of 250 milliseconds from stimulus to maximum output.

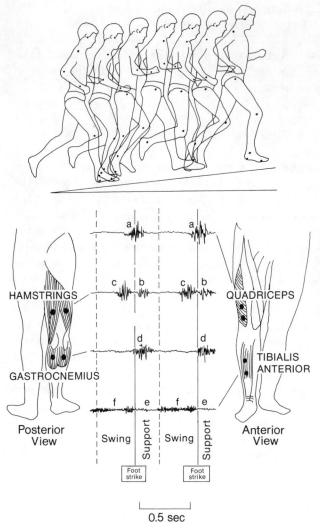

Figure 7–9. *Top:* Tracings from a cine film during uphill running on a treadmill (5 per cent grade at 13 km/hr).

Left and right below: Electrodes were placed over muscles principally involved in the action.

Center below: The brief phasic bursts of electrical activity during the running cycle signal the use of muscles, usually to oppose an existing movement and then to initiate a movement in the opposite direction. Two complete cycles are shown, with foot strikes and toe-off indicated by solid and broken vertical lines.

instance, the quadriceps muscles are therefore exerting a greater turning moment at the knee than are the hamstrings.

Up to this point we have discussed the body's performance of static tasks. When movement takes place, further properties of muscle have to be considered. A muscle that is shortening cannot develop as much tension as it can isometrically, but an active muscle being stretched (eccentric contraction) can develop tensions even greater than it can isometrically. This phenomenon is described by the force-velocity characteristic of muscle discussed in previous chapters. It is as common for muscles to resist or control movement as it is for them to produce movement. This realization has led to the incorporation of eccentric exercise as an integral part of many weight training programs.

NEWTON'S LAWS OF MOTION

Newton's Laws of Motion, which provide an essential link between the forces that arise during physical activity and the movements that are controlled or produced, are stated as follows:

First Law: A *body* continues in a *state of rest or uniform motion* unless acted upon by a *net force.*

Second Law: A body will change its *state of motion* at a rate proportional to the *applied force.*

Third Law: Action and reaction forces are equal and opposite.

The italicized words require some explanation. The *body* refers to any collection of matter, whether it be a baseball bat, a foot, the whole body, or a body holding a bat. The *state of rest or uniform motion* relates the center of gravity of the body to its environment. Motion indicates movement of the center of gravity relative to the environment. Usually the reference frame is the earth. Many forces may be acting on the body, as Figure 7–1 shows. No change of motion will occur unless these forces are unbalanced, producing a resultant, or *net, force* in some direction.

Motion, in Newton's language, means momentum, which is a vector quantity obtained by summing the products of the masses and the velocities of all particles in the body in a given direction; this is the same as the product of the total mass and the velocity of the center of gravity. For a solid body, the center of gravity can be located with little difficulty, although the quivering trunk of an obese person in motion, for example, may present difficulties of location.

If the body parts are treated as solid objects, the locations of their centers of gravity can be estimated with the help of data from anthropometric studies (measurements of body dimensions and properties in both living subjects and cadavers). It is then a simple matter to compute the location of the center of gravity of the whole body. This procedure is often applied to the analysis of sports activities through the use of high-speed cinematography.

It is important to realize that the center of gravity is not a fixed point in relation to the skeleton. This is illustrated in Figure 7–10 in which three instantaneous postures from a gymnastics routine are shown. The center of gravity moves from a position behind the gymnast, through his body, and out into space again. Perhaps the most

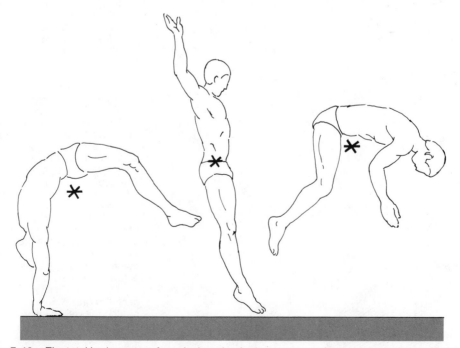

Figure 7–10. The total body center of gravity location in three postures from a gymnastics routine. Notice that the center of gravity is not fixed in relation to the body. In successive postures it falls behind, inside, and in front of the body.

dramatic example of shifting the center of gravity out of the body is to be found in a successful pole vault. The body passes over the bar while the center of gravity passes beneath it. This is an area in which the biomechanist can directly assist the athlete and his coach to develop a particular skill during training.

Rest and *uniform motion* imply states of zero and constant velocity, respectively, which are rarely found in the living body. They do not mean the same as "at rest" and "in steady movement" — terms that a layman might use to describe standing still or jogging at a steady rate. The latter are both the result of nonuniform motions that cancel out over a period of time. For this reason, Newton's First Law has less application in biomechanics than his Second Law, which states what happens when a net force does exist; that is, that the state of motion (momentum) changes at a rate proportional to the *force applied*. This relationship is stated in the familiar equations:

$$\begin{aligned} \text{force} &= \text{rate of change of momentum} \\ &= \text{mass} \times \text{rate of change of velocity} \\ &= \text{mass} \times \text{acceleration} \end{aligned}$$

Note that force produces acceleration that we do not see. Time must elapse before velocity builds up, and velocities must exist for a period of time before displacement is achieved.

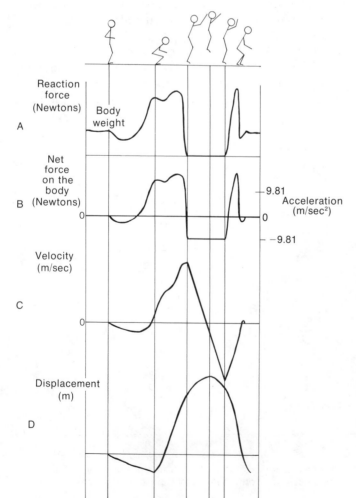

Figure 7–11. *A,* Vertical component of ground reaction force during a standing vertical jump performed with a counter movement, an initial downward movement before jumping. Notice that the reaction force was less than body weight during the counter movement. During flight the reaction force was zero.

B, Net force on the center of gravity is the reaction force minus body weight. The X axis is therefore moved to zero at the level of body weight. Since force equals mass × acceleration, the acceleration (right-hand axis) can be obtained by dividing force by mass. The acceleration during flight is -9.81 m/sec^2 — the acceleration due to gravity.

C, The velocity of the center of gravity is obtained by integrating the acceleration-time curve. The velocity is zero at the lowest point and reaches its peak slightly before takeoff.

D, The displacement of the center of gravity is found by integrating the velocity-time curve.

A force upon the body where contact is made with the environment is accompanied, according to Newton's Third Law, by an equal and opposite reaction upon the surroundings. The reaction is a force that can be measured.

Figure 7–11A shows ground reaction forces, as measured by a force platform, during the performance of a standing vertical jump. The net upward force on the body (Fig. 7–11B) is equal to the measured force minus the body weight. The result of the net force applied to the body is a change in velocity over a period of time (Fig. 7–11C). These changes cause the fluctuations in the height of the body relative to the ground (Fig. 7–11D). The velocity in Figure 7–11C was obtained by dividing the net force by body mass to give acceleration and then integrating with respect to time. (Integration is a mathematical technique for calculating the area under a curve.) The displacement record (Fig. 7–11D) is the integral of the velocity.

In addition to linear movements, a body may rotate about an axis through its center of gravity, independent of the motion of the center of gravity. If all the forces on the body are considered, and the distance of each force from an axis through the center of gravity is noted, the algebraic sum (sum having regard to sign) of the moments of these forces (force × distance) equals the rate of change of angular momentum. The reader will see the analogy between torque and *angular* movement on the one hand and force and *linear* movement on the other. The measurement of the reaction to a torque can lead to statements about a body's rotation; conversely, observations of angular acceleration can lead to deductions of the torques that must be acting.

A good example of the deduction of torque is seen in Figure 7–12 in which the motion of a golf club during the downswing, recorded with a high-speed camera, has been analyzed according to Newton's Laws. The analysis has been performed in the plane of movement of the club which is oblique to the plane that divides the body into two parts through the midline. The calculated torque that the hands applied to the club in order to produce this motion is shown in the figure.

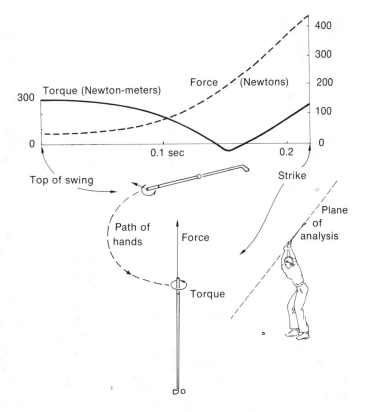

Figure 7–12. Golf: an analysis of the downswing of drive. Forces on the club are computed from the accelerations of the center of gravity. These data, combined with measurements of angular accelerations, are used to compute torques in the plane of motion of the club.

EXTERNAL FORCES

The internal forces that were discussed previously in the chapter cannot by themselves cause a net change in the position of the body's center of gravity. It is clear from the statement of Newton's Second Law that an external force must act for movement to occur. The environment on earth is dominated by the external force of gravity, which is always trying to accelerate the body towards the center of the earth. It has been seen from Newton's First Law that during quiet standing the ground exerts a force upwards on the feet equal to body weight, and so a static equilibrium exists. The vertical jump example demonstrated that as soon as muscle action causes the force at the feet to become either less than or greater than body weight, the center of gravity of the body will accelerate downward or upward, respectively. Since it allows statements to be made about the acceleration and subsequent velocity and displacement of the body the study of ground reaction forces is extremely useful — particularly if the ground reaction forces and gravity are the only external forces acting.

Figure 7–13 shows the ground reaction forces that act on the foot during the support phase of distance running. Although there is only one net force acting in one direction, it is usual to resolve the force into three components at right angles to each other. The force platform resolves the ground reaction forces automatically in the three directions shown in Figure 7–13.

The component of force F_x accelerates the body center of gravity in a side-to-side direction. After the initial peak when the body is being accelerated outward, a force tending to propel the body in the direction of the swinging limb predominates for the whole of the contact phase. Since a similar but opposite force exists during left foot contact, the center of gravity will continually oscillate from side to side about the mean direction of the run.

The component F_y in Figure 13 causes the body to slow down and speed up in the direction of progression. The force at first contact tends to slow the body down as control is gained during the early stages of support. The area under the force-time curve is called the *impulse,* and this area is an expression of how much speed the runner has lost since foot strike. When F_y becomes negative, the force tends to speed the body up to regain the velocity that has been lost. By this time the center of gravity is ahead of the point of support. If the negative impulse is less than the positive impulse, an overall loss of velocity will occur from touchdown to takeoff. Speeding up will occur if the negative impulse is greater.

The two positive peaks of the vertical force component F_z are characteristic of running, but they change their relative magnitudes as the speed of running changes. Within 0.50 sec after touchdown, the force becomes approximately one and a half times body weight. At this time, the center of gravity is travelling downward and this impact-force brakes downward movement. The second peak in F_z is of longer duration and greater magnitude. It is associated with the generation of enough vertical velocity for takeoff to occur.

Further analysis of the force platform data shown in Figure 7–13 can lead to statements concerning the instantaneous distribution of the reaction forces between the shoe and the ground. Figure 7–14 shows the resultant force vector and its point of application obtained from a group of subjects jogging across the force platform. Notice that the two peaks in the reaction force are applied to distinct regions of the shoe. The first peak is considerably anterior to the heel, and the second, as expected, is under the ball of the foot. These data serve as design information for running shoes, indicating the points where shock absorption is required.

Specific patterns of ground reaction force occur in different activities. People with injuries or abnormalities will exhibit unusual patterns, making the technique of measuring ground reaction forces potentially useful as a clinical tool.

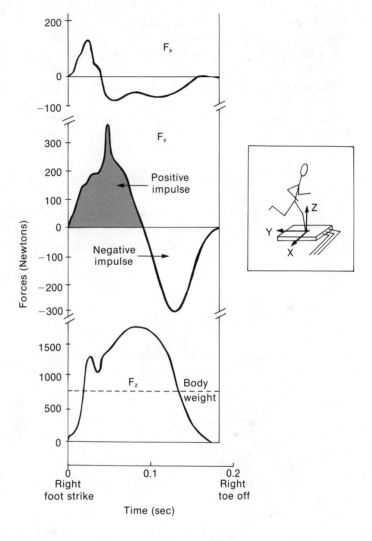

Figure 7–13. Ground reaction forces during contact with the right foot as a subject weighing 750 N jogs across the force platform (inset).

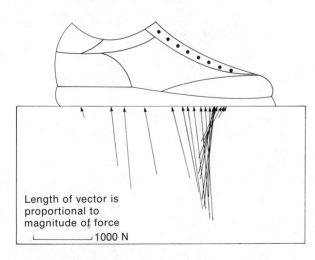

Length of vector is proportional to magnitude of force
⌊——————⌋ 1000 N

Figure 7–14. F_z and F_y from Figure 7–13 have been added vectorially and combined with pressure distribution data to show the magnitude, direction, and point of application of forces on the shoe during running. Notice how the first peak of impact is centered some distance in front of the heel and the second peak is applied to the ball of the foot. Also note that the force acts in a braking direction until the point of application is under the ball of the foot.

In many sports activities, external forces are applied to objects that consequently acquire velocity — unlike the earth, which moves only minutely as the runner contacts it. An example of forces applied by the hands to an object is shown in Figure 7–15. The subject lifts various weights onto a shelf as fast as possible. Liftoff (*arrow*) occurs when the subject exerts an upward force greater than the weight of the load. Note that in each case the impulsive force greater than the weight persists for only 0.3 sec. Although upward movement continues for the remainder of the lift, gravity is allowed to decelerate the load prior to placement. The skilled application and management of impulsive forces and of gravity are important elements in competitive weight lifting. In sports, impulsive forces are more common than steady force exertion.

OTHER ENVIRONMENTAL FORCES

The environments in which people move exert forces besides gravity; the most important of these in the context of sport activity is drag. A drag force occurs due to relative motion between a body and a fluid. In sports, the fluids are usually air and

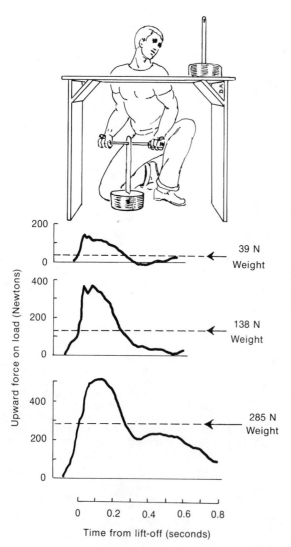

Figure 7–15. Upward forces involved in lifting various weights onto a table as quickly as possible. The handle of the weight contains an accelerometer so that the fluctuations of force applied to the handle may be recorded.

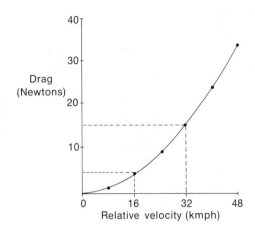

Figure 7–16. Drag forces acting on a cyclist during riding at various velocities. Notice that the force increases dramatically as the velocity increases. The force at 32 kmph is four times greater than the force at 16 kmph (direct square relationship).

water, which produce large drag forces for the cyclist and swimmer, respectively. Three major factors that control the magnitude of the drag force are frontal area, shape, and relative velocity.* The most critical of these in sports is relative velocity, since the drag force increases as the square of relative velocity (Fig. 7–16). For example, in a typical riding posture during cycling, the drag force may be 4 N at 16 kmph, but it rises to over 15 N at 32 kmph. During level cycling, drag is the single factor limiting increased speed, as is clearly demonstrated by world record speeds of over 160 kmph made behind vehicles equipped with wind shields. Although not quite so obvious, drag forces are important in other sports activities, such as running. It has been estimated that approximately 8 per cent of the distance runner's energy is used to overcome drag forces on a still day, while for the sprinter the figure may rise to 13 per cent.

In many throwing events, such as javelin and discus, another fluid force is of critical importance. This is the lift force similar to that exerted on an aircraft wing by the air. Lift tends to accelerate the object upward (Fig. 7–17), which is clearly useful since gravity is continually acting to pull the object toward earth. The magnitude of the lift force is determined by the orientation of the object, its shape, and its relative velocity. Careful attention to each of these factors can result in improved performance.

If an object moving through a fluid is spinning, additional forces will act during flight. Spin about a vertical axis will result in side forces, causing the object to deviate from a straight path. This phenomenon is used to advantage by pitchers, tennis players, and soccer players, but is often a source of frustration to golfers.

---

*Relative velocity takes into account the velocities of both object and fluid. For instance, the relative velocity is 30 kmph (kilometers per hour) if a cyclist is pedalling at 15 kmph into a 15 kmph headwind or at 30 kmph in still air.

Figure 7–17. Forces acting on a discus during flight. F_L, the lift force, tends to counter the effects of gravity, W, and is dependent upon the orientation of the discus, θ, as well as its shape. A drag force, F_d, acts to slow the discus down.

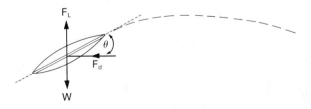

CONCLUSION

This chapter has provided a variety of examples of biomechanical analyses of sports movements. The field of biomechanics of sport is a young and vigorous one in which many sports activities remain to be studied. Indeed, 1977 was the first year in which the United States Olympic Committee made a concerted attempt to support biomechanics research, although such research has been an integral part of many European programs for some time.

If the student's interest has been aroused by the material presented here, coursework in biomechanics should be included in future study. A sound understanding of the biomechanics of movement will help all persons concerned with sports activities whether they participate, coach, design sports equipment, or are responsible for the welfare of the athlete.

SUMMARY

It has been the author's intention to show with the aid of numerous examples the distinct contribution that biomechanics can make to the understanding of athletic pursuits.

Commencing with static examples, the reader was introduced to the implications of muscle action and externally applied forces for the tissues of the body. This was followed by an enumeration of factors that influence muscle action and the means of studying them. Newton's Laws of Motion were set out as the basis for understanding dynamic activities, and examples of the major techniques of biomechanics as applied to running, jumping, cycling, and lifting were presented.

STUDY QUESTIONS

1. Give three reasons, other than fatigue, why the tension in the tendon of a fully active muscle may alter.

2. How quickly can a sportsman develop full output from an initially relaxed muscle following a command, and what mechanical changes would you expect as tension is developed?

3. Give three examples of muscles that change their mechanical advantage (leverage) at a joint as the posture of the joint changes.

4. If a weight lifter attempted to lift a barbell very slowly instead of using his usual technique, what limitations might he experience?

5. How can data on the direction and magnitude of ground reaction forces is running (Fig. 7–13) help in designing running shoes?

6. It was shown that during a continuous movement, such as running or walking, the major muscle groups are active for very brief periods of time. Explain this phenomenon in terms of Newton's First and Second Laws of Motion.

7. Draw free body diagrams to show the forces acting in the following situations:.
    a. A cyclist pedalling.
    b. The forearm and hand when lifting a weight under the action of the muscles shown in Figure 7–3A.
    c. The shank and foot at the moment of impact in kicking.
    d. A golf ball in flight spinning about a vertical axis.

FURTHER READINGS

Basmajian, J. V.: *Muscles Alive – Their Functions Revealed by Electromyography.* Baltimore, The Williams and Wilkins Company, 1967.

Grieve, D. W., Miller, D. I., Mitchelson, D., Paul, J. P., and Smith, A. J.: *Techniques for the Analysis of Human Movement.* Princeton, Princeton Book Company, 1976.

Hay, J. G., *The Biomechanics of Sports Technique.* Englewood Cliffs, N.J., Prentice-Hall, 1973.

International Congress on Biomechanics: *Biomechanics I–Biomechanics VI.* Baltimore, University Park Press, 1968–1978.

Miller, D. I., and Nelson, R. C.: *The Biomechanics of Sport – A Research Approach.* Philadelphia, Lea & Febiger, 1973.

Tricker, R. A. R., and Tricker, B. J. K.: *The Science of Movement.* New York, American Elsevier, 1968.

8

TEMPERATURE REGULATION

ETHAN R. NADEL, Ph.D.

The ability to regulate internal body temperature at a relatively high and constant level has endowed birds and mammals with a certain independence from the environment. Since the rates of most physical and chemical reactions are proportional to temperature, the body functions in general are likewise related to their local temperatures. The activity levels of temperature conformers (those animals that cannot regulate their temperature) are therefore largely subject to the environmental temperature. For example, lizards are much more effective hunters on warm days, when their body temperatures are relatively high, than on cool or cold days, when many cellular or organ system rates of reaction are slowed. On the other hand, those animals that regulate internal temperature are able to withstand considerable variation in environmental temperature and maintain a relatively consistent level of body function. Thus, a field mouse is as effective a hunter on a cool day as on a warm day. By providing for a relatively constant internal temperature, the temperature regulatory mechanisms have also provided an internal environment in which the rates of most reactions are relatively high and optimal with respect to one another.

In Chapter 1, the principles of cellular metabolism were described. In the presence of oxygen, fuels are degraded to produce chemically bound energy (ATP) and wastes. The chemically bound energy can subsequently be converted to electrical or mechanical forms, which provide for normal physiological activities such as muscular contraction. To prevent toxicity, the waste products must be transferred from each metabolically active cell through the body to the environment. The primary waste products are carbon dioxide and heat. Since the rates of waste production are closely related to the rate of metabolism (small differences can exist according to the type of fuel being oxidized), the problems associated with waste removal are increased during exercise, when the metabolic rate is increased. Accordingly, when the rate of energy production is ten times the resting metabolism, as it is in humans during moderately heavy exercise, the body's rate of heat production is also on the order of ten times greater than at rest. If the body had no special means for removal of this excess heat, it would burn up from the inside during prolonged exercise. Of course, this is not the case. The purpose of this chapter is to describe the mechanisms by which the body controls the rates of heat transfer from the sites of production to the environment, thereby regulating its internal temperature within fairly tight limits.

TEMPERATURE AND HEAT

What constitutes a normal body temperature? Or, to pose a more basic question, what is temperature? *Temperature* is a term that describes the feeling of relative warmth. Temperature gains a better definition when we have an objective, rather than subjective, measure — as with a thermometer. An evacuated capillary tube filled with mercury is the most widely used type of thermometer. When its bulb is immersed in ice water the mercury level is assigned a value, which is 0° on the *Centigrade* scale. When the bulb is immersed in boiling water (at sea level) the mercury expands and the new level is assigned a value of 100° C. According to Kleiber,[1] the Swedish botanist Linneaus was the first to describe this scale in 1740, two years before Celsius described a similar, but reverse scale. Thus, the *Celsius* scale reads from 100° to 0°. *Fahrenheit* devised a scale that attempted to place the human body temperature at 100° and the temperature of a freezing salt solution at 0°. The result was that melting ice has a value of 32° F and boiling water a value of 212° F. Scientists generally use the Centigrade scale, in which the normal body temperature is 37.0°. This value varies to some extent among individuals and in any individual over the course of the day (the circadian rhythm). Conversion from Fahrenheit to Centigrade is easily accomplished by using the following equation:

$$°C = (°F - 32) \times 5/9$$

Conversely, the Centigrade to Fahrenheit conversion is:

$$°F = (°C \times 9/5) + 32$$

It is easily seen that a change of 1.0° C is equivalent to a change of 1.8° F (Fig. 8–1). Thus, a fever of 102.2° F is the same as a 39.0° C fever.

The *kilocalorie* is the amount of energy that is required to raise the temperature of 1 kilogram of water 1 degree on the Centigrade scale. (The kilojoule (kJ) is the energy term favored by those who use the International System of units. To convert kcal to kJ, one must multiply by 4.187.) Since the specific heat of the body (defined below) is 0.83 kcal per kilogram (kg) and per degree, one can easily determine the amount of energy that a 75-kg individual would have to store in order to increase his body temperature by 1 degree:

$$0.83 \frac{kcal}{kg \, °C} \times 75 \text{ kg} \times 1°C = 62.25 \text{ kcal}$$

Since the heat production of a normal individual during moderate exercise can be on the order of 13 kcal per minute (this is determined by multiplying the oxygen uptake of 2.7 liters of O_2 per minute times 4.8 kcal* per liter of O_2), it is apparent that this individual would undergo a 1.0° C increase in body temperature about every five minutes if no temperature regulatory mechanisms were available. Since a marathon runner is able to sustain a much greater oxygen uptake than this for two to three hours,[2] with a body core temperature maintained between 39° and 41° C, it is evident that the temperature regulatory system is quite efficient.

The *heat content* of a system is related to its temperature, its mass (or volume), and its specific heat. The *specific heat* of any substance describes the ratio of the change in temperature of water to the change in temperature of that substance when equal

---

*The caloric equivalent of oxygen varies somewhat according to the fuel being oxidized. The value 4.8 kcal per liter is an average value that assumes the individual is metabolizing both fat and carbohydrate.

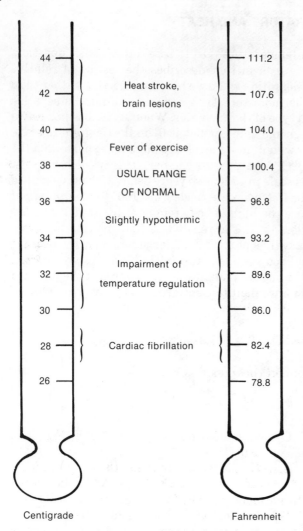

44 — 111.2

42 — Heat stroke, — 107.6
brain lesions

40 — 104.0

Fever of exercise

38 — USUAL RANGE — 100.4

OF NORMAL

36 — 96.8

Slightly hypothermic

34 — 93.2

Impairment of

32 — temperature regulation — 89.6

30 — 86.0

28 — Cardiac fibrillation — 82.4

26 — 78.8

Centigrade   Fahrenheit

Figure 8–1. The extreme range of internal body temperatures in humans, comparing the Centigrade and Fahrenheit scales. (Modified from DuBois, E. F.: *Fever and Regulation of Body Temperature.* Springfield, Ill., Charles C Thomas, 1948.)

volumes of the two are mixed. Practically speaking, this ratio gives the heating power of the substance per unit of mass and temperature change. If a substance has a high specific heat (as does water, which has a specific heat of 1.0 kcal per kilogram and per degree C), it takes a great deal more energy to change its temperature by 1.0° C than it does to change the same volume of a substance that has an extremely low specific heat, such as air. Another term that describes (and is numerically equivalent to) the specific heat of a substance is thermal capacity. The specific heat of the human body, which is largely made up of water, is taken to be 0.83 kcal per kilogram and per degree C.

The *latent heat* of any particular substance is that amount of heat required to change its state from solid to liquid or liquid to gas. Thus, the latent heat of vaporization of water, for instance, is the amount of heat necessary to evaporate a given amount of water, which comes to around 0.6 kcal per gram. This becomes important for any animal that regulates its body temperature, because a great amount of body heat can be dissipated by evaporation of water from either the respiratory tract or from the skin surface. This will be discussed in greater detail.

Specific heat and latent heat have been defined but thus far no definition of heat itself has been given. At present, *heat* is regarded as related to a random movement of molecules. The greater the molecular movement within a given substance, the greater are the collisions between the molecules and the greater is the heat of that substance.

With this definition, the terms heat and energy can be used interchangeably. Heat then can be treated as a characteristic of a substance that can flow from a warmer to a cooler area. Or, stated in another way, heat is that which can produce a change in temperature if added to a substance. It should be clear that the heat flow across a body is proportional to the difference in temperature when the mass and specific heat are constant. This can be represented as follows:

$$\text{heat flow} = (T_1 - T_2) \times M \times c$$

where $T_1 - T_2$ = the temperature difference across the body
             M = the mass or volume
             c = the specific heat

Practically speaking, in the human body where heat production occurs in the core, the heat must be transferred from core to skin down the temperature gradient, $T_1 - T_2$. Similarly, the heat produced in the core and transferred to the skin must be subsequently transferred from skin to environment. The dry heat transfer between the skin and environment also occurs along its temperature gradient. However, whereas the body temperature gradient is always from core to skin, requiring heat transfer in this direction, it is not unusual for the environmental temperature to exceed the skin temperature. In fact, during daylight hours on the desert, environmental temperatures of 45° to 50° C are not uncommon. In these cases, the dry heat transfer is from the environment to the skin because the temperature gradient is in this direction. However, humans and some other animals can maintain a net heat transfer from the skin to the environment in these conditions by making use of their ability to pant or sweat, thereby placing water on surfaces from which evaporation can readily occur. Evaporation is independent of the temperature gradient but related to the water vapor pressure gradient between the surface and the environment. In the following section, the modes of heat transfer and the specific rules that govern heat transfer will be discussed in some detail.

THE CONTROLLED SYSTEM

Energy Production Within the Body

As described in previous sections, the heat production within the body is directly related to the oxygen uptake and the type of fuel being oxidized. Ultimately, nearly all the total energy transformed must be accounted for as heat added to the body. The heat produced by metabolism can vary up to fifteen or more times the resting level during exercise, up to six times the resting level during brief bouts of intense shivering, and up to three times resting during prolonged shivering.

During rest, the oxygen uptake of any individual is on the order of 250 to 300 ml of O_2 per minute. This rate of oxygen utilization is necessary to provide the body with a rate of ATP resynthesis that will satisfy such minimal needs as maintenance of the cellular sodium pumps, activities of the respiratory muscles and heart, and resting metabolic activities of the other organ systems. Thus, using 4.8 kcal per liter of O_2 as the energy equivalent, one finds that the body produces between 72 and 86 kcal of heat per hour of sedentary activity. Using Systeme Internationale (SI) units, the equivalent energy production is between 84 and 100 watts during sedentary activity (1 watt is equivalent to 1.163 kcal per hour). In order to exactly balance the heat production, and therefore resist storing any of the heat that is being produced, the body must dissipate heat at a rate equivalent to that of heat production. When the heat storage is negligible, the internal body temperature is constant, in which case the body is in a thermal *steady state*.

Energy Transfer Within the Body

Figure 8–2 is a schematic diagram that shows the pathways of heat transfer from the body core to the skin to the environment. As stated above, maintenance of a relatively constant internal body temperature is dependent upon a fine balance between the rate of heat production and the factors that govern the rates of heat transfer from core to skin and from skin to environment. Should the rate of heat production increase dramatically, as it does during exercise, the body must make adjustments in the heat loss pathways to attempt to regain the steady state of internal temperature. If this were not done, the internal temperature would continue to increase at a rate in proportion to the increased heat production.

The heat transfer from core to skin occurs by two means. Heat is transferred by *conduction* directly across the body tissues. Conduction of heat is passive and fixed according to the insulative value of the tissues and, of course, the temperature gradient. The insulative value from core to skin is directly proportional to the layer of

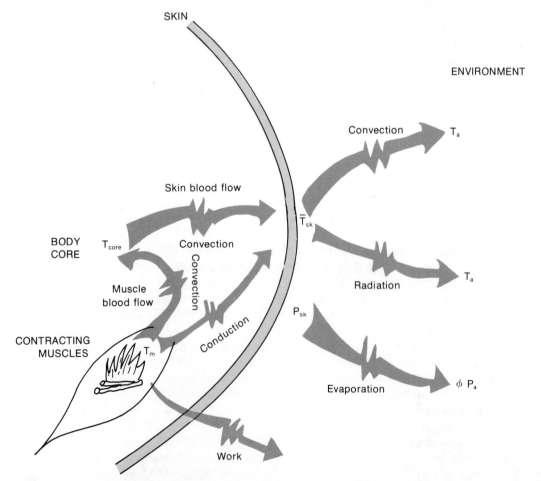

Figure 8–2. A schematic representation of the pathways of heat transfer from the sites of production to the skin and subsequently to the environment. See text for definition of terms.

subcutaneous fat, which has a relatively low thermal conductivity. Thus, the rate of heat transfer from core to skin by conduction is lower in fat people than in thin people. This fact becomes especially important during water immersion, when the object is to keep the heat within the body core and away from the skin. Normally, however, transfer of body heat to the skin by conduction is relatively unimportant in terms of the total heat flux.

The other means for heat transfer within the body is *convection*. Convective heat transfer is related to the velocity and density of the medium that carries the heat away from the warmer area. Within the body, heat is transferred from warmer areas to the blood stream, carried in the venous return to the heart, and finally directed to the skin surface in the cutaneous (skin) circulation. Since the rate of skin blood flow is under nervous system control, the rate of heat transfer from core to skin by convection can vary considerably between vasoconstricted and vasodilated conditions. Also, the net convective transfer of heat is related to both the rate of skin blood flow and the temperature difference between core and skin. Thus, even when skin blood flow is high, the heat flow may be relatively limited if the core to skin temperature gradient is low. Normally, however, the convective heat transfer within the body is proportional to the skin blood flow. Thus, the ability to control skin blood flow is a primary means for promoting or restricting heat transfer from the body core to the skin in different conditions.

Energy Transfer from the Body

The delivery of body heat to the skin surface would be of little value if there were no means for transfer of the heat to the environment. The avenues of heat transfer between the body and the environment are shown in Figure 8–2. Whereas the production of heat within the body is the consequence of chemical reactions, the transfer of the heat from the body to the environment is dependent upon physical laws. It should be obvious that all heat exchanges between the skin surface and the environment can be drastically reduced by placing increasing layers of clothing over the skin. The discussion of heat exchanges will consider only those between the exposed skin surface and the environment.

As with heat transfer from core to skin, heat can be transferred from skin to environment by conduction and convection. Conductive heat transfer depends upon the body's being in direct contact with its environment as well as upon the temperature difference and the thermal capacities and insulations of the two bodies. Because the thermal capacity of air is so low, heat transfer by conduction between the skin and the air is low and is usually combined with the convective component.

Heat transfer by convection is also dependent upon the thermal physical characteristics of the exchanging bodies, but is primarily related to the relative movement of the two bodies with respect to one another. In practical terms, convective heat exchange is related to the air velocity. When wind speed is greater, the heat loss by convection is accordingly greater (if skin temperature is higher than air temperature). When running, the effective air velocity is greater than when standing (unless of course one is running with the wind), and it follows that the heat exchange by convection is also greater. It should be emphasized, however, that heat losses by convection can rarely exceed 30 kcal per hour per degree of temperature difference between skin and environment in a nearly nude individual. Thus, to give an extreme example, when environmental temperature is relatively low, for example, 10° C (50° F), the mean temperature of the skin may be 25° C and the resulting heat loss due to convection will be 450 kcal per hour — about half the heat production during moderate running. Usually, convective losses are much less than this because the skin to ambient temperature gradient is less than 15° C. In any case, even in these conditions, in order to attain a steady state the bulk of the heat production must be dissipated by means other than convection.

One of these other means for energy transfer is *radiation*. Radiant exchange involves the transfer of thermal energy by means of electromagnetic waves. In a nearly nude person at rest in a moderate environment with no air movement, about 50 to 60 per cent of the heat produced is eliminated from the body by radiation to the environment. However, since radiative exchanges are independent of ambient conditions such as air velocity and relative humidity, the percentage of heat exchanged by radiation is reduced during exercise when both heat production and convective and evaporative losses are increased.

The thermal exchanges by radiation and convection can be mathematically represented as follows:

$$R + C = h_{r+c} \times (\overline{T}_{sk} - T_a)$$

where
$R + C$ = heat exchange by radiation and convection in kcal per hour and per m² of body surface.

h_{r+c} = combined *heat transfer coefficient* for radiation and convection. The value of h_{r+c} has been experimentally determined to be 7.4 kcal/(hour × m² × °C) at rest in still air. The heat transfer coefficient is dependent upon the thermal physical characteristics of the environment.

$(\overline{T}_{sk} - T_a)$ = the skin to environment temperature gradient, in °C.

Usually this description is normalized to the body surface area available for energy exchange. This description emphasizes that the primary factor that both determines the "dry" heat exchange and is under physiological control is the $\overline{T}_{sk}$. A high skin blood flow under given conditions results in an increase in $\overline{T}_{sk}$ and a widening of the $T_{sk} - T_a$ gradient (when $\overline{T}_{sk} > T_a$). This enhances the heat transfer by convection and radiation.

As mentioned before, the most potent avenue for heat dissipation is via *evaporation*. Evaporation is the process by which a substance changes from the liquid to gaseous phase. This conversion requires a certain amount of energy, termed the latent heat of vaporization. When water is placed onto the skin surface, it will evaporate at a rate determined by the water vapor pressure gradient between skin and environment. Each gram of water that evaporates removes 0.6 kcal from the skin. During heavy sweating conditions, an individual can produce around 20 grams of sweat per minute over the skin surface. If all of this is evaporated, the heat loss will be 12 kcal per minute, or 720 kcal per hour. Add to this another 2 grams per minute evaporated from the respiratory tract, and the evaporative rate can be around 800 kcal per hour, accounting for the greatest fraction of the heat loss from the body.

In a manner similar to the description for the dry heat exchanges, the evaporative exchange can be represented mathematically:

$$E = h_e (P_{sk} - \phi P_a) \times A_w/A_D$$

where
E = heat loss due to evaporation in kcal/(hr × m²)

h_e = heat transfer coefficient for evaporation, which is proportional to h_c and therefore related to the air velocity, in kcal/(hr × m² × mm Hg)

$P_{sk} - \phi P_a =$ water vapor pressure gradient between skin and air in mm Hg

$A_w/A_D =$ the fraction of the body with exposed wet skin

This description emphasizes two factors. The first is that to enhance the water vapor pressure gradient, water must be added to the skin surface. This is done via the sweating mechanism, which is under physiological control. The second factor is that the ambient humidity can have a great effect upon the evaporative rate. In dry desert conditions the gradient is large and all the water reaching the skin surface evaporates readily. However, in humid conditions the gradient may be small and evaporation will occur more slowly. The placing of clothing between the skin and the environment has the effect of increasing the humidity of the air directly over the skin surface and reducing the A_w/A_D ratio. Evaporation will occur only from the outer surface of the wet garment, and the cooling effect on the body is minimal. Therefore, in conditions of body heating, one should discard clothing to enhance evaporative cooling.

The Energy Balance Equation

Once the avenues of energy exchange are monitored, one can add up all the heat gains to the body and heat losses from the body and complete the energy balance equation. In the thermal steady state, when there is no change in the mean body temperature, the equation is written as follows:

$$M = E \pm (R + C) + (\pm W)$$

where

$M =$ rate of energy metabolism

$E =$ rate of evaporative loss

$R + C =$ rate of radiant and convective loss, when the sign is positive

$W =$ work rate, where $+W$ represents work energy done on an external system and $-W$ represents work energy absorbed by the body. Values of W are usually small with respect to M.

If there is an unsteady state and a gain or loss in mean body temperature, the two sides of the equation will balance only if a heat storage term (S) is included, as follows:

$$S = M - E \pm (R + C) - (\pm W)$$

The storage term then accounts for the change in mean body temperature with time. Most of the change in mean body temperature is reflected by a change in the body core temperature. Thus, a positive value of heat storage indicates an increasing internal body temperature.

THE CONTROLLING SYSTEM

Herein lie the elements that separate the temperature regulators from the temperature conformers. This complex negative feedback system provides the body with the abilities to (1) sense its thermal profile, (2) integrate and analyze this thermal information from the various loci of the body, and (3) direct an integrated reflex that constantly provides for fine adjustments in heat flow in such a way as to correct for deviations from the "desired" temperature profile. In other words, the temperature regulatory mechanism defends a specific body temperature or group of temperatures. From animal studies,[3] we know that the "desired" or reference temperature signal is set within the hypothalamus, a tiny group of specialized neurons at the floor of the brain. As noted earlier, the reference temperature of humans is around 37.0° C, a value that varies by about 0.5° C over the 24-hour cycle.

The only exception to this tightly prescribed reference occurs during the events leading to a fever. By events not yet understood, the activity of pyrogens released during infection results in an upward displacement of the body thermostat. The consequence of this resetting of the reference is that a higher internal body temperature becomes defended and the regulatory mechanism acts to achieve and maintain the new condition. This is the reason one experiences a "chill," and perhaps even active shivering, just prior to a fever; the increase in heat production is the body's attempt to minimize the "error" between the actual hypothalamic temperature and the new, elevated reference temperature. Conversely, when a fever "breaks," a common experience is a massive outpouring of sweat. In this case, the reference temperature has been readjusted to the normal level, and the internal temperature, which had been previously regulated about an elevated level, is subsequently sensed as too high. The appropriate thermoregulatory response to correct for this error is an activation of the heat dissipation mechanisms. These events are portrayed in Figure 8–3.

Temperature Sensors

In order to effectively assess its thermal profile, the body should have temperature sensors distributed over a wide range. Temperature-sensitive free nerve endings have been found in abundance over the skin surface[4] and in the preoptic area of the hypothalamus.[5] It is of considerable importance to have these two sets of temperature receptors relaying signals to the brain. The temperature sensors on the skin surface are ideal for providing the integrating center with information about the ambient temperature. The temperature sensors in the hypothalamus detect the absolute level of temperature at this important site, thereby providing the thermoregulatory center with information about the overall heat balance of the body. The skin receptors act as an early warning system, allowing the body to make adjustments in heat flow that are necessary to meet the demands of the environment and thereby maintain a constant internal temperature. The hypothalamic receptors, although incapable of sensing

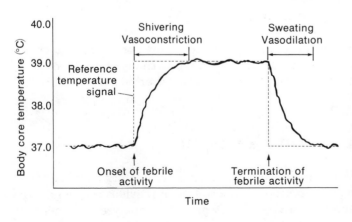

Figure 8–3. The events of a febrile episode. The fever occurs during a period in which the rate of heat production exceeds the rate of heat dissipation. The temperature is then regulated about the new elevated level. The fever breaks when the rate of heat dissipation exceeds the rate of production. The hypothetical reference temperature signal appears as a dotted line. (Modified from Brengelmann, G. L. *In* Ruch, T. C., and Patton, H. D. (eds.): *Physiology and Biophysics.* Philadelphia, W. B. Saunders Company, 1965.)

changes in ambient temperature, are necessary to detect the increased blood temperature that results from the increased heat production of exercise. Without internal temperature sensors, the body would burn up from the inside before the skin temperature sensors would be activated. There is some recent evidence that temperature sensors also exist in the spinal cord; they may act as auxiliary sensors of body core temperature. The information from the skin and core temperature receptors is integrated within the central nervous system, providing an accurate evaluation of the body's total thermal state.

Effector Organs

The primary organs that provide for adjustments in heat flow in humans are the sweat glands, vasomotor smooth muscle, and skeletal muscle. According to Kuno,[6] there are on the order of three million sweat glands in the human skin. These vary over the skin surface, with the face having the greatest density (approximately 350 glands per cm^2) but the trunk having the most glands (about 180 glands per cm^2). The absolute number of glands is fixed prior to birth. There are relatively few differences in density of sweat glands between the sexes and among races. Differences in sweating capabilities between individuals are probably related to factors such as sweat gland training, which will be discussed below.

Most of the sweat glands in human skin are *eccrine glands,* which are distributed over nearly all of the body surface, whereas *apocrine glands* are found primarily in the underarm and pubic regions. Eccrine glands are under thermoregulatory control and secrete a relatively dilute hypotonic sweat. Apocrine glands are thought to secrete in response to emotional stress. Each eccrine gland consists of a tightly coiled basal segment, which is the site of secretion of the sweat, and a straight segment, which is the duct extending to the epidermis. The secretory segment is innervated by the sympathetic nervous system; sweat secretion is stimulated by the release of acetylcholine* from the preglandular nerve terminals and subsequent reception of this neurotransmitter by the gland itself. It is generally thought that the rate of glandular secretion is proportional to the rate of nervous system activity. Thus, the greater the drive from the temperature regulatory center in the central nervous system, the greater the rate of release of acetylcholine at the neuroglandular junction and the greater the secretory activity of the sweat glands.

The ability to adjust the tone of smooth muscles around the small arterioles of the cutaneous vascular bed provides the means for enhancing or restricting the transport of heat from core to skin. The cutaneous vasculature of the hands and feet is innervated by adrenergic sympathetic vasoconstrictor nerves. Increased nervous activity reduces skin blood flow, while an absence of activity allows the blood flow to remain at a maximum level. Over most of the skin, however, the blood flow is modulated by an active vasodilator mechanism, with acetylcholine the probable neurotransmitter.

Increased heat production can be achieved by either voluntarily activating the skeletal muscles or undergoing involuntary shivering contractions. Voluntary movement, such as running or jumping, is accompanied by increased air movement and therefore an increase in the convective heat transfer coefficient, with a subsequent increase in heat loss from the skin. Shivering contractions are mediated by the autonomic nervous system and are not accompanied by significantly large increases in heat loss.

---

*The neurotransmitter associated with most sympathetic nervous system activity is norepinephrine. Eccrine sweat glands provide an exception to this general rule.

The Integration Center

As stated above, the integration between the thermal stimuli and the efferent (outgoing) responses occurs within the hypothalamus. The hypothalamus sorts out the thermal stimuli, compares notes with other regulatory centers that share information (such as the circulatory regulatory center in the medulla), and directs the appropriate efferent activity to maintain the hypothalamic temperature at its reference temperature signal.

To investigate the characteristics of the integrator, physiologists have attempted to develop experiments in which the internal and average skin temperatures are varied independently and one or several of the efferent responses are monitored. In this way, the effect of a given change in internal or skin temperature upon the response could be quantitatively described. The basis for this type of experiment rests with the classic 1938 study of Marius Nielsen.[7] Nielsen found that in any individual the internal (rectal) temperature is proportional to exercise intensity. Therefore, by asking subjects to perform different levels of exercise under controlled conditions, a range of internal temperatures can be obtained. If these exercise bouts are repeated under several different ambient temperature conditions, a range of average skin temperatures can be obtained. Results from this type of experiment are shown in Figures 8-4 and 8-5.

Several important findings are evident.[8,9] First, driving up the internal temperature* results in a proportional increase in skin blood flow and sweating rate once the response thresholds have been attained. These linear relationships are valid up to the point at which response capabilities are maximal. Second, the effect of modifying the mean skin temperature is to shift the internal temperature threshold for both heat dissipation responses without changing the slope of the relationship once the response

---

*Temperature measured in the esophagus is the closest noninvasive estimate of hypothalamic temperature in humans. Tympanic membrane and rectal temperatures have also been used, but they respond more slowly to a change in the thermal load.

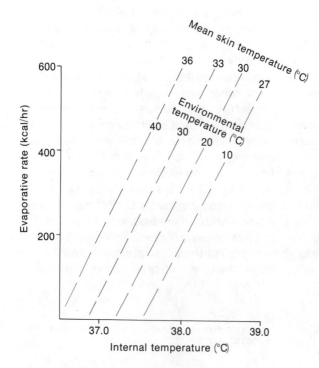

Figure 8-4. Relation between evaporative rate and internal temperature at different levels of mean skin temperature. (Modified from Nadel, E. R., et al.: J. Appl. Physiol. *31*:80–87, 1971.)

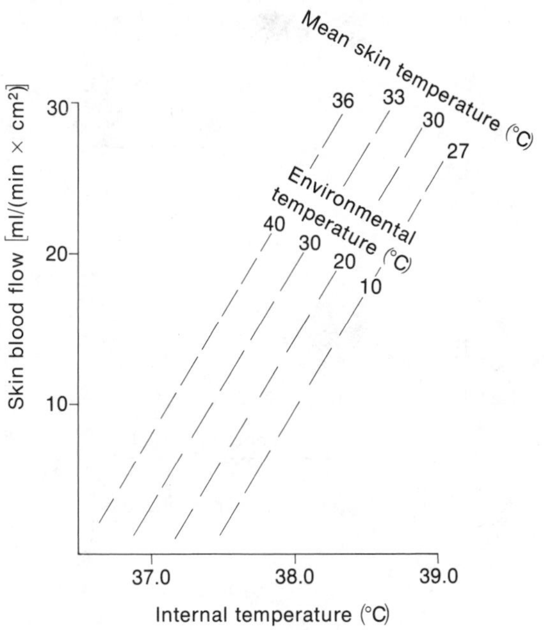

Figure 8–5. Relation between rate of skin blood flow and internal temperature at different levels of mean skin temperature. (Modified from Wenger, C. B., et al.: J. Appl. Physiol. *38*: 58–63, 1975.)

is initiated. An increase in mean skin temperature lowers the internal temperature threshold for both sweating and vasodilation by approximately the same amount. Third, the effect of a change in internal temperature per unit of response is about ten times that of a similar change in skin temperature. That is, the integrator sees a change in its own temperature as being an order of magnitude more important than the same change in the average skin temperature. These generalities also hold for the control of shivering metabolism, although the experimental evidence is much less complete.

A brief scenario of the thermal events occurring during exercise, then, goes as follows: Accompanying muscular contraction, there is an increase in heat production in the muscle that is related to the intensity of exercise. The venous blood draining the muscle distributes this excess heat throughout the body core. Thermal sensors in the hypothalamus increase their activity in response to the higher blood temperature. The hypothalamic integrator then compares its temperature with a reference temperature signal, finds an error between the two, and directs nervous system activity toward the appropriate effector organs. As internal temperature rises, the vasodilatory and sweating thresholds, which are functions of the mean skin temperature, are attained. Once the response thresholds have been surpassed, skin blood flow and sweating rate increase in proportion to the increase in internal temperature, enhancing heat flow from the body and thereby slowing the rate of internal temperature rise. (The absolute rates of skin blood flow and sweating are functions of both the internal and mean skin temperatures.) Finally, the rate of heat dissipation by radiation, convection, and, most importantly, evaporation balance the rate of heat production.

At this point the internal temperature becomes steady at a new, elevated level (Fig. 8–6). This new steady state of internal temperature is *not* being regulated at an elevated level, as occurs during a fever. Rather, the regulatory mechanism attempts to return the internal temperature to the reference level of 37.0° C but is incapable of doing so in the face of the elevated heat production. If, for instance, the sensitivity of the sweating response were increased, the increase in sweating rate per unit of internal temperature rise would be greater and the steady state in internal temperature would be achieved at a lower internal temperature than before. This is one

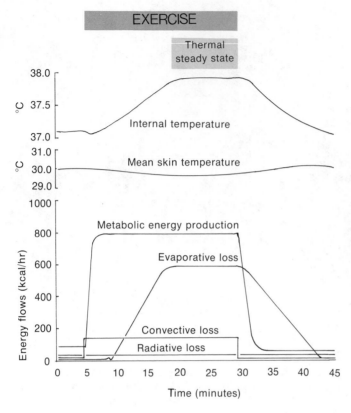

Figure 8–6. Thermal and energy events occurring during 25 minutes of exercise in a 20°C environment. At the beginning of exercise, prior to the thermal steady state, the energy production exceeds the energy losses, heat is stored, and internal temperature rises. During the steady state, the energy production is equal to the energy loss. At the termination of exercise, the energy production falls below the energy losses, heat storage is negative, and the internal temperature is able to return to its regulated level.

beneficial effect of a physical fitness program: one is able to train the sweating mechanism by repeated bouts of exercise. Sweat gland training causes an increased sensitivity to a change in internal temperature and results in a lower internal temperature during a given intensity of exercise.[10] This provides for a greater margin of safety between operating temperature and limiting temperatures and is accompanied by lower demands on the circulatory system as well.

EXERCISE IN THE HEAT

Problems with Fluid Balance

Water is the solvent in which all of the body's organic and inorganic solutes are dissolved. Because the body's normal activities depend upon a precise regulation of many of these solutes (e.g., plasma concentrations of Na^+, K^+, HCO_3^-), it follows that disturbances in the amount of body water could have a profound effect upon normal function. The net turnover of water averages around 2.0 to 2.5 liters per day. The balance is the consequence of water intake in foods and fluids, with subsequent absorption in the gut, and water output from the kidney, gastrointestinal tract, and the evaporative surfaces. On the output side, only the renal activity is directed toward regulation of body fluid balance. On the input side, the relatively imprecise sensation of thirst controls drinking behavior. It should be obvious that any great disturbances on one side of the daily fluid balance equation would require compensatory adjustments on the other side. This is the case in heavy sweating conditions.

It is not unusual for an individual to lose 10 to 15 liters of water during excessively heavy sweating conditions. This is five times the normal turnover, far outside the range where normal regulatory activities would be expected to compensate. The thirst mechanism is undoubtedly called into play, but this control system must be augmented by voluntary drinking. Renal activity is diminished by the activation of antidiuretic hormone, or, as it is also known, vasopressin. The body must also replace its sodium (Na^+) losses. Although normal sweat is hypotonic with respect to plasma (Na^+ concentration in sweat is around 60 milliequivalents per liter, compared with 142 milliequivalents of Na^+ per liter of plasma), the Na^+ that is delivered to the skin surface in the sweat is lost from the body. Loss of electrolytes can have an effect upon cellular activity (such as the muscle cells). The proper balance of water and electrolyte concentrations requires movement of these substances out of the body tissues when no other sources are available. Replacement must be accomplished primarily by ingestion of electrolytes in the diet. Most balanced diets take care of this replacement within a day or two, but individuals who are continuously exposed to heavy sweating conditions may need a dietary supplement. Sodium retention is also promoted in these conditions by enhanced reabsorption from the renal tubule, mediated by the hormone aldosterone.

The temperature regulatory system has its own mechanism that acts to conserve body water in heavy sweating conditions. Experiments have shown that dehydration results in a higher internal body temperature during exercise than occurs during normally hydrated conditions.[11] It is likely that this elevation in internal temperature is the consequence of a reduction in the sensitivity of the sweating response per unit of internal temperature increase. In this case, the rate of sweating required for a given thermal steady state would be achieved at a higher internal temperature. This is shown in Figure 8–7. Unfortunately, this mechanism is a two-edged sword, because in reducing the amount of sweating at any given internal temperature, the body temperature is forced up to a level that may in itself stimulate breakdowns in other control systems. In these conditions, exercise should be terminated and rehydration with a balanced solution should be promoted.

Maintenance of Central Circulation

Another problem encountered during exercise in warm conditions is the maintenance of the central circulating blood volume. Heat-induced syncope, or fainting, is the consequence of a reduction in cardiac filling pressure, and subsequent reduction in

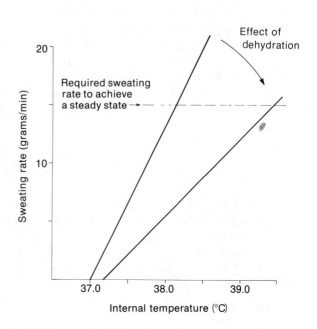

Figure 8–7. Effect of dehydration upon the linear relation between sweating rate and internal temperature at a constant skin temperature. Dehydration causes a reduction in the sensitivity of this control system, resulting in an increase in the steady state internal temperature from 38.1°C to 39.4°C in these hypothetical conditions.

cardiac output, caused by the uncompensated decrease in the venous return to the heart. A marked decrease in the central circulating blood volume occurs during exercise in warm conditions because a number of simultaneous demands are placed on the circulatory system. Because of the high skin blood flow brought about by high internal and skin temperatures, the skin blood volume rapidly increases to its maximum. There is a concurrent loss of plasma to the extravascular spaces in the muscle, which may exceed 15 percent of the plasma volume in extreme conditions. Accompanying these reductions in circulating blood volume, there is an additional movement of fluid to supply the sweating mechanism. The body is able to compensate for these losses to some extent by reducing blood flow to metabolically inactive areas, like the splanchnic or renal beds, but in extreme conditions the compromise may limit extended exercise.

Limitation of exercise may be the result of circulatory or thermoregulatory breakdown. In warm conditions, the capabilities of the thermoregulatory system may be exceeded and the body cannot dissipate the combined thermal load from exercise and environment. In this case, internal temperature continues to rise until the person stops exercising due to discomfort, heat cramps, or heat exhaustion. The circulatory breakdown is the consequence of the inability to maintain the simultaneous demands for high blood flow from the contracting muscles and the skin in the face of the reduced circulating blood volume. In order to maintain cardiac output at its elevated level, the body must maintain heart rate and stroke volume. When the venous return is compromised, the cardiac filling pressure is reduced and stroke volume is likewise reduced (Starling's Law). Because of the baroreflex, the heart rate will increase to compensate for the transient fall in carotid artery pressure (which itself is the result of the transient fall in cardiac output) and thereby act to return the cardiac output to the level that is sufficient to meet the demands of the periphery. Breakdown occurs when heart rate approaches its maximum in these conditions; this can happen at exercise intensities that are considerably less than maximal in cool conditions. At one time or another, most persons have experienced this tachycardia (high heart rate) during exercise in a hot environment.

The competition for blood flow is minimized in trained individuals. Athletes usually have lower thresholds for sweating and vasodilation and a more sensitive sweating response. Maintenance of lower thermoregulatory profile via a heightened sweating sensitivity provides for a lower circulatory strain than would otherwise develop from increased skin circulatory demands and increased reductions in plasma volume. Furthermore, the trained individual has the capability to maintain cardiac output at a given intensity of exercise by relatively higher stroke volumes and relatively lower heart rates than the untrained individual. Perhaps the circulatory benefits result from an enhanced ability to maintain central circulating blood volume. At any rate, the adaptations that occur in both the temperature regulatory and circulatory regulatory systems provide the trained individual with a greatly improved tolerance to exercise in the heat.

HEAT INJURY*

Heat injury results when the demands of the environment exceed the capabilities of the body's regulatory mechanisms. Although heat-induced injury is usually reversible, heat stroke and death occur often enough to make one aware of the consequences of uncompensated breakdowns in physiological regulatory systems.

The primary cause of the heat injury syndrome is the *hyperthermia,* or high internal temperatures, that can occur during exercise in a hot or warm, humid environ-

---

*This subject is also discussed in Chapter 21.

ment. Increases in internal temperature of 2° to 3° C generally do not have any ill effects upon normal body functions. However, when internal temperature rises to 40° to 41° C, central nervous system dysfunction may occur. This is manifested as a feeling of malaise, nausea, dizziness, and general inability to think rationally or orient oneself. Above 41° to 42° C convulsions may occur, with a loss of consciousness. Above 42° to 43° C there may be denaturation of cellular material, severe brain damage, and, ultimately, death.

On the other side, an excessive decrease in internal body temperature, *hypothermia,* can result from excessive cold exposure without proper insulation. Below an internal temperature of 36.5° C or so, maximal vasoconstriction and shivering occur. If the increased heat production is insufficient to prevent a fall in internal temperature, as is the case during prolonged immersion in cold water, progressive hypothermia will ensue. Central nervous system activity becomes increasingly depressed with body cooling, and when internal temperature is around 33° C, there is a loss of consciousness. Below 30° C many regulatory systems are lost, and fibrillation of the heart occurs around 28° C. Most of the deaths from accidental immersion following shipwreck occur from hypothermia, not drowning.

Prevention

To prevent overheating, a maximum surface area should be exposed for evaporation (i.e., clothing shed). Once the body's water loss becomes excessive, the sweating mechanism will gradually shut down (reduce its sensitivity) and internal body temperature will begin to climb. The two most obvious treatments in this case are to remove onself from the conditions producing the heat load (i.e., stop exercising, find shade, a cool room, or a lake) and drink water or a balanced electrolyte solution. These are essential treatments for survival in extreme conditions. It is readily seen that the circulatory failure leading to syncope in these conditions is actually a protective mechanism, requiring the individual to stop exercising and assume a supine position in which heat production is minimal and cardiac filling pressure is maximal.

Similarly, during extreme cold exposure, the first objective is to increase insulation between skin and environment. If this is insufficient to prevent body cooling, one should attempt to escape from the environment. In the case of cold water immersion, the most well-insulated individual will resist hypothermia best. In this case it is beneficial to be fat.

SUMMARY

The temperature regulatory system provides for physiological control of the body's heat flows in such a way as to attempt to balance heat production and heat loss. Temperature sensors on the skin surface and in the hypothalamus constantly appraise the regulatory center, also in the hypothalamus, of the body's thermal profile. If, because of thermal disturbances, the thermal profile deviates from a "desired" condition, the regulatory center directs an efferent response to correct for this deviation. Efferent organs are the skeletal muscles for elevations in heat production, the smooth muscles of the arterioles for control of heat transfer within the body, and the sweat glands for increases in heat dissipation. During exercise when heat production is high, the body achieves a new, elevated steady state of internal temperature that is related to the exercise intensity in any individual. This is not a new "regulated" temperature, but a steady state determined by the rate at which the heat dissipation responses were activated to the level at which they balanced the heat production.

STUDY QUESTIONS

1. Define temperature, heat, specific heat, and latent heat.

2. Describe the means by which heat is produced in the body.

3. Describe the means by which heat is transferred from the sites of production to the environment.

4. How does the body modify these rates of heat transfer?

5. How does the body's control system evaluate the body's thermal state and make appropriate adjustments?

6. Describe the sweating system and elaborate upon why this is the most effective means for dissipation of heat.

7. What are the specific problems presented to the temperature regulatory system by heavy exercise? How are these solved?

8. What are the specific problems presented to the circulatory system by heavy exercise? How are these solved?

9. Why is a trained athlete better able than an untrained individual to tolerate heavy exercise in the heat?

FURTHER READINGS

Burton, A. C., and Edholm, O. G.: *Man in a Cold Environment*. Edward Arnold Ltd., London, 1955.
Cabanac, M.: Temperature regulation. Ann. Rev. Physiol. *37*:415–439, 1975.
Hammel, H. T.: Regulation of internal body temperature. Ann. Rev. Physiol. *30*:641–710, 1968.
Hardy, J. D.: Physiology of temperature regulation. Physiol. Rev. *41*:521–606, 1961.
Nadel, E. R. (ed.): *Problems with Temperature Regulation During Exercise*. New York, Academic Press, 1977.

REFERENCES

1. Kleiber, M. *The Fire of Life*. New York, John Wiley & Sons, Inc., 1961.
2. Adams, W. C., Fox, R. H., Fry, A. J., and MacDonald, I. C.: Thermoregulation during marathon running in cool, moderate and hot environments. J. Appl. Physiol. *38*:1030–1037, 1975.
3. Fusco, M. M., Hardy, J. D., and Hammel, H. T.: Interaction of central and peripheral factors in physiological temperature regulation. Am. J. Physiol. *200*:572–580, 1961.
4. Hensel, H., Iggo, A., and Witt, I.: A quantitative study of sensitive cutaneous thermoreceptors with C afferent fibers. J. Physiol. (London) *153*:113–126, 1960.
5. Nakayama, T., Hammel, H. T., Hardy, J. D., and Eisenman, J. S.: Thermal stimulation and electrical activity of single units of the preoptic region. Am. J. Physiol. *204*:1122–1126, 1963.
6. Kuno, Y.: *Human Perspiration*. Springfield, Ill., Charles C Thomas, 1956.
7. Nielsen, M.: Die Regulation der Korpertemperatur bei Muskelarbeit. Skand. Arch. Physiol. *79*:193–230, 1938.
8. Nadel, E. R., R. W., Bullard, and Stolwijk, J. A. J.: Importance of skin temperature in the regulation of sweating. J. Appl. Physiol. *31*:80–87, 1971.
9. Wenger, C. B., Roberts, M. F., Stolwijk, J. A. J., and Nadel, E. R.: Forearm blood flow during body temperature transients produced by leg exercise. J. Appl. Physiol. *38*:58–63, 1975.
10. Nadel, E. R., Pandolf, K. B., Roberts, M. F., and Stolwikj, J. A. J.: Mechanisms of thermal acclimation to exercise and heat. J. Appl. Physiol. *37*:515–520, 1974.
11. Greenleaf, J. E., and Castle, B. L.: Exercise temperature regulation in man during hypohydration and hyperhydration. J. Appl. Physiol. *30*:847–853, 1971.

9

ENDOCRINE SYSTEMS

RONALD L. TERJUNG, Ph.D.

In order to survive, humans must maintain the internal environment of the body within fairly narrow limits — a process called homeostasis. Adjustments must be made in response to conditions that cause perturbations. Inability to maintain this homeostasis can lead to impaired physiological function and even death. For example, the loss of insulin results in altered energy metabolism, taxed renal function, cardiovascular collapse, and ultimately coma and death. Although certain voluntary actions can be important in this process, a myriad of "unconscious" adjustments occur continuously within the body to help maintain homeostasis. These responses can be as immediate as the cardiovascular responses necessary to combat the effects of gravity when getting up in the morning, or as gradual as metabolic adaptations established through the induction of a slowly synthesized enzyme. Early studies of these homeostatic processes identified two important control systems, the autonomic nervous system and the endocrine system.

The classical definition of a hormone required that it be produced by a specialized tissue and transported in the blood to a distant site where its effect could be manifest. Thus, removal of an endocrine tissue and subsequent replacement of the extracted compound was the classical evidence of a hormonal effect. More recently, however, the definition of a hormone has been viewed more liberally owing to the identification of systems that do not precisely fulfill the requirement of being produced by specialized cells, that are not transported in the systemic circulation, or that are not moved a great distance to produce their effect. Indeed, $3',5'$ adenosine monophosphate (cyclic AMP) has been referred to as an intracellular "hormone," since it has been found to mediate many hormonal effects in target cells. In addition, the presumed distinction between the nervous system and the endocrine system has not been borne out. The pituitary, which once was considered to be the master endocrine gland, is now known to be controlled by the adjacent portion of the brain, the hypothalamus. A further complication is that biologically active compounds may have multiple roles. For example, some compounds that are neurotransmitters (e.g., norepinephrine) may also exert a biological effect at some distant target tissue after transport through the blood. This more encompassing view of endocrine function has led to greater recognition of the important role that hormones have in maintaining homeostasis.

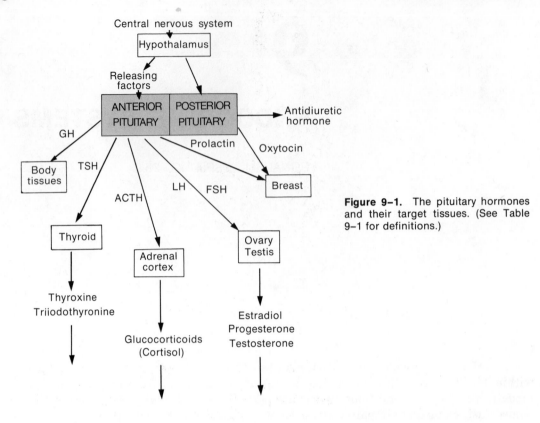

Figure 9–1. The pituitary hormones and their target tissues. (See Table 9–1 for definitions.)

ENDOCRINE ORGANIZATION AND HORMONE FUNCTION

Many of the endocrine systems have a common link through the pituitary gland (Fig. 9–1). As pointed out, the release of these hormones is a function of the hypothalamic influence. Most of the pituitary hormones act specifically on other endocrine glands as their target tissues, and these glands, in turn, release hormones that exert many of the functions to be described below. In addition, there are a multitude of other hormonal systems that function independently of the pituitary gland. As a general reference, a summary of many of the endocrine systems is given in Table 9–1. The reader is referred to a general textbook of endocrinology for a thorough discussion of these and other hormonal systems.

Hormone Control Systems

The ability of the endocrine systems to integrate physiological responses is indeed great. The process of normal growth and development is ample proof of this, when one considers the complexity of the human body with its assortment of highly specialized tissues. Such a level of integration requires that certain physiological responses occur in the appropriate tissue, at the right time, and in the correct magnitude. This may be the result of a single hormonal response or of synergistic actions of several hormones. This high level of organization suggests that fairly elaborate control systems must be operating. Indeed, it is generally found that either insufficient or excessive hormonal action leads to dysfunction. Thus, control processes must have sensitive checks to avoid significant deviations in either direction. This control is generally accomplished

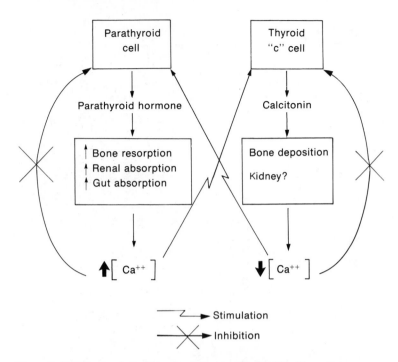

Figure 9–2. The control of blood calcium levels. (Modified from Tepperman, J.: *Metabolic and Endocrine Physiology,* 3rd ed. Chicago, Year Book Medical Publishers, 1973.)

through a negative feedback circuit in which the end result of a hormonal action exerts an influence to diminish the production of the hormone.

Figure 9–2 gives an excellent example of a simple feedback circuit for the control of plasma calcium levels. In this case, however, the control of plasma calcium is two-sided: one hormone (PTH — parathyroid hormone) acts to increase plasma calcium, while the other (calcitonin) acts to decrease it. This provides an exquisite control whereby a deviation (e.g., an increased plasma calcium level) is corrected by two actions: first, a withdrawal of PTH, whose action contributes to the deviation, and second but more importantly, the stimulation of calcitonin, which acts directly to diminish the deviation. The management of blood glucose levels also involves a similar control system. Other hormonal control systems are much more complex and involve multiple feedback sites.

Hormone Specificity

The extent of hormone action may range from the specific, with a target tissue responding uniquely to the hormone, to the encompassing, with a generalized effect accomplished in nearly all tissues. The hormone's action is specific because the target tissues contain a receptor that permits that tissue to "recognize" that particular hormone. The recognition of a receptor for its hormone is so specific that even slight modifications of the hormone molecule can result in complete loss of hormonal activity. This specificity is important, since the hormone circulates in the blood and is available to many other tissues. The encompassing type of hormonal response also depends on a specificity imparted by the cellular receptor. However, the receptor has such a widespread distribution that nearly all the cells in the body may respond. Thus, the

TABLE 9–1. A SUMMARY OF ENDOCRINE SYSTEMS AND THEIR FUNCTIONS

Hormone	Origin	Stimulating Factors	Target Tissue	Action
Oxytocin	Neurohypophysis (posterior pituitary)	Neural influence ?	Mammary gland	Milk production, feeding young
Antidiuretic hormone (ADH) (also called vasopressin)	Neurohypophysis (hypothalamus)	↓ Blood volume, hypertonic plasma	Kidney, vascular smooth muscle	Water retention, possibly vasoconstriction during hemorrhage
Growth hormone (GH)	Adenohypophysis (anterior pituitary)	Neural influence: generalized stress	All cells	Growth and development, free fatty acid release
Thyroid-stimulating hormone (TSH)	Adenohypophysis	Neural influence: ↓ blood thyroxine	Thyroid gland	Production and release of the thyroid hormones
Thyroxine (T_4) Triiodothyronine (T_3)	Thyroid	TSH	All tissues	↑ Basal metabolic rate, necessary for normal growth and development, lipid metabolism
Adrenocorticotropin (ACTH)	Adenohypophysis	Neural influence: generalized stress	Adrenal cortex	Production and release of the glucocorticoids (e.g., cortisol)
Glucocorticoids (cortisol)	Adrenal cortex	ACTH, generalized stress	Liver, all tissues	Promotes gluconeogenesis, muscle protein breakdown, anti-inflammatory
Mineralocorticoids (aldosterone)	Adrenal cortex	↓ Blood Na^+	Kidney	Na^+ retention
Luteinizing hormone (LH)	Adenohypophysis	Neural influence: stimulated by estrogen, inhibited by progesterone	Male: testis Female: ovary	Androgen production Estrogen production, follicular development
Follicle-stimulating hormone (FSH)	Adenohypophysis	Neural influence: ↓ estrogen stimulates ↑ estrogen inhibits	Male: testis Female: ovary	Spermatogenesis, follicular development

Hormone	Source	Stimulus	Target	Action
Estrogens (estradiol)	Ovary, placenta	LH	Uterus, mammary gland, others	Uterine development, secondary sex characteristics, Ca^{++} and Na^+ retention
Progesterone	Ovary, placenta	Dependent on LH, FSH	Uterus, mammary gland	Uterine development, mammary gland growth
Androgens (testosterone)	Testis	LH	Seminal vesicles, prostate, muscle, bone	Supports spermatogenesis, secondary sex characteristics, general anabolic function
Parathyroid hormone	Parathyroid	↓ Blood Ca^{++}	Bone, kidney	Increases blood Ca^{++} level, enhances Ca^{++} reabsorption
Calcitonin	Thyroid C-cells	↑ Blood Ca^{++}	Bone	Decreases blood Ca^{++} level
Insulin	Pancreas β-cells	↑ Blood glucose	All tissues	Decreases blood glucose, increases fat deposition, is protein anabolic
Glucagon	Pancreas α-cells	↓ Blood glucose ↑ Blood amino acids	Liver, other tissue	Increases blood glucose, is gluconeogenic, glycogenolytic, lipolytic
Epinephrine Norepinephrine	Adrenal medulla Sympathetic nerve endings	Sympathetic activation	All tissues	Increase blood glucose, free fatty acid mobilization, enhanced cardiac performance, vasomotor control
Erythropoietin	Kidney, other tissues ?	Hypoxia	Bone marrow	Promotes red blood cell production

CELL MEMBRANE

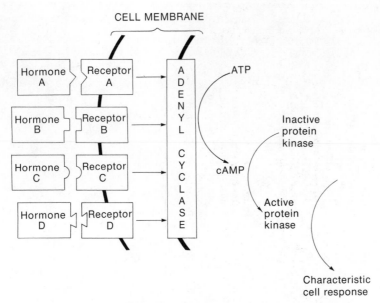

Figure 9–3. Schematic diagram of hormone-membrane receptor interactions that activate adenyl cyclase. (Modified from Tepperman, J.: *Metabolic and Endocrine Physiology,* 3rd ed. Chicago, Year Book Medical Publishers, 1973.)

function of cellular receptors is an integral part of the mechanism of hormone action.

Hormones initiate their actions on the cell through binding to the outside of the membrane alone or by entry into the cell, or both. The extracellular binding of a hormone can influence membrane permeability characteristics; this, in turn, alters the interaction between the cell and its environment. For example, the uptake of electrolytes, glucose, amino acids, and other compounds may be greatly accelerated. This action of a hormone can involve both a direct effect on the membrane itself as well as a secondary response that changes membrane components.

One consequence of many hormones binding to their extracellular receptors is the activation of the membrane-bound enzyme adenyl cyclase (Fig. 9–3). This enzyme functions to increase the production of cyclic AMP, which then catalyzes the production of another enzyme, protein kinase, to its active form. The active protein kinase, in turn, interacts with other cell processes to yield the characteristic action of the hormone.

Several hormones may cause a similar response. For example, fat cells break down triglycerides in response to epinephrine, norepinephrine, adrenocorticotropic hormone (ACTH), and glucagon. Thus, any hormone that increases cyclic AMP in fat cells stimulates lipolysis. The response of a cell to increased cyclic AMP is determined by its protein kinase system. For example, epinephrine increases cyclic AMP in liver, skeletal muscle, and fat cells. However, the response in liver and muscle is to increase glycogenolysis, whereas in the fat cell lipolysis is accelerated. Thus, a particular hormone action can involve both a specificity of the membrane receptor and a specificity within the cell to the hormone-receptor response.

As stated previously, some hormones also enter cells to exert their influence. Intracellular recognition of the hormone occurs through the binding to receptors. These receptors are specific to the target cells and function to translate the hormonal message into cellular action. For example, a hormone may bind to the intracellular receptor and be taken up by the nucleus, where it "turns on" protein synthesis through the production of RNA (ribonucleic acid).

ENDOCRINE RESPONSES TO EXERCISE*

Catecholamines

The release of the catecholamines epinephrine and norepinephrine occurs with the activation of the sympathetic nervous system. The greater the activation, the greater the increase in blood levels. Although norepinephrine functions primarily as a neurotransmitter, it becomes blood-borne and can influence other tissues. In contrast, epinephrine is released directly into the blood by the adrenal medulla, especially at higher degrees of sympathetic activation. This response brings about a multitude of physiological changes that are needed to accommodate a general acceleration of bodily functions. The end result is greatly enhanced cardiac performance (an increase in both heart rate and contractile strength), a shunting of blood to areas of prime need, increased glycogenolysis in liver and muscle, and the stimulation of adipose tissue lipolysis. These responses not only "turn on" the body to meet an increased energy expenditure but also promote the mobilization of substrates needed to support energy metabolism. Thus, sympathetic activation has become synonymous with the "fight or flight" phenomenon.

It is not surprising, therefore, that exercise brings about an increase in epinephrine and norepinephrine levels in the blood. This response is clearly dependent on the intensity of exercise (Fig. 9–4). The norepinephrine levels rise gradually as the work

*See Table 9–2.

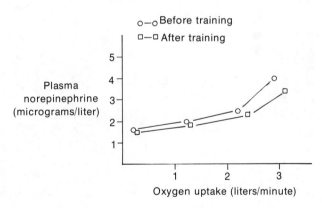

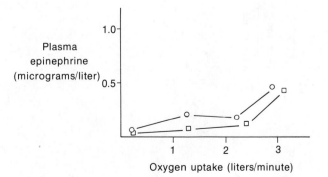

Figure 9–4. The influence of increasing workloads on plasma norepinephrine and epinephrine levels before and after training. (Modified from Hartley, H., Mason, J. W., Hogan, R. P., et al.: Multiple hormonal responses to graded exercise in relation to physical training. J. Appl. Physiol. 33:605, 1972.)

TABLE 9–2. A SUMMARY OF HORMONAL CHANGES DURING EXERCISE

Hormone	Exercise Response	Special Relationships	Probable Significance
Catecholamines	Increase	Greater increase with intense exercise, norepinephrine > epinephrine, increase less after training	Increased blood glucose
GH	Increases	Increases more in unfit person, declines faster in fit person	?
ACTH-cortisol	Increase	Greater increase with intense exercise; increase less after training with submaximal exercise	Increased gluconeogenesis in liver (kidney)
TSH-thyroxine	Increase	Increased thyroxine turnover with training but no toxic effects evident	?
LH	No change	–	–
Testosterone	Increases		?
Estradiol-progesterone	Increase	Increase during luteal phase of cycle	?
Insulin	Decreases	Decreases less after training	Decreased stimulus to utilize blood glucose
Glucagon	Increases	Increases less after training	Increased blood glucose via glycogenolysis and gluconeogenesis
Renin-angiotensin-aldosterone	Increase	Same increase after training in rats	Sodium retention to maintain plasma volume
ADH	Expected increase	–	Water retention to maintain plasma volume
PTH-calcitonin	?	–	Needed to establish proper bone development
Erythropoietin	?	–	Would be important to increase erythropoiesis
Prostaglandins	May increase	May increase in response to sustained isometric contractions—may need ischemic stress	May be local vasodilators

intensity increases and become disproportionately elevated at heavy workloads. In contrast, epinephrine increases little at light and moderate workloads but increases greatly during heavy exercise. The duration of exercise can also influence the blood catecholamine levels. Epinephrine levels increase beyond those expected for the work intensity as the exercise duration progresses to the point of exhaustion. This can probably be attributed to an apparent increase in the work effort associated with fatigue.

The importance of the sympathetic nervous system for normal exercise performance is well documented. The direct neural sympathetic influence on certain tissues is most important. Removing its influence, by a variety of means, results in diminished exercise performance. For example, the rapid adjustments of the cardiovascular system are lost, and mobilization of free fatty acids is impaired. Nonetheless, sympathetic-deficient animals survive well and even show many (but not all) of the typical adaptations to training.[2] The role of the circulating catecholamines during exercise, however, is less clear. It is possible that they influence energy substrate provision by enhancing lipolysis in the fat cells and glycogenolysis in the liver. The lipolytic effect on fat cells is probably secondary to the direct influence of sympathetic nerves. The glycogenolytic effect in the liver could be direct or through the release of glucagon, or both (see further on in this chapter). The role of catecholamines in increasing muscle glycogenolysis is probably of little importance, since muscle contains its own sensitive system to break down glycogen in response to muscle contraction.

Following training, there is a diminished sympathetic activation during exercise. This may not be surprising in view of the feeling of greater ease in performing a given work task after training. The reduced sympathetic discharge is easily seen in the lower heart rate found during exercise and is also evident in the blood catecholamine levels (Fig. 9–4). Both epinephrine and norepinephrine levels are less elevated after training. Thus, chronic physical activity brings about adjustments that render a person less "excitable" to work tasks.

Growth Hormone

Growth hormone is the only known anterior pituitary hormone that does not function through a specific target organ. Rather, growth hormone affects virtually all the cells of the body. This generalized effect is necessary for normal growth and development. Inadequate production of growth hormone in a juvenile leads to dwarfism, whereas hypersecretion results in giantism. The importance of growth hormone is well recognized, but it has been found to be most effective when acting in conjunction with the thyroid, adrenal, and gonadal hormones. This synergism is not uncommon among the endocrine systems. Among the many anabolic effects of growth hormone, increased bone growth and accelerated protein synthesis and muscle growth are probably the most notable.

These effects are most dramatic during the adolescent years and seem less necessary during adulthood. Nevertheless, growth hormone is secreted by the anterior pituitary throughout life. The exact function of growth hormone in the adult is not well understood. However, some of its effects play an important role in normal body function. For example, even though overt growth has ceased in the adult, cellular turnover always occurs, with the breakdown of cell components requiring a coincident replacement through protein synthesis. Thus, the need for protein synthesis is never lost. In addition, growth hormone exerts a direct influence on fat cells to increase triglyceride breakdown, thereby supplying the blood with free fatty acids. This increased free fatty acid level in the blood causes a shift to fatty acid oxidation in other cells, thus conserving blood glucose.

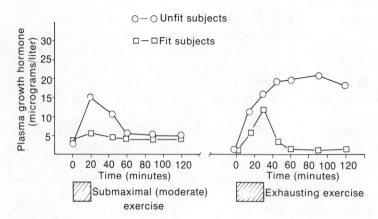

Figure 9–5. The influence of submaximal and exhausting exercise on plasma growth hormone levels in fit and unfit subjects. (Modified from Sutton, J. R., Young, J. D., Lazarus, L., et al.: The hormonal response to physical exercise. Aust. Ann. Med. *18*:85, 87, 1969.)

The influence of exercise on growth hormone levels in the plasma has been studied by many investigators. All studies show that the blood levels of growth hormone increase during physical activity. As might be expected, the increase is not instantaneous with the onset of exercise; nonetheless, it can be dramatic, reaching many times the resting value within 30 to 60 minutes (Fig. 9–5). This large increase in blood levels indicates that a release of growth hormone from the anterior pituitary has occurred, since a change in the removal rate from the blood could not account for such a large increase in such a short time. The growth hormone level in the blood seems to increase with the length of exercise up to about one hour; however, during prolonged mild running (five to seven hours) the blood levels decrease somewhat and become quite variable. The exercise response depends upon the fitness of the subject.[3, 4] A light to moderate workload causes a considerable increase in levels of plasma growth hormone in sedentary individuals, while little change is found in trained individuals (Fig. 9–5). Furthermore, exercise training results in a distinct lowering of the growth hormone response to heavier workloads. This lesser response in trained individuals should not be surprising, since the work task is more easily performed and less taxing. Thus, the adjustments necessary to accommodate the exercise should be less intense for the trained person.

Another factor that separates trained from untrained individuals is the growth hormone response after exhausting exercise. Although the growth hormone level in the blood is greatly elevated in both, the hormonal levels return quickly to normal in the trained individual, whereas they remain greatly elevated in the unfit person (Fig. 9–5). This reinforces the importance of growth hormone release by the anterior pituitary during exercise and suggests that chronic physical activity establishes a difference in the control processes of this hormone.

Although the response of growth hormone to exercise is similar to its response to a variety of other conditions that provide a generalized stress signal, the purpose of the altered growth hormone levels has not been established. It was originally thought that growth hormone might be important in mobilizing free fatty acids during exercise. The appearance of growth hormone during exercise, however, is too delayed to account for the increased free fatty acid release, and the enhanced lipolysis is in fact due to activation of the sympathetic nervous system.

Adrenocorticotropic Hormone and Cortisol

The pituitary adrenocorticotropic hormone (ACTH), whose release is controlled by the neural influence exerted by the hypothalamus, stimulates the release of the glucocorticoids from the adrenal cortex. The most important glucocorticoid, cortisol, exerts a general effect on metabolism. One important influence is the increased production of glucose from smaller carbon fragments, a process called gluconeogenesis. Thus, cortisol is antagonistic to the action of insulin (see further on). Cortisol not only directly accelerates the rate of hepatic gluconeogenesis but also increases the capacity of this pathway by inducing the synthesis of several key enzymes. To support this enhanced gluconeogenesis, cortisol stimulates the breakdown of protein to amino acids, especially in skeletal muscle, to provide the necessary substrates. This response is particularly important during starvation, when muscle is converted into necessary glucose.

Cortisol is secreted in significant quantities in a wide variety of situations. Its stimulation by such conditions as fright, pain, and physical trauma attests to the neural control of the hormone. Even the anxiety associated with taking an examination or the anticipation of a competitive athletic event can cause the blood levels of cortisol to increase. Moderate to heavy exercise invariably causes an increase in blood cortisol levels. However, since physical activity is often accompanied by anxiety, it is difficult to pinpoint the precise effect of exercise. Thus, it is not surprising that prior exercise experience can result in a diminished cortisol response to light to moderate workloads. Nonetheless, blood cortisol levels increase considerably with heavy to severe workloads, regardless of any prior exercise experience.

One aspect of cortisol's action may be physiologically important during exercise: its effect on gluconeogenesis could prove beneficial by enhancing glucose provision. This action would be most important during prolonged submaximal exercise, when a significant fraction of the glucose released from the liver is obtained from gluconeogenesis. This action to increase gluconeogenesis would support the effects of glucagon (see further on). It has been recognized for some time that glucocorticoid deficiency has a detrimental effect on exercise performance. Thus, a normal cortisol secretion is essential. However, the exact significance of the extra cortisol released during exercise is not known.

Insulin and Glucagon

The proper control of blood glucose levels, which is critically important for normal brain function, is established by the pancreatic hormones, insulin and glucagon. Glucose is supplied to the blood through intestinal absorption after meals and by release from the liver. The liver supplies glucose by breaking down its stored glucose (glycogen) by a process called glycogenolysis or through gluconeogenesis. The latter process is especially important during fasting or when dietary glucose is inadequate. Insulin, which is secreted by the β-cells of the pancreas, acts on all body tissues to increase glucose utilization, thereby decreasing blood glucose levels. It specifically acts to increase glucose transport into the cells (which otherwise occurs minimally), enhance glycogen deposition, and encourage fat deposition. As would be expected, insulin is released in response to elevated blood glucose levels, for example, after a meal. This action of insulin, however, represents only one side of the control process, since a diminution of insulin levels does not itself increase the release of glucose into the blood. This action is accomplished by glucagon.

Glucagon is secreted in response to low blood glucose levels by the α-cells of the pancreas. It acts on the liver to increase the provision of glucose through glycogenolysis and gluconeogenesis. Glucagon release occurs during fasting, when no glucose is ingested, or during enhanced glucose utilization, when an increased glucose supply is necessary. The catecholamines can also rapidly increase glucose provision from the liver during times of stress. In addition, the catecholamines can stimulate the release of glucagon. Apparently, the catecholamines aid in the immediate increase of glucose, while glucagon provides a long-term stimulus that includes gluconeogenesis.

Although the uptake and utilization of glucose by the body tissues depends upon the presence of insulin, muscle contraction has a specific effect of increasing the glucose uptake in the active muscles. Thus, it is not surprising that blood glucose utilization increases with physical activity. This is not to say that blood glucose represents the major energy substrate during exercise; the importance of fatty acid oxidation and, at higher workloads, of muscle glycogen has been well established (see Chapter 1). Nonetheless, exercise causes an increased glucose turnover that, in turn, requires a response to enhance glucose provision. This response must be sufficient to maintain near normal glucose levels so as not to impair brain function. In fact, prolonged submaximal exercise can tax the body's glucose stores sufficiently to result in dangerously low blood glucose levels (hypoglycemia). Indeed, hypoglycemia may be one factor that contributes to the severe fatigue of prolonged physical activity. The advisability of moderate glucose ingestion under such conditions is obvious.

Since blood glucose utilization is increased with physical activity, it is not surprising that a moderate decline in blood insulin levels occurs during exercise (Fig. 9-6). Thus, the hormonal stimulus for glucose uptake is abated to some degree. On the other hand, glucagon levels increase during exercise. This would provide a stimulus for both glycogenolysis and gluconeogenesis. The increase in glucagon is apparently rapid enough at the onset of exercise to stimulate glucose release adequately, since blood

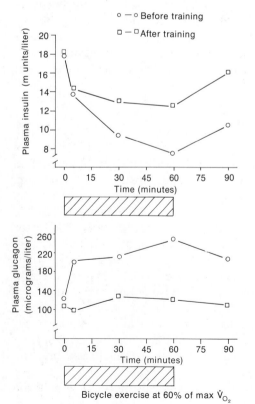

Figure 9-6. The influence of exercise on plasma insulin and glucagon levels before and after training. (Modified from Gyntelberg, F., Rennie, M. J., Hickson, R. C., and Holloszy, J. O.: Effect of training on the response of plasma glucagon to exercise. J. Appl. Physiol. 43:304, 1977.)

glucose levels show little decline in the first few minutes of exercise. In fact, an increase can be found. This process, however, is probably aided by sympathetic stimulation, which causes glycogenolysis.

Besides the continued action to increase glucose supply through glycogenolysis, glucagon initiates a process that has more prolonged effects. Since the amount of glycogen in the liver is finite, the supply of glucose from glycogenolysis is somewhat limited. Thus, the activation of a significant rate of gluconeogenesis is important to sustain an adequate glucose supply. Estimates of liver gluconeogenic function indicate that this pathway of glucose supply increases progressively during prolonged moderate exercise to account for approximately one half of the glucose released from the liver. This glucose is synthesized from lactic acid, pyruvic acid, glycerol, and amino acids extracted from the blood by the liver. The lactate, pyruvate, and some of the amino acids are released from the muscles, whereas the glycerol comes from the fat cells as a result of the triglyceride breakdown needed for fatty acid release. Thus, this gluconeogenic pathway represents a system in which the liver recycles other metabolites to glucose for the maintenance of blood glucose levels.

An interesting change in this exercise response occurs after physical training: the hormonal changes described above are greatly reduced in their magnitude (Fig. 9–6). The decline in insulin is not so great, whereas the increase in glucagon may be nearly absent.[5] Nevertheless, glucose levels are maintained at normal levels. Several other training responses are worth mentioning in this regard. As described previously, the increase in blood catecholamines during a work task is less after training. This may contribute significantly to the less intense insulin-glucagon response, since these sympathetic amines activate the release of glucagon and inhibit the release of insulin. In addition, it should be recalled that during submaximal exercise, trained individuals obtain a greater fraction of their energy output from fatty acid oxidation. This places a lesser demand on glucose reserves. Evidence from animal studies demonstrates that training significantly reduces the loss of liver glycogen during prolonged exercise. Thus, the altered exercise response of glucagon and insulin seems to be part of a coordinated training effect that increases work tolerance during prolonged moderate exercise.

Thyroid Function

The hormones of the thyroid gland, thyroxine and triiodothyronine, are critically important to normal cell function and metabolism. The actions of these two hormones are similar except that triiodothyronine is more potent and rapid-acting. These hormones have an overwhelming effect on all cells. Virtually no physiological process escapes their influence. Sufficient thyroid hormones are needed to permit normal growth and development, brain function, cardiovascular function, muscle function, energy metabolism, protein synthesis, and lipid metabolism, to mention just a few. Insufficient thyroxine (hypothyroidism) generally produces a dulling or suppression of these functions. Excessive thyroxine (hyperthyroidism) greatly accelerates many processes, is catabolic, and is progressively degenerative. The obvious need for a balanced thyroid hormone secretion is met by a fairly complicated feedback circuit involving the hypothalamus and thyroid-stimulating hormone (TSH), which is produced by the anterior pituitary.

The production of thyroxine is greatly increased in trained individuals.[6] The blood levels in athletes, however, are not chronically elevated, since an enhanced degradation of thyroxine occurs to match the greater amount produced. Thus, it is the turnover of thyroxine that is affected. It may be that the enhanced blood clearance of thyroxine represents the stimulus for the increased thyroxine turnover. However, the provision of thyroxine to the tissues seems to be increased during exercise.[7] This probably encourages thyroxine removal from the blood, especially by the liver.[8] The physiological significance of this greater thyroxine turnover is not well understood. It is clear, however, that even though this thyroxine secretion rate is similar to that found in many hyperthyroid patients, athletes show no clinical signs of hyperthyroidism. Even the basal metabolic rate, which is characteristically elevated with hypersecretion of thyroxine, is not altered by training.[9] Chronic physical activity, therefore, seems to influence thyroxine metabolism in a manner that is free from the toxic effects produced by an oversecretion of this hormone.

Androgens and Estrogens

The primary androgen, testosterone, is secreted by the Leydig's cells of the testes in response to luteinizing hormone (LH) from the anterior pituitary. The influence of testosterone is particularly apparent at puberty, when masculine development begins. Testosterone is generally anabolic, leading to bone thickening and development of muscle mass. In addition, testosterone is necessary for spermatogenesis and the onset of secondary sex characteristics. Loss of adequate androgenic influence results in sterility. Testosterone also promotes epiphyseal closure of the long bones, which prevents any further bone elongation.

Because of the anabolic actions of this hormone, considerable interest has been generated with regard to its possible influence on physical performance. Although little information is available concerning the influence of exercise on androgen function, it has been found that treadmill running or cycling does increase plasma testosterone levels.[10, 11] This reaction, however, appears to be dissociated from LH, since blood levels of this hormone do not change.[3, 11] No physiological significance has been established for this response. A matter of greater attention, however, is whether exogenous androgen treatment will enhance strength and muscle mass development. Although the results of many studies are equivocal, it appears that short-term androgen treatment can promote gains in lean body mass and strength when the subjects are on a high-protein diet and participate in an intense weight lifting program. The extent of benefit, however, is quite variable and is generally greatly overestimated by the participants involved. This is recognized by many researchers as the so-called "placebo" effect, which often results from the subjects' belief that they are benefiting by taking the hormone.

Clinical studies have shown that anabolic steroid administration can cause serious undesirable side effects. One major concern is the development of a type of liver damage that results in biliary obstruction and jaundice. Another complication is the possibility of depressed spermatogenesis and sterility, since gonadotropin (FSH and LH) and testosterone production by the body are suppressed. Although these clinical complications are dose-dependent, the quantity of anabolic steroids commonly used is not much below that needed to cause these toxic effects. Furthermore, long-term studies have not been carried out to show that sustained androgen treatment, even at minimal levels, is free from side effects. Thus, use of these steroids seems ill-advised.*

The hormonal interactions involved in the female reproductive cycle are exceedingly complex. As we have seen with other hormone systems that involve the pituitary gland, the central nervous system can exert an overriding influence by modulating the

---

*Effects of anabolic steroids on the female are discussed in Chapter 20. See also Appendix B, "The Use and Abuse of Anabolic-Androgenic Steroids in Sports."

hypothalamic releasing factors. Thus, it is not surprising that environmental factors and psychological stress can alter the cyclic nature of menstruation. The blood levels of estradiol, the most important estrogen, vary in a regular biphasic manner during the typical 28-day menstrual cycle. An initial sharp peak reaching eight times the level found at the beginning of the cycle occurs just prior to rupture of the ovarian follicle (ovulation). Ovulation culminates the first half (follicular phase) of the cycle, during which LH and follicle-stimulating hormone (FSH) have produced ovum maturation. In the second half (luteal phase) the circulating level of estradiol remains elevated by approximately fivefold. In addition, progesterone, which is another steroid hormone secreted by the ovary, increases steadily to very high values. Both estradiol and progesterone act to inhibit further FSH release from the pituitary; thus, follicular growth that leads to ovulation is delayed. Coincident with these events in the ovary, the uterus undergoes preparation, under the influence of estrogen and progesterone, to support implantation of an embryo. However, if fertilization does not occur, menses ensues and another cycle is initiated. Besides this important function in the menstrual cycle, estradiol produces the secondary sex characteristics at the onset of puberty. These include accelerated growth of the uterus, vagina, pelvis, and breasts, as well as the characteristic subcutaneous fat deposition.

The circulating levels of both estradiol and progesterone tend to rise with physical activity. Although the exercise response was hardly evident during the mid-follicular phase, there was a significant increase in the mid-luteal phase.[12] This increase is apparently related to the intensity of exercise. It is difficult to evaluate the significance of this response in the luteal phase, since at that time the blood levels of these hormones are normally so great that additional increases due to exercise may be ineffectual. Further research is needed to clarify the potential influence of physical activity on the female reproductive hormones.

Parathyroid Hormone and Calcitonin

The control of blood calcium levels represents another homeostatic process that is finely tuned. Again, changes in either direction produce dramatic abnormalities in bodily functions. Most notably, decreased plasma calcium levels lead to hyperexcitability of nerve and to tetany, whereas increased calcium results in cardiac arrhythmias. These effects are attributed to the complex interactions between calcium and nerve membranes. Control of the plasma calcium concentration is accomplished by the actions of two reciprocal hormone systems (Fig. 9-2). As we have seen, increased parathyroid hormone (PTH) secretion increases calcium levels, while increased calcitonin secretion decreases calcium levels. Release of these hormones is directly stimulated by changes in plasma calcium levels that are opposite to their respective actions. Thus, an increase in plasma calcium will stimulate the release of calcitonin and diminish the release of PTH. The converse is also true. This dual hormonal system establishes a highly sensitive control, since a deviation of plasma calcium levels in either direction brings about a positive action to correct the abnormality.

When bones are subjected to particular strain forces, an increase in bone deposition occurs. This process adjusts bone thickness and density to meet the support needs of the skeleton. An example of this is the greatly enlarged little finger of a laborer who had the misfortune of losing his other fingers years previously. In contrast, disuse of skeletal structures, especially those critical to antigravity support, results in bone resorption. Thus, prolonged bed rest leads to an enhanced calcium mobilization from bone and elevated urinary excretion. It would seem, therefore, that increased physical activity could play a major role in calcium metabolism. Evidence for this, however, is not convincing. For example, one study found that simply standing for three hours per day was effective in reversing the calcium mobilization caused by prolonged bed rest, whereas cycling in the supine position each day was not.[13] Thus, normal daily activity may be sufficient to maintain normal bone integrity. If this is correct, then moderate amounts of added physical activity would not greatly affect normal bone metabolism. Nevertheless, a powerful type of physical activity may have quite an important effect on the particular bones involved.

Electrolyte and Water Metabolism

The body must constantly respond to stresses that tend to alter the cardiovascular fluid volume. For example, body water is continuously lost through evaporation from the skin and lungs and through sweat and urine flow. The control systems involved must be particularly sensitive to decreases in fluid volume, since cardiovascular collapse could result. These control systems manage both plasma electrolytes and water. The most important electrolyte in this regard is sodium, since it is the major cation in the extracellular fluid. Ingestion of excessive sodium results in renal excretion, whereas sodium depletion results in retention of this ion by the kidney. This process is directly controlled by the hormone aldosterone, which is secreted by the adrenal cortex. Uncompensated loss of this hormone leads to sodium depletion and death. In view of its importance, the release of aldosterone involves a responsive control system that is sensitive to sodium content and fluid volume. This control is effected by special cells in the kidney (juxtaglomerular cells) that release a proteolytic enzyme called renin in response to a sodium loss, a blood volume decrease, or an activation of the sympathetic nervous system (Fig. 9–7). Renin, in turn, acts on a circulating plasma protein to form angiotensin I. This compound is readily converted to angiotensin II, which then causes the release of aldosterone. The other part of the fluid volume control system involves the management of water loss through the kidney. This is accomplished by means of a hormone aptly called antidiuretic hormone (ADH).* ADH is actually produced by brain cells in the hypothalamus but is released

*Diuretic: increasing the secretion of urine.

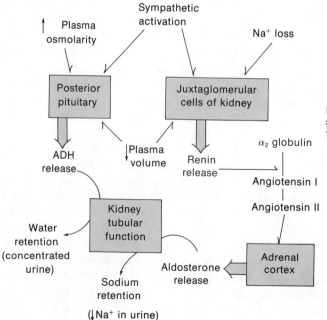

Figure 9–7. Hormonal changes associated with exercise that help maintain the circulating fluid volume.

from the posterior pituitary. This close neurological link explains the responsive release of ADH to neural sensing of decreases in fluid volume and increases in osmotic pressure. ADH is also released during a general discharge of the sympathetic nervous system. This hormone acts on the distal nephrons and collecting ducts of the kidney to enhance water reabsorption, which results in a concentrated urine.

Since the release of both renin and ADH is influenced by the sympathetic nervous system, the reader should have already anticipated the exercise response. The processes of both sodium retention and water retention are activated during exercise (Fig. 9–7). The increase in plasma osmotic pressure and decrease in plasma volume provide the stimulus. In the case of renin release, a direct involvement of the sympathetic system was demonstrated when prior treatment with a sympathetic antagonistic drug (propranolol) completely eliminated the increase typically induced by exercise.[14] An added stress to this system occurs during prolonged exercise, especially in the heat, when considerable amounts of sodium and, to a greater degree, water are lost in the sweat. Fluids and electrolytes need to be replaced during prolonged endurance events or during moderately sustained activity in the heat.

Erythropoietin

This hormone is produced in the kidney and increases red blood cell production (erythropoiesis) in bone marrow. The increased erythropoiesis that occurs with anemia or altitude exposure can be related to a greater secretion of erythropoietin. Thus, hypoxia seems to be one factor regulating red blood cell production. There is some evidence to indicate that exercise produces a slightly larger circulating red blood cell volume.[15] One might expect this to come about because of an increased bone marrow stimulation by erythropoietin. Although this is speculation, it can be noted that moderate to heavy exercise does decrease renal blood flow. This might provide a hypoxic situation that could promote erythropoietin release.

Prostaglandins

The prostaglandins are a class of biologically active compounds, the first of which was isolated from seminal fluid. They have since been identified in a wide variety of tissues, including the pancreas, kidney, brain, and muscle. In addition to their widespread distribution, the prostaglandins exhibit a great variety of biological effects. One action is a very profound vasodilation, which may be involved in the reactive hyperemia (increased blood flow) that follows intense muscle contraction.[16] This is suggested by the fact that a drug that blocks prostaglandin production also reduces the enhanced blood flow following sustained muscle contractions. This vasodilation response would be localized to the area where the hormone is released and would not spread to the systemic circulation, since the prostaglandins are readily inactivated while passing through the lungs. Thus, this supposed reaction would serve to increase blood flow where most needed — in the local muscle tissue.

SUMMARY

The endocrine systems provide important control processes that help maintain body homeostasis. These systems integrate cellular function to support the life of the person. Appropriate amounts of secretion of each hormonal system are established by fairly elaborate feedback controls, which diminish a hormone's secretion when it is excessive or increase it when insufficient. Since exercise causes such an extensive acceleration of bodily processes, many homeostatic mechanisms are stressed to their limit. It is not surprising, therefore, to find such a variety of endocrine responses during exercise (see Table 9–2). Although the importance of some of the hormonal changes is not well understood, it is clear that many hormonal responses help the body adjust to exercise and support the high rate of metabolism through substrate supply.

STUDY QUESTIONS

1. What is homeostasis and why is it important?

2. Why should hormonal changes be important during exercise?

3. What mechanisms account for the fact that there seems to be a strong neural influence on many endocrine systems?

4. Describe a simple negative feedback control process.

5. Explain the specificity of hormone actions.

6. Why is cyclic AMP so important?

7. What endocrine systems are involved in the "fight or flight" phenomenon?

8. What hormones alter blood glucose and how?

9. Why is gluconeogenesis important during prolonged moderate exercise?

10. Is free fatty acid release from fat cells important during exercise?

11. Why is water balance important in exercise?

12. What general influence does training seem to have on the hormonal responses to exercise?

FURTHER READINGS

Bloom, S. R., Johnson, R. H., Park, D. M., Rennie, M. J., and Sulaiman, W. R.: Differences in the metabolic and hormonal response to exercise between racing cyclists and untrained individuals. J. Physiol. 258:1–18, 1976.

Booth, F. W., and Gould, E. W.: Effects of training and disuse on connective tissue. Exercise Sports Sci. Rev. 3:83–112, 1975.

Felig, P., and Wahren, J.: Fuel homeostasis in exercise. N. Engl. J. Med. 293:1078–1984, 1975.

Gollnick, P. D., and Ianuzzo, C. D.: Acute and chronic adaptations to exercise in hormone deficient rats. Med. Sci. Sports 7:12–19, 1975.

Hartley, L. H.: Growth hormone and catecholamine response to exercise in relation to physical training. Med. Sci. Sports 7:34–36, 1975.

Lamb, D. R.: Androgens and exercise. Med. Sci. Sports 7:1–5, 1975.

Tepperman, J.: Metabolic and Endocrine Physiology. Chicago, Year Book Medical Publishers, 1973.

Terjung, R. L., and Winder, W. W.: Exercise and thyroid function. Med. Sci. Sports 7:20–26, 1975.

Tharp, G. D.: The role of glucocorticoids in exercise. Med. Sci. Sports 7:6–11, 1975.

Vranic, M., Kawamori, R., and Wrenshall, G. A.: The role of insulin and glucagon in regulating glucose turnover in dogs during exercise. Med. Sci. Sports 7:27–33, 1975.

REFERENCES

1. Hartley, L. H., Mason, J. W., Hogan, R. P., Jones, L. G., Kotchen, T. A., Mougey, E. H., Wherry, F. E., Pennington, L. L., and Ricketts, P. T.: Multiple hormonal responses to graded exercise in relation to physical training. J. Appl. Physiol. 33:602–606, 1972; Hartley, L. H., Mason, J. W., Hogan, R. P., Jones, L. G., Kotchen, T. A., Mougey, E. H., Wherry, F. E., Pennington, L. L., and Ricketts, P. T.: Multiple hormonal responses to prolonged exercise in relation to physical training. J. Appl. Physiol. 33:607–610, 1972.
2. Paynter, D. E., Tipton, C. M., and Tcheng, T. K.: Response of immunosympathectomized rats to training. J. Appl. Physiol.: Respir. Environ. Exercise Physiol. 42:935–940, 1977.
3. Sutton, J. R., Young, J. D., Lazarus, L., Hickie, J. B., and Maksvytis, J.: The hormonal response to physical exercise. Aust. Ann. Med. 18:84–90, 1969.
4. Rennie, M. J., and Johnson, R. H.: Alteration of metabolic and hormonal responses to exercise by physical training. Eur. J. Appl. Physiol. 33:215–226, 1974.
5. Gyntelberg, F., Rennie, M. J., Hickson, R. C., and Holloszy, J. O.: Effect of training on the response of plasma glucagon to exercise. J. Appl. Physiol.: Respir. Environ. Exercise Physiol. 43:302–305, 1977.
6. Irvine, C. H. G.: Effect of exercise on thyroxine degradation in athletes and non-athletes. J. Clin. Endocrinol. Metab. 39:313–320, 1967.
7. Terjung, R. L., and Tipton, C. M.: Plasma thyroxine and thyroid-stimulating hormone levels during submaximal exercise in humans. Am. J. Physiol. 220:1840–1845, 1971.
8. Winder, W. W., and Heninger, R. W.: Effect of exercise on tissue levels of thyroid hormones in the rat. Am. J. Physiol. 221:1139–1143, 1971.
9. Terjung, R. L., and Tipton, C. M.: Exercise training and resting oxygen consumption. Int. Z. Angew. Physiol. 28:269–272, 1970.
10. Sutton, J. R., Coleman, M. J., Casey, J., and Lazarus, L.: Androgen responses during physical exercise. Br. Med. J. 1:520–522, 1973.
11. Galbo, H., Hummer, L., Petersen, I. B., Christensen, N. J., and Bie, N.: Thyroid and testicular hormone responses to graded and prolonged exercise in man. Eur. J. Appl. Physiol. 36:101–106, 1977.
12. Hall, J. E., Younglai, E. V., Walker, C., Jones, N. L., and Sutton, J. R.: Ovarian hormonal responses to exercise. Med. Sci. Sports 7:65, 1975.
13. Rodahl, K., Birkhead, N. C., Blizzard, J. J., Issekutz, B., and Pruett, E. D. R.: Physiological changes during prolonged bed rest. In Blix, G. (ed.): Nutrition and Physical Activity. Stockholm, Almqvist and Wilksell, 1967, p. 107.
14. Leon, A. S., Pettinger, W. A., and Saviano, M. A.: Enhancement of serum renin activity by exercise in the rat. Med. Sci. Sports 5:40–43, 1973.
15. Scheuer, J., and Tipton, C. M.: Cardiovascular adaptations to physical training. Ann. Rev. Physiol. 39:221–252, 1977.
16. Morganroth, M. L., Young, E. W., and Sparks, H. V.: Prostaglandin and histaminergic mediation of prolonged vasodilation after exercise. Am. J. Physiol. 223:H27–H33, 1977.

10

PRINCIPLES OF INFECTION

THOMAS P. STOSSEL, M.D.*

A misconception of our antiseptic age is that health is freedom from germs. Quite the contrary, we are, as John Donne said, ". . .bits of excremental jelly," teeming with microorganisms. Although from birth on we are always *infested* with microbes, they usually do not make us ill, that is, *infect* us. This state of health reflects our capacity to maintain a truce with these creatures. The factors that determine this truce — the nature of the microorganisms, how they cause disease, and how we defend against them (Fig. 10–1) — are the subject of this chapter.

MICROORGANISMS AND THEIR MECHANISMS OF INFECTION

Viruses

Viruses are the smallest and most primitive bits of living matter, life being defined as the capacity to reproduce. The virus, too small to see with conventional optical microscopes, is a total parasite, insofar as it can reproduce only inside the cells of higher organisms. The virus is a tiny piece of the chemical matter called nucleic acid, which contains the genetic information that can reproduce and a bare minimum of other organic molecules needed to cover up the nucleic acid and permit the virus to perform its few activities. These activities include the capacity to attach to and enter a host cell and, in some cases, to "program" the host cell actually to devote its own synthetic mechanism to making more viruses from the virus's genetic material. This action may result in a number of possibilities. (1) The virus is produced in such massive quantities that the cell dies and literally bursts, widely dispersing virus. (2) A virus can be produced and bud from the cell with little or no detriment to the cell. (3) The virus is reproduced in small amounts or not at all and persists within the cell. In (1) and (2), the continuous generation of viruses makes it possible for ongoing infection of more and more cells to occur, unless the cycle is broken.

 *Supported by a grant from the Webster Foundation, Boston, Massachusetts.

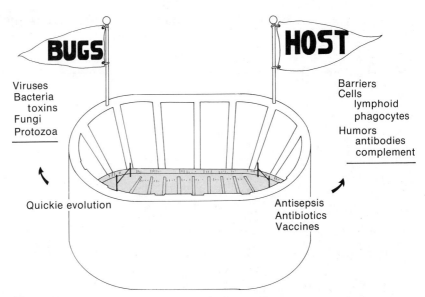

Figure 10–1. Overview of the "game of survival." Shown are the lineups in the battle between microorganisms (contemptuously called "bugs") and the human host. The invaders seek a pleasant place to live. As a backup, they can call on "quickie evolution" (rapid mutation) to confound the host. Host defenses repel or contain the invaders by a variety of means and can be aided by antisepsis, antibiotics, and vaccines.

Bacteria

Bacteria are much smaller than animal cells but are visible in the optical microscope after being stained with certain dyes. They usually have three principal shapes: balls (called cocci) occurring in clumps, doublets, or chains; rods (bacilli); or corkscrew-shaped objects (spirochetes). The balls do not actively move about, but the rods and spirals have hairlike projections (flagellae) with which they propel themselves. The bacteria are classified according to their appearance, staining reaction, ability to grow in different nutrients, and the products they make (for example, sulfurous gases that waft over polluted rivers or stagnant ponds). Unlike viruses, bacteria reproduce on their own. Bacteria reside in great quantities in the human—on skin, in the mouth, and in the large intestine (by the pound!). The vast bulk of bacteria in the world is not ever harmful to humans, and most of the bacteria that live in people become harmful only under unusual circumstances. A few are always potentially dangerous if they are encountered (Table 10–1).

Fungi, Protozoa, and Worms

Fungi (for example, molds and yeast) are like bacteria but differ in their life cycles and chemical composition. Most are never harmful (pathogenic) unless something is wrong with the host. Protozoa are primitive free-living cells like the amoebas that inhabit ponds, and many have complex life cycles involving multiple hosts. A few are pathogenic (Table 10—1). The parasite of malaria is the most common infecting agent in the world. Worms are multicellular organisms that can cause infection, the most familiar being pinworms, tapeworms, and hookworm. In the tropics and other warm places, worms can be a serious health problem. The schistosome, a parasite that infects the bladder, liver, and lungs, is a major public health problem in the Orient and Middle East.

TABLE 10–1. SOME MICROORGANISMS THAT CAUSE DISEASE

Microorganism	Disease	Transmission	Vaccination Available
Viruses			
Rhinovirus	Common cold	Airborne in droplets	No
Adenovirus	Influenza	Airborne in droplets	Yes
Enterovirus	Paralytic polio	Airborne, water	Yes
Herpesvirus	Chicken pox, cold sores, shingles	Airborne, venereal	No
Arbovirus	Yellow fever, dengue fever	Mosquitoes, flies	Yes
Bacteria			
Staphylococci	Boils; rarely pneumonia and other serious infections	Ubiquitous	No
Streptococci	Skin and throat infections	Ubiquitous	No
Salmonella (a bacillus)	Typhoid fever, dysentery	Water; contaminated eggs, meat	Yes
Pasteurella (a bacillus)	Bubonic plague	Lice on rodents	Yes
Treponema pallidum (a spirochete)	Syphilis	Venereal	No
Gonococcus	Gonorrhea	Venereal	No
Clostridium (a bacillus)	Tetanus	Ubiquitous	Yes
Fungi			
Histoplasma	Histoplasma pneumonia	Airborne spores	No
Trichophyton	Skin inflammation	Ubiquitous	No
Protozoa			
Malarial parasite	Malaria	Mosquito	No
Amoeba species	Amoebic dysentery	Water	No
Larger Organisms: *Worms*			
Tapeworm	Intestinal parasitism	Contaminated, uncooked food	No
Trichinella	Trichinosis (muscle inflammation)	Contaminated, uncooked pork	No
Hookworm	Anemia due to intestinal bleeding	Soil	No
Schistosoma	Schistosomiasis	Snails and water	No

THE BODY'S DEFENSE AGAINST MICROORGANISMS

The human body utilizes nonspecific and specific defenses. The nonspecific defenses are not directed against any particular microorganism and do not change in response to infection. In contrast, specific defenses are active against particular classes of microorganisms and amplify the response to infection.

Nonspecific Defenses

The nonspecific defenses are barriers, secretions, flow, filters, and phagocytes. Most of the microorganisms that infect humans live on the outer surface of the skin and on the inside lining of the mouth and large intestine (*mucosal surfaces*). The skin and mucosal surfaces constitute a physical barrier to the ingress of microorganisms and also have materials that keep these organisms from rapidly multiplying. The skin secretes waxy substances that inhibit growth of certain bacteria. The saliva, tears, and intestinal secretions contain substances that actively destroy various microorganisms. Acid produced by the normal stomach kills many swallowed microorganisms. Finally, the constant flow principle upon which the various tracts of the body operate (most of the gastrointestinal system and all of the urinary system) helps to flush out microorganisms. Therefore, the small intestine and the kidneys, bladder, and external urinary drainage system are usually sterile, that is, free of microorganisms. The large intestine becomes highly infested because of its "holding tank" function.

No defense is perfect, and microbes do gain access to the inner recesses and channels of the body. The principal fluid conduits of the body are the blood and lymphatic circulatory systems. The blood circulates through certain organs, mainly the spleen and liver, that serve, among other functions, as filters. The organization of these organs is such that blood flows through very fine passageways lined with voracious cells whose job it is to snare foreign matter, such as microorganisms. These cells have the capacity to bind and, like amoebas, actually engulf and kill the microbes. (Cells with such properties are called *phagocytes* — eating cells. There are a number of cell types that can act as phagocytes.) These particular phagocytes are large cells with single round nuclei and are called *macrophages* (large eaters). The macrophages must recognize microbes to eat them, and indeed can do this in many instances. However, certain organisms have surfaces that intrinsically resist recognition. In many cases of this sort, a series of proteins called *complement,* which are found in the blood serum (the fluid, as opposed to the cellular fraction of the blood), will coat microbes, making them recognizable to the phagocytes (Fig. 10–2). In other cases, described further on, an element of specific immunity is required for this coating to occur.

Macrophages also remove microbes from the lymphatic circulation. They are concentrated in filters called *lymph glands,* of which more will be said later on. The tonsils and adenoids are examples of these structures, which also exist in the armpits, groin, neck, and many other locations. The clearing function of macrophages presumably occurs constantly. It has been stated that every time we chew food, a multitude of microbes gains access to the circulation.

However, when microbes penetrate the barriers, they do not always enter the circulatory systems, but may take up residence in the local tissues. The body deals with these invaders by deploying an army of mobile phagocytes called *polymorphonu-*

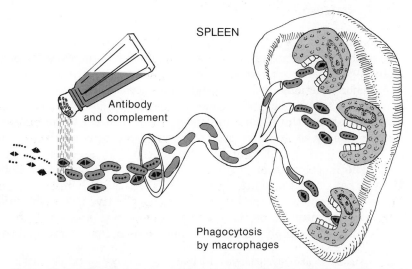

SPLEEN

Antibody and complement

Phagocytosis by macrophages

Figure 10–2. Normal defenses against infection. These include antibodies and complement, which react with microorganisms and either dissolve them or coat them to make them attractive to macrophages for phagocytosis in the filter organs (spleen, liver, lymph nodes). (Modified from Stossel, T. P.: How to manage the patient with recurrent infections. Medical Times *105*(9):30, 1977.)

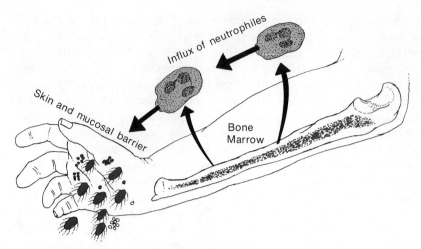

Figure 10–3. Leukocytes on guard. We are constantly infested with potentially pathogenic organisms. These organisms are normally kept at bay by mucosal and skin barriers and by a constant influx of wandering phagocytes – the polymorphonuclear leukocytes generated by bone marrow. (Modified from Stossel, T. P.: How to manage the patient with recurrent infections. Medical Times *105*(9):32, 1977.)

clear leukocytes (white blood cells with lobulated nuclei) (Fig. 10–3). Polymorphonuclear leukocytes, unlike the fixed macrophages, are in transit in the blood stream and have the capacity to sense the presence of microbes, principally bacteria and fungi. The signal heralding the invasion of microbes is, again, complement proteins, which become altered in the presence of microorganisms. These altered proteins diffuse from the site of tissue invasion into nearby blood vessels, where polymorphonuclear leukocytes subsequently stick, penetrate, and crawl actively toward the source of the inciting event. On arrival, these travelling phagocytes engulf and kill the invading organisms.

Specific Defenses

As indicated previously, recognition of microorganisms is a vital aspect of defense. One of the most remarkable elements of biology is the capacity of higher organisms, including humans, to make specific serum proteins called *antibodies*. Antibodies have four major functions: first, they bind to microorganisms and thereby promote their recognition by phagocytes; second, some antibodies interfere with the functions of microorganisms; third, some antibodies can also cause complement proteins to be altered rapidly so as to amplify the generation of recognition factors; fourth, antibodies react with and neutralize toxic products secreted by certain microorganisms. The mechanism of antibody production is incompletely understood, but it is known that a kind of white blood cell called the B-lymphocyte* makes antibodies. These cells circulate in the blood but are most active in lymph glands. In response to infection, the number of B-lymphocytes increases and antibody production ensues (explaining why lymph glands near infections become large and sometimes painful).

---

*The names B- and T-lymphocyte arise from experiments with animals that have identified the organs vital for the production of these cells during fetal development. Removal of an epithelial outgrowth, the bursa of Fabricius, from the fetal bird leaves the bird without cells able to make antibodies. Similarly, removal of the thymus gland (an organ in the chest) from fetal mice and humans prevents development of cells capable of producing immunity against viruses and tubercle bacilli. Hence the terms B- (from bursa) and T- (from thymus) lymphocytes.

Upon the first threat of infection, these cells take about a week to make significant amounts of antibody. After controlling infection, these cells are programmed to recall the inciting stimulus (or antigen) and can, on reencountering the microbes, very quickly produce antibody.

The specific defense against certain kinds of microbes, especially viruses and the bacteria that cause leprosy and tuberculosis, involves another kind of lymphocyte called the T-lymphocyte.* This defense is complicated by the fact that these parasites live inside as well as outside host cells. Therefore, eradication of infection may require that host cells bearing the pathogens be destroyed, as well as the pathogens themselves. T-lymphocytes have the capacity to do this by methods that are not clearly known. After exposure to microbes, memory T-cells that can quickly respond to another call also arise.

HOW INFECTION CAUSES DISEASE

The most straightforward mechanism for disease and infection occurs when tissues serve as nutrients for microbes that actually eat the host alive. This happens rarely. One example is a form of tularemia, a bacterial infection carried by rodents (the disease has been called "rabbit fever") in which the organism is inhaled and destroys lung tissue.

A much more common mechanism for disease occurs when the illness results from a combination of the presence of the microorganism and the body's reaction to it (or *inflammation*). When staphylococci (a common staph infection) breaks the initial defense barriers, the nonspecific defense mechanism results in the collection of polymorphonuclear leukocytes around the microorganisms. The staph germs are very difficult for the polymorphonuclear leukocytes to kill, and a sort of stand-off ensues. The infection becomes walled off by a mass of live and degenerating polymorphonuclear leukocytes, and the decaying polymorphonuclear leukocytes are what constitutes pus. The infection, called a boil, carbuncle, or abscess, is tender, painful, and swollen.

In some instances, the consequences of infection are more far-reaching. When bacteria (various forms of cocci) invade the lungs, the pus may fill so much of the lung that respiration may be seriously impaired. Streptococcal infections of the skin or throat usually evoke only a local inflammation, but they can spread to the blood and lymphatic streams. If *clearance* is not highly effective, the microorganisms multiply rapidly and, by their very presence, play general havoc with the body's metabolic processes. The upheaval may be so chaotic that the heart ceases to function and death results. In some infections, the defensive reaction may persist long after the microorganisms are dead or dormant. Syphilis is an example in which the inflammatory reaction becomes inappropriately directed against host tissues—the heart, blood vessels, and brain — causing circulatory problems, dementia, and death. Occasionally, the immune response to streptococcal infection can damage the heart valves or kidneys. Therefore, inflammation engendered by the defense is a two-edged sword.

Some microorganisms cause little inflammation and do little damage to tissues locally, but secrete highly toxic materials. The bacteria of diphtheria produce a potent toxin that inhibits neurological functions. The tetanus bacillus makes another nerve toxin that causes severe muscle spasm (the origin of the term lockjaw).

---

*See footnote on facing page.

CONTROL OF INFECTIONS

Antisepsis

Complete freedom from microorganisms is not a normal requirement for health, but some microorganisms are intrinsically more troublesome (virulent) than others. Therefore, it is advisable to try to avoid or eradicate them.

The bacteria that cause tuberculosis, typhoid, typhus, and cholera almost always cause infection and disease of varying severity when exposure to them occurs. Although effective treatment is now available for tuberculosis, the incidence of the disease declined prior to availability of this treatment. This decline was the result of improvements in housing conditions and of surveillance to identify sufferers of the disease and isolate them, thereby rendering them unable to transmit the disease further. Improvements in plumbing and sewer technology have largely eradicated typhoid and cholera as public health problems in the Western world. Eradication of domestic rats that carry typhus and the species of mosquito that transmit yellow fever and malaria have eliminated these scourges from the continental United States. Hence, social forces and plumbing can be considered important aspects of antisepsis. However, one difficult problem that complicates such infection control is the *carrier* of pathogenic microorganism who is not ill. The immune systems of carriers and the infection have arrived at a stand-off whereby the pathogens (examples are the typhoid bacillus and a virus that carries hepatitis) are alive and excreted by the host but do not make him sick.

Simple antisepsis has a role in preventing the spread of less lethal but more common diseases. For example, hand-washing, screening of food handlers, and control of sewage disposal facilities can prevent the transmission of viral hepatitis, a debilitating liver infection prevalent in many societies, including our own.

Antisepsis is also important to prevent initiation or spread of infection by microorganisms that are usually of low virulence but that get out of control when defense barriers break down. This is why it is advisable to wash superficial wounds and abrasions with soap and water and to protect them initially with sterile dressings. In preparation for surgery, areas of skin to be cut are cleansed with a strong antibacterial substance (iodoform solution, for example). Instruments used in surgery are sterilized, and personnel in the operating room wear sterile gloves, masks, and gowns — all maneuvers designed to minimize the number of microorganisms that get into the surgical wound. These procedures help the body's own defenses, which can deal with a small number of microbes much more effectively than with a large number.

Vaccination

The ability of microorganisms to invade often exceeds the capacity of nonspecific defenses to hold them in check. Specific immune mechanisms are then usually required for the host to win. However, after a first encounter with microorganisms, at least seven days may be needed for an effective specific response, which may occasionally be too late. In the case of toxins like diphtheria toxin, even a small exposure may be lethal.

A strategy first applied by Jenner in the eighteenth century against smallpox, and amplified a century later by Pasteur for rabies and anthrax, is to expose the host to a *vaccine* of weakened or killed microorganisms that cannot cause disease but does generate an immune response — either antibodies or primed T-lymphocytes. One can also vaccinate with chemically inactivated toxins (called toxoids), which are harmless but elicit neutralizing antibodies. This process of active *immunization** has been highly successful in reducing the incidence of former scourges — diphtheria, whooping cough, tetanus, polio, and measles — in developed countries and has nearly eradicated smallpox from the earth.

Vaccination fails as a panacea for a number of reasons. First, even in well-developed countries, complacency and uneven health care policies result in failure to immunize universally. Sporadic infection therefore occurs and prevents the eradication of the microorganism. Second, it is not always possible to obtain microorganisms in the proper state for making an effective vaccine. Third, microorganisms have a powerful resource, the ability to undergo rapid mutations. The changes can involve surface properties that are those recognized by the immune system. Therefore, many microorganisms, especially viruses, change so rapidly (the "quickie evolution" indicated in Fig. 10–1) that no vaccine covers them all.

Antibiotics

The major advance in modern times against infection has been the discovery of drugs that selectively kill microorganisms or inhibit their growth without being overly toxic to humans. These drugs operate on the basis of subtle differences in metabolism between microorganisms and mammalian cells. Antibiotics are particularly valuable in controlling infection in the interval before specific immunity develops, especially in young children and debilitated persons, or when the infection is severe.

Unfortunately, antibiotics have their limitations. First, antibiotics are primarily effective against bacteria. There are some that work against protozoa and fungi, but in the latter case they are often not very potent. Antibiotics are virtually useless against viruses, although some experimental drugs may turn out to be helpful. Second, the mutability of bacteria ("quickie evolution") permits them to stay ahead of the drug chemist. The microorganism can develop resistance to antibiotics and, perversely, the very use of antibiotics speeds the development of such resistance. Third, the antibiotics are not totally free of toxicity to the host. Finally, antibiotics alone are usually incapable of controlling infection. The immune system of the host must be able to join the fray.

SOME SPECIFIC ASPECTS OF INFECTION PERTINENT TO ATHLETES

Stress and Fatigue

Pasteur showed that ducks partially immersed in cold water fared worse in response to inoculation of virulent bacteria than ducks not so treated. But little is known, aside from this historic experiment and from folklore, about the relationship between stress and susceptibility to infection. Certain hormones released during "stress" have the capacity to inhibit immune responses, but the practical consequences of these effects are not clear. There is no reason to believe that the stresses of athletic endeavor predispose at all to susceptibility to infection.

---

*Passive immunization is the administration of serum or white blood cells from an actively immunized animal or human to a patient suffering from or exposed to a serious infection to which he is known not to be immune. Passive immunization is inefficient and fraught with various complications.

The other issue is whether exercise will exacerbate preexisting infection. There is little reliable data on this point. Studies with military personnel fail to show that enforced rest or exercise makes much difference in the outcome of viral hepatitis. However, some viruses can (rarely) adversely affect the heart. It is sensible to avoid strenuous exercise when fever or significant infection of any kind is present.

Infections Associated with Athletics

Most infections in athletes are the usual viral and bacterial infections that plague young adults — the common cold, infectious mononucleosis (a viral infection of the white blood cells), and hepatitis. Bacterial infections arise from surface trauma, skin abrasions, burns, or incorporated foreign bodies that become infected. The role of cleansing has been discussed. Additional treatment, such as incision and drainage of abscesses, use of antibiotics, and reimmunization against tetanus, would depend on the nature of the injury, the status of the individual's immunizations, and the discretion of attending physicians. Superficial fungal infections can arise in warm, moist areas of the body, especially the groin and between the toes. These infections respond well to treatment of the surface with antibiotics.*

Some unusual infections associated with athletics have been encountered. A Swedish sport called orienteering involves a form of cross-country running in which the participants may receive cuts on their legs from thorns and brambles. Viral hepatitis was spread in epidemic fashion among such individuals who passed the infection from their blood to other individuals by using communal bath water.

SUMMARY

Microorganisms that can infect the body include viruses, bacteria, and fungi. The body's nonspecific defenses include barriers, secretions, flow, and filters (spleen, liver, lymph nodes) containing phagocytes. Certain white blood cells (polymorphonuclear leukocytes) travel into tissue to surround and kill invaders. Specific defenses include antibodies and T-lymphocytes. The body's defenses can be aided by the use of antiseptics, antibiotics, and vaccination.

STUDY QUESTIONS

1. Once a virus has infected a cell, what are the possible results?

2. List three diseases caused by bacteria.

3. Is the urinary system usually sterile? Is the gastrointestinal system, or any part of it, usually sterile?

4. How are microorganisms removed from the blood?

5. Why do lymph nodes in the groin sometimes become enlarged when the foot is infected?

6. What is the function of complement?

7. What is the composition of pus?

---

*See Chapter 16.

8. Give several functions of antibodies.

9. How can one decrease the number of microorganisms contaminating a superficial wound?

10. How does vaccination act to prevent a specific disease?

11. Against which type of microorganism are antibiotics generally effective? Against which microorganisms are they ineffective?

FURTHER READINGS

Dubos, R.: *Mirage of Health.* New York, Harper & Row, Publishers, 1971.
Thorn, G. B. (ed.): *Harrison's Principles of Internal Medicine.* New York, McGraw-Hill Book Co., 1977.
Zinsser, H.: *Rats, Lice, and History.* Published by Atlantic Monthly Press. Boston, Little, Brown & Co., 1935.

SPORTS INJURIES AND MEDICINE

Section 3 contains the core of sports medicine. The goals of this section are to teach the student how to recognize sports medical problems, when to send the athlete to a health professional, what limitations in activity to expect, and how to prevent problems whenever possible. Illustrations of the human skeleton appear in Appendix A.

11

INJURIES TO SOFT TISSUES

THOMAS B. QUIGLEY, M.D.

GENERAL CONSIDERATIONS

Any young man or woman participating in organized sports today under the auspices of a school, college, or university has certain rights. He or she is entitled to good coaching, good equipment, and good medical care. If these cannot be provided, an athletic program should not be attempted. Good medical care requires planning and organization, including arrangements for the prevention, diagnosis, and treatment of injuries that are inevitable.

Preparticipation Examination

The preparticipation physical examination is absolutely essential. A few individuals will be found for whom participation in any sport is impossible: for example, those with certain serious heart diseases or marginal renal function. However, most persons with disabilities can participate in appropriate sports and physical activities.

The loss of one of a set of paired organs was viewed as an absolute prohibition to participation in contact or collision sports by the American Medical Association Committee on the Medical Aspects of Sports more than 20 years ago. It was felt that no athletic activity was worth the risk of blindness, castration, or death. Every year since then, this rule has produced a small group of disappointed young men and women. In general, however, this rule has been felt to be wise, and there have been very few instances of litigation or proposals to shift the responsibility for participation from the institution or its doctor to the student or his parents. Interestingly, in these 20 years, to the author's knowledge, no instance of blindness, castration, or death has occurred when athletes with missing eyes, testes, or kidneys have been allowed to participate in contact or collision sports. The reason for this record probably is that most athletes and parents have accepted the rule concerning lost organs. Therefore, the chances for disaster must be very small indeed.

Other disabling disorders, such as epilepsy, diabetes, and musculoskeletal deformity, should be evaluated by appropriate consultants in special fields of medicine. Every athletic program should have such consultants. No team or school doctor can know everything. In all but the most remote communities, specialists in orthopedic surgery,

179

neurosurgery, ophthalmology, and other fields are reasonably available. Often they can be made members of the team, in a sense, by giving them free tickets to contests. A surprising number of doctors have participated in sports in their high school or college days and continue to be interested. Close association with a hospital and a well-functioning transportation system are essential for the high school, college, or university with any sort of athletic program.

Facilities

A warm, quiet room must be available so that the injured player can be examined immediately and carefully. In a large university program where literally thousands of athletes may be performing at one time, the room can be expanded to include facilities for minor surgery and x-rays. The importance of immediate x-rays in establishing definitive diagnoses of fracture, dislocation, and ligament rupture cannot be over-emphasized. Whenever the budget of the sponsoring organization permits, such x-ray facilities should be made available. It is of course assumed that the doctor on duty knows how to read the films and does not have to wait for the weekly visit of the radiologist for their interpretation.

Records of the preparticipation clinical examination and of subsequent injuries must be kept, whether the program is in a small high school or a major university.

INJURY, HEALING, AND TREATMENT

A contusion (bruise) is a crush injury of soft tissue that results from a direct blow that does not break skin or bone. Sprain, strain, and fracture are discussed in the following chapters. The progression of events that leads to healing is similar in many injuries. Bleeding occurs from capillaries, arteries, and veins broken open by the injury. A hematoma (collection of blood) is formed, the size of which is limited by the clotting mechanism of blood and the pressure of the intact soft tissues about the point of bleeding. Within hours, white blood cells — the scavengers of the body — begin to carry away the debris of damaged tissues. Within days, fibroblasts — the cells from which the basic supporting structures of the body are derived – appear and replace the injured tissues with scar.

Healing is an orderly and remarkable process. We still have very little knowledge of how it is initiated or what brings it to a halt. When these mysteries have been unravelled, an enormous step will have been made toward understanding many biological processes, including those of cancer.

The basic principle of treatment of contusions, sprains, and strains is to assist nature. The immediate application of *cold* in the form of an ice pack will constrict the blood vessels involved in the injury and minimize bleeding. *Compression* by appropriate bandaging also decreases bleeding and, in addition, helps to disseminate blood that has appeared at the site of injury and facilitate its absorption. *Elevation* of the affected part above the level of the heart diminishes bleeding and facilitates the return of venous blood, thus minimizing swelling. *Rest* is necessary until normal painless function has returned. This is achieved by the application of appropriate splints or, when injury is confined to a lower extremity, by the use of crutches or a cane. Rest is instinctive throughout the animal kingdom. A dog or horse, for example, will not bear weight on an injured extremity. However, humans at times do so. The result is always an increase in the trauma and the period of disability.

COMMON INJURIES NOT INVOLVING
THE MUSCULOSKELETAL SYSTEM

Skin

Injuries to the skin are different from injuries to any other soft tissue, since the skin is the body's armor against infection. When the armor is broken, bacteria can enter. Nature's repair mechanism involves not only the replacement of injured tissue, but also the defeat of bacterial invaders.

Blisters result from repetitive rubbing of the skin, as from poorly fitting shoes. A layer of skin is separated and raised by the exudation of clear, watery fluid from the blood and lymph. The skin below the blister is intact. When activity or equipment can be altered so that no further rubbing or pressure occurs, the blister should be left unbroken to act as an excellent sterile dressing, and the fluid may resorb. However, attempts to preserve this fluid-filled bubble until nature has replaced the lifted layer of skin with new skin are often futile in athletes. The blister frequently bursts. Treatment then consists of opening the blister along the edge with sterile scissors or scalpel after cleansing the skin gently with soap or detergent and painting it with an antiseptic solution. A protective substance such as tincture of benzoin can then be introduced into and all over the blister, immediately producing a tough, protective sheath. Appropriate measures can then be taken to protect this artificially toughened area of skin from further rubbing.

Abrasions occur when the skin is subjected to scraping, as in a fall on gravel. Bits of dirt can be driven into the skin. Treatment consists of cleansing with a gentle detergent or bland soap and, if necessary, with a soft brush to remove the embedded gravel and dirt. At times a magnifying glass and sterile instruments may be necessary. If all the dirt is not removed, the skin will become inflamed,* and disability may be prolonged considerably. After cleansing, the raw area can be dressed with sterile, no-stick gauze, with or without antibiotic ointment.

Lacerations are breaks in the continuity of the skin caused by direct blows from objects of varying degrees of sharpness or sometimes by stretching, as in a fall on the knee or elbow when the skin is literally pulled apart. The treatment of lacerations requires the direct supervision of a doctor of medicine. All lacerations should be carefully cleansed and irrigated. Irritating antiseptic solutions such as tincture of iodine should never be placed in them. Ragged lacerations must be made clean by excision of the dead tags of tissue hanging from their edges. Clean, fresh wounds are closed with sutures or, sometimes, with special strips of adhesive tape. Wounds that are more than a few hours old or that are contaminated significantly are not closed because of the high probability of wound infection.

All breaks in the skin in athletes raise the question of protection against *tetanus*. Tetanus spores live in the earth of playing fields. However, today almost every student in high school or college has had basic immunization against tetanus. A booster dose of tetanus toxoid may be needed to assure complete protection from this potentially fatal disease. Antibiotics are almost never necessary as a preventive measure in this age group.

Eye

It is truly remarkable how infrequently the eye is seriously injured in sports. The instinctive reflexes of closing of the lids and moving the head from a threatening blow,

---

*Inflammation is characterized by pain, swelling, redness, and warmth.

together with the protection afforded by the bony orbit, are very effective. The blow from a boxing glove or large ball can produce bleeding under the skin around the eye ("black eye"), but the eye itself is rarely injured. However, small objects such as golf balls and squash balls can produce very serious injuries, since they are smaller in diameter than the orbit.

Examination of the injured eye should be carried out with the patient lying on a table and the examiner at the patient's head with a good light and a magnifying glass at hand. The only injury to the eye that should be treated by anyone other than an ophthalmologist is the foreign body (speck of dirt) caught underneath a lid. The lid can be turned over a matchstick and the foreign body whisked away by the very gentle use of a cotton swab. All subjective disturbances of vision, obvious abrasions, contusions, or lacerations of the eye itself should be referred promptly to a specialist.

Ear

Bruises of the ear produce bleeding between the cartilage framework and the thin overlying skin. Left untreated, these hematomas do not dissipate as they do elsewhere in the body but remain as masses of unsightly scar, the familiar "cauliflower ear." Dissemination of the hematoma by pressure is made very difficult by the complex convolutions of the ear. Even if a resilient pad can be fitted, the pressure itself can be very uncomfortable. Treatment therefore is daily removal of blood with a sterile needle after careful preparation of the overlying skin. The amount of fluid that reaccumulates diminishes over the course of a week to 10 days, after which usually no more than slight residual thickening remains, rather than an ugly mass.

The complex and delicate structures of hearing and balance that constitute the inner ear are extremely well protected by nature and are almost never injured in sports. If dizziness or loss of hearing occurs, the injured player should be seen at once by a qualified expert.

Nose

The familiar "bloody nose" occurs most frequently from an injury to the septum (central dividing portion) of the nose. Often there is a fracture of the bones or cartilage plates, which give the nose its shape. Occasionally a tiny artery will burst when the systemic blood pressure rises during active sports. In either case, bleeding generally stops within a few minutes when an ice pack is placed on the nose of the injured player, who should be sitting up rather than lying down.

If bleeding continues for more than a few minutes, the point of injury must be determined and the bleeding controlled, either by a pressure pad in the nose or by the application of a cauterizing chemical. This requires a good light and a source of suction to clear the nostril of blood, as well as technical skills. These items are rarely found in field houses but are always present in hospital emergency rooms.

Fractures of the nasal bones can be obvious, with marked deformity, or subtle, with no deformity and only partial blocking of the flow of air through a nostril. If there is visible deformity or appreciable decrease in the exchange of air through a nostril, prompt examination and correction by a doctor with appropriate skills is indicated. If this is not done, permanent difficulty in the exchange of air may result from deformity and deviation of the septum between the two nostrils.

Mouth and Teeth

A blow against the cheeks or lips can produce laceration of their inner surfaces or of the tongue. Such lacerations can produce alarming bleeding for a few moments. Suturing is required only occasionally. Healing without perceptible scar is the rule.

Injury to the teeth, however, is a serious matter. Before the general use of protective devices in collision sports, more money was paid out by insurance companies for injuries to teeth in athletics than for any other single type of trauma. All loosened or otherwise injured teeth should be seen promptly by a dentist. A tooth that has been knocked out intact (including the root), should be rinsed with tap water and replaced immediately in its socket. The dentist who deals with this emergency may be able to reimplant the tooth.

When a piece of tooth is missing and if the injured player is coughing, an x-ray of the chest may well reveal the tooth fragment in a lung. Its removal by bronchoscopy is indicated to prevent the development of a localized infection.

Chest

The heart and lungs are well protected by the rib cage, and serious direct injury, even in collision sports, is very rare. However, bruising of the lung can occur, most often associated with fractures of rib, and coughing of blood can result. The diagnosis and subsequent resolution of pulmonary (lung) contusion can be seen in serial x-rays. There is no specific treatment other than rest. Permanent disability does not occur.

Pneumothorax is the escape of air into the space between a lung and the rib cage, with associated lung collapse. This can occur simply from strenuous exertion; a direct blow is not necessary. An air sac at the lung surface simply breaks through the overlying layer of pleura into the pleural space. The athlete feels varying degrees of shortness of breath and vague discomfort on the side of the pneumothorax. The diagnosis can be made with a stethoscope and is confirmed by x-rays. No specific

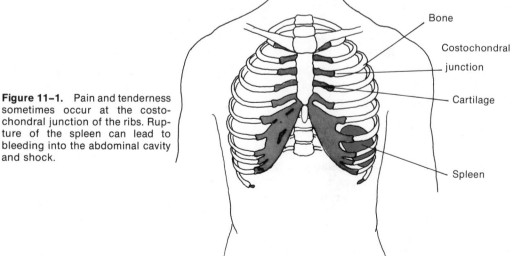

Figure 11–1. Pain and tenderness sometimes occur at the costochondral junction of the ribs. Rupture of the spleen can lead to bleeding into the abdominal cavity and shock.

Bone

Costochondral junction

Cartilage

Spleen

treatment, other than rest until the trapped air disappears, is indicated, unless the break in the lung surface acts like a valve and air builds up under pressure. This can completely collapse the lung and even displace the heart to the other side of the chest. Prompt release of pressure by the insertion of a needle or a tube into the affected side is necessary.

Occasionally, air will escape from the lung into the space between the heart and the sternum (breastbone). The result can be pain over the heart of a sort that raises the question of a myocardial infarction ("coronary"). The diagnosis is easily made by listening to the heartbeat with a stethoscope. With each beat, the trapped air produces a sloshing sound unlike any other sound made by the heart. The diagnosis can be confirmed by an appropriate lateral x-ray. No particular treatment is indicated.

In the age group of high school and college athletes, ribs are very resilient and fractures are unusual. However, the junction of the ribs with their cartilages on the front of the chest (costochondral junction, Fig. 11–1), is a common site of annoyingly uncomfortable injury. There is tenderness at this junction and occasionally a little swelling. No abnormality is seen on x-rays because the cartilage is transparent to x-rays. Treatment is simple protection by appropriate padding. Symptoms on exertion may persist for several weeks.

Abdomen

A blow to the upper abdomen can be very disabling for a few moments. In boxing this is known as a "solar plexus punch." In other sports the recipient is said to have his "wind knocked out." The recipient of the blow finds breathing difficult for 20 to 30 seconds but then recovers completely. What happens as a result of this injury is not known, but it is theorized that the diaphragm is temporarily paralyzed.

The organ within the abdomen that is injured most frequently from a direct blow is the spleen (Fig. 11–1). A spleen that is enlarged from mononucleosis is particularly susceptible to rupture. From the moment of injury, there is little doubt that the injured player has suffered serious trauma. There is pain in the left upper abdomen, and as blood escapes from the cracked spleen, it can irritate the adjacent diaphragm and produce pain in the shoulder referred through the phrenic nerve. As further bleeding occurs within the abdomen, the victim becomes pale, the pulse rate increases, and the blood pressure drops. (See also Chapter 15.) This is an immediate surgical emergency that can be evaluated and treated only in a hospital by a surgeon competent to remove the injured spleen if necessary.

Occasionally, after a blow to the abdomen, the area of the spleen remains sore for several days. The athlete should not return to sports until the soreness is gone because the damaged spleen may rupture up to three weeks after the original injury has occurred.

A hernia is a weak place in the abdominal wall through which intestine or other abdominal contents can extrude. The weakness in the abdominal wall is present at birth, and herniation can develop at a later time. Theoretically, a hernia might result from the stress of athletics or from blows on the abdomen that increase intra-abdominal pressure. However, such an occurrence is unusual.

Genitourinary System

The kidneys (Fig. 11–2) lie behind the abdominal cavity, in front of the powerful paravertebral and flank muscles. They are thus very well protected, but a direct blow

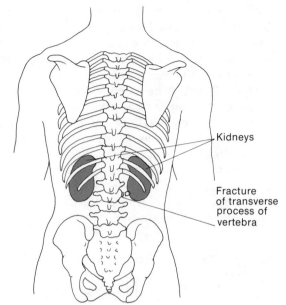

Figure 11–2. A blow to the flank can injure the kidney or fracture a transverse process of a vertebra.

Kidneys

Fracture of transverse process of vertebra

to the flank can produce serious injury. As in the case of injuries to the spleen, there is little doubt that the injured player is seriously hurt if the kidney is lacerated. Bleeding, as with the ruptured spleen, can increase the pulse rate, lower the blood pressure, and produce paleness and deep shock. The urine is usually bloody or blood-tinged. This injury, like spleen injury, must be evaluated promptly in a hospital.

Lesser injuries to the kidney produce pain and tenderness over the flank and are often associated with fracture of a transverse process of a vertebra (Fig. 11–2). Again, urine may be bloody, and it is very important that the injured player not be allowed to urinate without recovering a specimen of urine for examination. The bleeding may not be grossly visible in the urine but may be apparent on microscopic examination. Treatment will depend on the degree of injury and should be evaluated by a competent specialist. Certainly the player should not return to sports until healing is complete.

Rupture or other injury to the urinary bladder has never been known to occur in athletics. The reason is very simple. The last thing any athlete does before competing or practicing is to empty his bladder, and the empty bladder is almost impossible to injure.

Injuries to the scrotum and its contents are not to be taken lightly. A bruise of the testis can produce swelling that could interfere permanently with its function. Also, in some individuals the testes are free from their normal attachment to the scrotum and are subject to twisting from relatively minor trauma. This twisting cuts off the blood supply and causes pain and swelling. If not treated promptly, the testis will be destroyed. Any pain in, or swelling of, a testis following injury in sports should be carefully observed. If symptoms are not gone within an hour, the individual should be evaluated by a qualified surgeon.

SUMMARY

The preparticipation medical examination helps to identify potential problems. Persons with disabilities usually can participate in appropriate sports. Those who have lost one of a pair of organs should not take part in contact or collision sports.

Blisters should be left unopened if further trauma can be avoided. Otherwise, the blister can be opened widely near the base. Abrasions should be cleaned well and covered initially with a nonadherent dressing. Suturing of lacerations, when required, should be performed within a few hours of injury.

All eye problems, except for a speck of dirt in the eye, should be treated by an ophthalmologist. A hematoma of the ear may require removal of blood by needle for several days in order to prevent "cauliflower ear." Nosebleeds usually can be stopped by having the person sit upright with an ice pack on the nose. A nasal fracture may be present and will require treatment. All damaged teeth should be examined promptly by a dentist.

A blow to the abdomen may rupture the spleen, which results in bleeding into the abdomen and shock. Kidney injury can also produce shock and often is associated with blood in the urine. Injuries to the testis should be seen by a surgeon if symptoms are severe or persist longer than one hour.

STUDY QUESTIONS

1. Describe briefly the general process of healing following injury.

2. Give two possible treatments for a blister.

3. Why must abrasions be cleaned particularly thoroughly?

4. Why is a laceration not sutured after a delay of 12 hours?

5. Which eye injuries should be seen by an ophthalmologist?

6. How is "cauliflower ear" avoided once the initial injury has occurred?

7. What is the immediate treatment for a bloody nose?

8. What should be done when a whole tooth is knocked out?

9. What is the treatment for tenderness at the costochondral junction?

10. What symptoms are associated with serious spleen injury? What course of action should be taken if such symptoms are present?

11. Of what significance is visible blood in the urine?

12. What are two signs or symptoms of significant damage to a testis?

FURTHER READINGS

Dunphy, J. E., and Way, L. W.: *Current Surgical Diagnosis and Treatment.* Los Altos, Calif., Lange Medical Publishers, 1973, pp. 96–106.
O'Donoghue, D.: *Treatment of Injuries to Athletes.* Philadelphia, W. B. Saunders Company, 1976.
Thorndike, A.: *Athletic Injuries.* Philadelphia, Lea & Febiger, 1956.

12

AN INTRODUCTION TO ORTHOPEDICS*

JAMES G. GARRICK, M.D.

The injuries sustained by athletes are not much different from those suffered by people in other activities. A dislocated patella (kneecap), for example, involves injury to the same structures whether it is the result of a misstep on a balance beam or of slipping on a supermarket floor. The diagnosis and treatment of injuries, however, is somewhat different in a population made up of participants in sport or recreational activities. The athlete as a patient is usually in good physical condition at the time of the injury and highly motivated to return to his previous activity level. Indeed, he may be so highly motivated that he becomes his own worst enemy during recovery. Contrary to the belief often expressed by athletes and coaches, the athlete's muscles, tendons, and bones do not heal any more readily than those of nonathletes of the same age.

The vast majority of injuries to athletes involve the musculoskeletal system, that is, bones, joints, ligaments, and musculotendinous units. These injuries can be divided into two major categories: traumatic disruptions, such as sprains, strains, and fractures; and overuse syndromes, such as shin splints. Traumatic disruptions are seen more frequently in team sports, particularly in contact sports, whereas overuse syndromes occur more often in timed events that require specific repetitive motions.

Injuries to sport and recreational participants generally involve soft tissues. Fractures occur but are far less frequent than sprains and strains. Soft tissue injuries do not show up on standard x-rays. X-rays may be required to make sure that there is no bone injury, but a good history and physical examination is extremely important in making a diagnosis.

Sport and recreational injuries often present diagnostic problems because the circumstances under which they occur may be unfamiliar to the examiner. Indeed, a person who has pain in the Achilles tendon only after running 5 miles is not considered to have a serious impairment under most circumstances. However, if he is a marathon runner, this problem is as devastating as if he could not run at all. Thus, problems that might never surface in sedentary individuals may prove to be "impossible" diagnostic or treatment problems in high-performance athletes.

Generally, athletic injuries have another common characteristic: that is, if ignored, they often become more disabling. Unfortunately, the athlete frequently has to

---

*Orthopedics is the branch of surgery that is specially concerned with the preservation and restoration of the musculoskeletal system.

find this out for himself because a common response to an injury is denial. Attempting to continue in spite of symptoms, even though they are only slightly disabling, often results in the use of compensatory mechanisms that may alter gait or activity. Such changes may cause problems that are worse than the original injury.

INJURY DETERMINATION: SHOULD PARTICIPATION BE CONTINUED?

Whether an individual is responsible for a group of athletes, as their coach or trainer, or is simply responsible for himself, it is important to have guidelines regarding continuation of activity following injury. Obviously, a set of rules that cover every eventuality in sports would be encyclopedic. There are injuries that "don't follow the rules," — for example, severe injuries that do not hurt and minor injuries that are very painful. However, guidelines that allow appropriate decisions in the vast majority of cases have been established.

Once a sport or recreational participant has been injured, three questions must be answered appropriately before the individual returns to participation:

1. Exactly what happened? (What is the diagnosis?)
2. Will continued participation make the injury more severe?
3. Will continued participation increase the likelihood of another type of injury?

To answer these questions, one must have a fair amount of knowledge regarding not only the diagnosis of athletic injuries but also the demands placed on various structures by specific sport and recreational activities. The athlete may know about the demands but often cannot make a diagnosis; the opposite is frequently true of a physician. Thus, because of the knowledge gaps in both groups, this particular system of answering the preceding three questions lends itself to reasonably conservative management of athletic injuries. Stated another way, less knowledge regarding the diagnosis or the demands of the sport, or both, results in more conservative management of injuries, for example, longer periods of rest than may be necessary before returning to sports.

Deciding whether or not an injury has occurred is often a problem. The aches and pains that accompany athletic participation — particularly an unaccustomed level of participation — should not be considered athletic injuries. There should be some guidelines for deciding what is "expected" as a result of sport participation and what is an "injury." The following is a list of characteristics, any one of which usually indicates a true injury (Fig. 12–1). In most cases, the injured person should not return to participation until evaluated — usually by a physician — to determine whether further participation would be harmful. Evaluation sometimes can be completed at the sideline of a game.

Signs and Symptoms of Injury

1. Unconsciousness. A simple rule is that an individual who reacts inappropriately (or not at all) for more than ten seconds — the time required for someone to realize that a participant is down — is (or has been) unconscious. He or she should not return to participation until the preceding three questions can be answered appropriately. The assistance of a physician is usually required. (See also Chapter 15.)
2. The presence of any neurological abnormality such as "needles and pins" sensation, numbness, tingling, a sense of weakness, and so forth.
3. Obvious swelling. Although some injuries that are not severe can cause swelling (usually the result of bleeding), this is the exception rather than the rule. The presence of swelling following an injury usually indicates that it is reasonably severe.

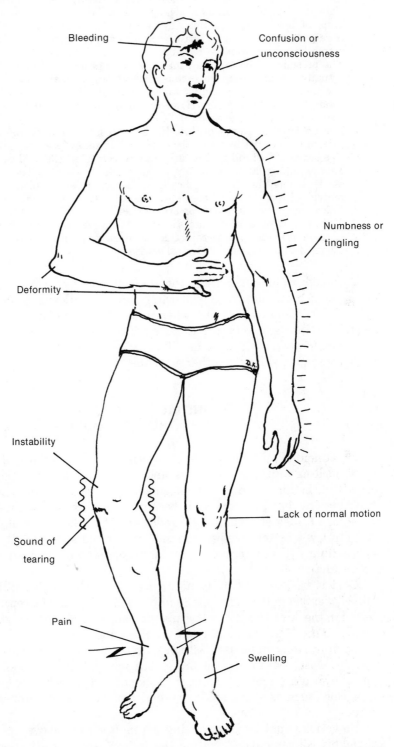

Figure 12–1. Signs and symptoms of injury. (A symptom, such as pain, is felt by the victim; a sign, such as swelling, can be observed by another person.)

4. Presence of pain through the normal range of motion. If there is any question about what the normal range of motion is, the opposite extremity can be used to find out, for example, "how far that elbow bends or straightens out" compared with the injured side.

5. Lack of normal motion (for any reason). The individual may be unable to extend (straighten out) the knee, wrist, shoulder, and so on, not because the part is "hurt" but rather because motion is "blocked."

6. The presence of bleeding. In many cases, injuries that bleed appear worse than they actually are, and when the area is cleansed only a small abrasion or laceration is found. Frequently, an injured individual can continue to participate after appropriate first aid treatment has been given. However, when bleeding occurs, the three questions listed previously must be answered.

7. The presence of any deformity. If, as the result of injury, one side of the body or one extremity does not look like the other side or other extremity, it should be evaluated.

8. The sense of instability. The athlete who comes off the field or court complaining of a knee or ankle that feels "wobbly" or "unstable" or one that "bends the wrong way" should not be ignored but, rather, should be thoroughly evaluated. More often than not, this individual has assessed his condition accurately even in the absence of pain.

9. The sound or sensation of something "tearing," "ripping," "going out of place," and so forth. Again, the athlete's assessment of these events is more often valid than that of the examiner. If the athlete says that something is out of place in his knee, it must be assumed to be so until proven otherwise.

Although rigid adherence to this decision model will result in some unnecessary forfeiture of participation, it will rarely, if ever, allow significant worsening of an injury. Thus, it places priorities where they should be placed. The athlete may not be able to recall the score of a particular match or game 15 years from the time of injury. He or she, however, will have no difficulty remembering the ignored injury that now precludes tennis, skiing, or other activities.

INITIAL MANAGEMENT
OF ATHLETIC INJURIES

Treatment of athletic injuries can involve as little as the application of a Band-Aid or as much as multiple operations and months of rehabilitation. Regardless of the severity of the injury, initial management (treatment) includes some simple common denominators that are important because they accomplish the following: (1) lessen discomfort, (2) lessen swelling, (3) reduce the likelihood of making the injury worse, and (4) allow a better examination to be performed subsequently because of less pain and swelling. *Cold, compression, rest,* and *elevation* are appropriate for virtually every fresh athletic injury.

Cold is best applied by using an ice bag or plastic bag filled with crushed ice applied over the injured area for 30 minutes. This should be repeated every four to six hours for the first two days. If a plastic bag is used, the ice should not be applied directly to the skin (e.g., put a wet towel around the ice bag).

Compression can be used with or without ice. While icing, the bag can be held in place by elastic wrap applied firmly but not tightly. Between icings, the wrap is applied over a compress. A donut or U-shaped compress should be used over any bony protrusions such as at the ankle in order to place pressure around, not on, these bony points.

Elevation usually means raising the injured area above the level of the heart (if reasonably convenient). Elevating the injured area usually results in resting it as well.

With acute injuries, one should *never* (1) apply heat, (2) wrap tightly enough to cause skin discoloration beyond the wrap or cause any numbness or tingling, or (3) attempt to "walk or run off the injury."

Once 36 to 48 hours have passed and the injury has stabilized (stopped swelling), treatment may take one of many forms. The fact that some authors advocate heat and others cold (after two days) may be confusing, but has nothing to do with the *initial* management, which *always* involves the use of cold.

FRACTURES

A fracture is a broken bone. Fractures are unique among injuries because they heal with the same kind of tissue (bone) that was originally injured, and thus the structure regains its preinjury strength. All other tissues heal by scar, which does not have the same characteristics as the uninjured material (muscle, tendon, ligament). Fractures can be described, somewhat confusingly, by their location (fractured femur); by the direction of the break (transverse); by the number of pieces (comminuted: more than two pieces); or by the mechanism of injury (avulsion: torn off). A fracture can even be named for the person who described it (Colles).

A fracture is generally associated with a deforming force (being kicked or stepped on), pain, the sound or sensation of something breaking or snapping, a grinding sound (crepitation) with continued motion, tenderness to the touch, deformity, or evidence of a fracture on x-ray, or any combination of these factors. Occasionally, the two pieces of bone lie in relatively normal positions (an undisplaced fracture) so that the break is difficult to see on x-ray.

Characteristics of bone change with growth and age. Generally, fractures heal more rapidly in children than in adults. Cancellous (spongy) bone generally heals faster than does cortical (more dense) bone. Fractures that are rigidly immobilized (in casts or sometimes by an operation) heal more quickly than fractures that continue to move (which may not heal at all). Fractures heal better and more quickly if the pieces are in contact than if another material such as muscle is interposed between them. Although any healing bone can remodel, that of the child has more remodelling capabilities. Thus, a fracture that appears to have been "set crooked" will "straighten out" with subsequent growth and present no problems. Although some disease states negatively influence fracture healing, athletic activity generally does not. Thus, athletes do not need extra calcium, increased amounts of milk, or protein supplements to aid healing.

The treatment of a fracture depends on the healing characteristics of the bone, the location of the fracture, the circumstances surrounding the injury, the forces involved, and other factors. Most of the common fractures in athletes are not complicated and can be dealt with in a straightforward manner. There are no hard and fast rules for the treatment of all fractures. It is important to realize that no matter what one does (proper diet, rehabilitation exercises, etc.) there are few, if any, fractures that will heal in less than four to six weeks. Some require three to four months.

The most common fractures in sports are those of the hand and fingers. Often these injuries can be splinted to allow continued participation without compromising the final result. However, it is important to make the diagnosis and reduce (set) the bone properly because a small degree of deformity can impair hand function for life. Fractures often involve the joints and, if ignored or improperly cared for, can result in loss of motion, instability, or acceleration of wear and tear causing subsequent arthritis.

Rib fractures are also reasonably common. They are generally treated symptomatically; that is, those activities that can be performed comfortably are allowed. The muscles surrounding the ribs splint the fracture. The ribs and clavicle (collarbone) are examples of bones that do not require rigid immobilization. They move with every breath, yet heal well. Sometimes the chest is strapped to decrease discomfort caused by motion.

The third most common type of fracture in sport and recreational activities is the avulsion fracture, occurring most often at the ankle. Such fractures are actually severe sprains and are discussed in the following section.

SPRAINS

Ligaments are bands of fibrous tissue that stabilize joints by attaching one bone to another. A sprain is an injury to one or more ligaments. Compared with muscle, ligaments have little elasticity. If a ligament is stretched beyond its elastic limit, it will remain longer permanently or may even rupture (break).

Ligamentous injuries (sprains) are among the most common injuries in sports. They happen most frequently in team sports, particularly contact sports, but can occur in almost any athletic activity. Sprains result when a joint is forced to move in a direction that is abnormal, that is, one for which it was not designed. This differs from a strain, which involves a muscle or its tendon and is usually the result of an unaccustomed amount of force. Most sprains occur to hinge joints, that is, joints that are designed to function in one plane. The knee and ankle, which function approximately as hinges are the most frequently sprained joints.

Often something in the environment causes or contributes to a sprain. For instance, this factor may be part of the individual's equipment, such as cleats that are too long and do not allow the foot to come free when struck or twisted or a long lever arm fastened to the foot as in skiing. The environment may also provide another individual to strike the region around the joint, such as occurs in the "clip" in football.

Sprains can be classified by degree of severity (Fig. 12–2). Grade 1 sprains (mild) involve a minimal amount of tearing of the ligament and no instability or abnormal motion of the joint. Grade 2 sprains (moderate) involve an appreciable amount of tearing and thus some instability of the joint. Anywhere from about 5 per cent to 99 per cent of the fibers of the ligament may be ruptured. A grade 3 sprain (severe) involves a complete rupture of the ligament, thus permitting an abnormal plane of motion in the joint. Such a sprain may allow dislocation of the joint (being "out of joint"). A grade 3 sprain can also involve an avulsion fracture, in which the ligament pulls loose a piece of bone rather than rupturing itself.

Diagnosis of the sprain depends partially upon the severity of the injury. The less severe sprains are usually less dramatic with regard to the presence of a "snapping" or "popping" noise, the sensation of something "letting loose," and the amount of pain present. Most injuries hurt as they occur, but often the less severe injuries (grade 2) may continue to be quite painful, while the more severe injuries, particularly those around the knee, may become painless in a few minutes. As long as any of the ligament remains intact, testing the stability of the ligament (attempting to stretch it) will usually cause pain, particularly during the first few days after injury. In the case of a complete tear of the ligament, this pain may be absent and the injured athlete may allow an examination that will reveal grossly abnormal motion without any evidence of discomfort. Bruising (discoloration of the skin) or rapid swelling in the region of a sprain usually indicates a severe injury. A good test of injury is palpation (pressing with fingers) because the torn place in the ligament is tender.

Treatment of the sprain depends not only on the degree of severity but also on the joint involved. Generally, the main goal of treatment is to protect the ligament until it has an opportunity to grow back together. It does not grow back together with more ligamentous tissue but rather heals with scar,which has different characteristics. In

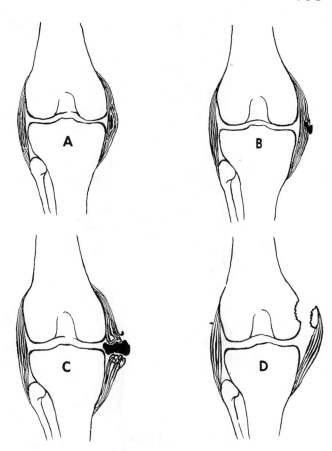

Figure 12–2. Knee joint, showing various types of sprain. *A,* Grade 1 (mild) sprain, in which only a few fibers of the ligament are separated. *B,* Grade 2 (moderate) sprain, in which greater tearing of the ligament occurs. *C,* Grade 3 (severe) sprain, in which the ligament is ruptured. *D,* Sprain-fracture. The ligament has torn loose a piece of bone rather than rupturing itself. (From O'Donoghue, D.: *Treatment of Injuries to Athletes.* Philadelphia, W. B. Saunders Company, 1976.)

some cases, it is desirable to repair the torn ligament surgically. The goal of surgical repair is not so much to make the structure stronger by introducing foreign material (stitches) but rather to bring the broken ends together so that a shorter distance has to be spanned by scar, which is a less than ideal material.

Protection of the injured ligament while it is healing is usually necessary. Often this protection can be provided by muscles that cross the same joint as the injured ligament. External means such as a cast or brace must be used if the individual is unable to provide the protection by his own musculature. Ligaments require a long period (up to six months) to heal to the point of regaining nearly normal strength. Obviously, most sprains are not protected until healing is complete. External means are used only until the healing ligament is moderately strong and the muscles can be rehabilitated to assist in protection. External protection is often necessary initially because the injury has resulted in some dysfunction of the structures that would normally protect that joint.

The three areas of the body most frequently sprained are the ankle; the knee; and the hand, wrist, and fingers.

Knee

The most frequently injured structure of the knee is the medial collateral ligament (Fig. 12–3). Such injuries occur most often in contact sports in which a blow is

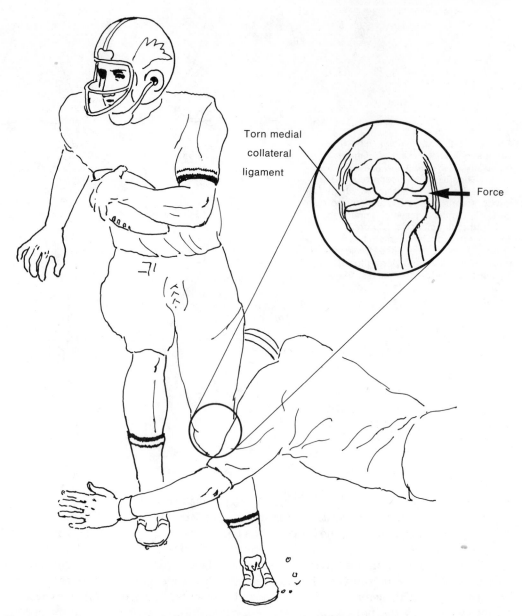

Figure 12–3. The medial collateral ligament is torn when a force on the outside of the knee causes the inside (medial) part of the knee joint to spread apart.

delivered to the outside of the knee by another participant, especially in football and wrestling, but also in basketball, soccer, rugby, lacrosse, and so on. The medial collateral ligament is also injured in skiing accidents during a twisting fall in which the binding fails to release.

In a medial collateral ligament injury it is of foremost importance to recognize the complete tear because it usually requires surgical repair in order to avoid a devastating problem. The injury may be painful for only a moment and then may result in a painless, unstable joint. The injured athlete often seeks aid not because the knee hurts but rather because it "bends the wrong way" or "feels wobbly." This description of the situation should never be ignored. Such individuals frequently do not have significant swelling but later may get bruising over the injury. Paradoxically, less severe knee sprains may be more painful than complete ruptures.

Ankle

The lateral (outside) ligaments of the ankle are most frequently injured, usually when the foot is bent inward. This commonly happens in basketball but also occurs in other running and jumping sports, particularly those practiced on an irregular surface. The individual frequently feels a crunching or tearing sensation as the foot rolls under. Swelling is often rapid and appreciable, but does not necessarily indicate the severity of the injury.

Initial treatment of the ankle may include the use of a plaster cast, taping, wrapping, or crutches, or any of these. Regardless of how the sprain is treated, the aim is to restore a normal gait, a normal range of motion, and at least normal strength of those muscles crossing the ankle. Complete rehabilitation is critical. The injured extremity (limb) will be "favored" until it becomes comfortable, and such favoring may result in other problems. It is the author's observation that far more people have long-term disability from a lack of normal flexibility and strength at the ankle than from instability.

Finger

With the exception of the thumb, most joints of the fingers are hinge joints. The collateral ligaments, on each side of the joint, are responsible for this function. When a hinge joint is bent perpendicular to its normal plane of function, the collateral ligaments are often injured. These injuries sometimes cause avulsions of small fragments of bone, which may break the joint surface. Thus, the badly sprained finger should be x-rayed in most cases so that fractures can be discovered and treated. The dislocated finger that is "put back" by the coach or trainer should be evaluated further for the stability of the surrounding ligaments because the loss of stability, particularly when it involves the pinch (use of thumb and index finger), can be disabling indeed.

STRAINS

A strain (pull) is a tearing injury of a muscle or its tendon. The musculotendinous unit — like a ligament — connects bone to bone but is elastic and can contract. Injuries to the musculotendinous unit are most common in timed sports (e.g., running, swimming). The injuries are generally dynamic; that is, they do not require outside intervention, as is often the case with sprain injuries, for which a hostile environment is partially responsible. Indeed, the individual usually causes the injury himself.

Any place in the musculotendinous complex can be injured: bone-tendon interface, tendon, tendon-muscle junction, or muscle. In the young athlete, the muscle and tendons are stronger than the bond between the tendon and bone, so the attachment to bone may fail under excessive tension. The older athlete, on the other hand, often injures tendons because they have become the weakest link.

As with ligament sprains, there are three degrees of strains. Grade 1 (mild) strains involve a minimal amount of tearing of fibers. They usually are not the result of a single muscle contraction and, in most cases, heal without disability. Mild strains require only protection such as wrapping so that failure to use the muscle properly during the healing phase does not cause further injury. Grade 2 (moderate) strains involve significant tearing, although some continuity remains. The musculotendinous unit is weakened, and continued use can make the injury worse. Individuals require not only symptomatic treatment but also reestablishment of strength and flexibility, both of which are lost during healing. Grade 3 (severe) strains involve a complete loss in continuity of the musculotendinous unit. They are often painless initially, usually occur with a single muscle contraction, and are frequently accompanied by dramatic sensation or sound. Indeed, the injured athlete often feels that he or she has been struck in the region of the injury by a racket or ball.

Bruising is a reasonably good indicator of the severity of a strain. More significant injuries are generally accompanied by greater dysfunction; the amount of pain, however, may not be commensurate with the degree of dysfunction. If the injury occurs within the tendon and is unaccompanied by much bleeding and soft tissue swelling, pain may not be a good indicator of severity. Some of these injuries are virtually painless.

The ultimate goal in treatment of musculotendinous injuries is the reestablishment of continuity of the muscle-tendon unit as well as the restoration of strength and flexibility. Because so much muscular dysfunction results from the injury, the muscle is often kept partially contracted (unstretched) and relatively immobilized until the pain disappears. The result is an atrophic (wasted) shortened muscle. There are two schools of thought on the treatment of musculotendinous injuries. One group feels that the muscle-tendon unit should be stretched actively throughout the entire healing phase so that it does not "heal shortened" and thus lead to an increased possibility of subsequent injuries. The other group feels that the muscle-tendon unit should first be allowed to heal (painful activity of any sort prohibited), then gradually stretched to its normal length, and finally restrengthened. Both groups have a number of proponents, and both claim better results. In the long run, it matters little what method is used to attain normal strength and flexibility as long as the results are successful.

Acute musculotendinous injuries in athletes occur most frequently in the hamstrings, quadriceps, and calf muscles (Fig. 12–4). Hamstring injuries, occurring most often in runners, frequently result from the runner's attempt to accelerate beyond his capabilities. They usually occur after the individual has started running and not with the first few steps. The more severe injuries cause instant disability, with the athlete often falling on the track. The less severe injuries may occur over a space of two or three steps or even an entire workout but result in pain and disability later on the day of injury or on the following morning. The same comments might be made for quadriceps injuries. A big difference is that defects of the portion of the quadriceps most frequently torn (the rectus femoris) do not seem to impair performance much. Defects in hamstrings, on the other hand, are more frequently associated with recurrent injuries and diminished performance ability.

In the serious athlete, hamstring or quadriceps injuries occur most often at the musculotendinous junction. In the younger athlete, before growth centers (epiphyses and apophyses) have closed, large amounts of bone may be pulled free with the tendon at the proximal tendon-bone junction. These complete (grade 3) strains usually put an end to that particular season of competition but, if properly managed, should not preclude subsequent competition.

Ruptures of the calf muscle mechanism can occur in young athletes (under 25 years) but the Achilles tendon itself (Fig. 12–4) rarely ruptures. When it does, the rupture usually follows a period of inflammation (tendinitis), as is often the case in the older athlete. The individual most likely to rupture the Achilles tendon is an athlete in his 30's or 40's who is involved in a running or jumping sport or in one that requires frequent starting, stopping, and changing direction. The individual often feels that he

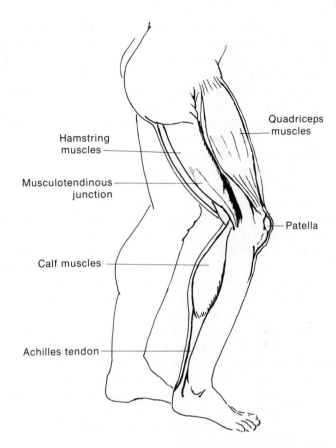

Figure 12–4. Muscles and tendons of thigh and leg.

has been struck in the lower calf by a ball or kicked by another player. Although burning may be present initially, pain is not usually a predominant factor, and disability may not be as extensive as might be imagined. Diagnosis, rather than treatment, is a major problem with injuries involving the Achilles tendon. Good results are reported with both surgical and nonsurgical treatment. However, most orthopedists would choose to operate on the injuries in the younger, more active, individual and reserve nonoperative treatment for those who are older.

DISLOCATIONS

A dislocation is the displacement of a bone at a joint (Fig. 12–5). In general, dislocations cause significant damage to surrounding ligaments, which are stretched

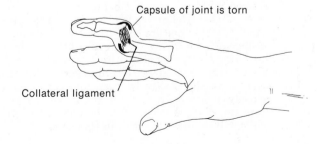

Figure 12–5. Dislocation of finger.

or broken when the joint is forced into an abnormal position. If a dislocation is only partial, it is usually referred to as a subluxation. Dislocations are named for the joint involved (dislocation of the shoulder) or for the two bones concerned (acromioclavicular dislocation).

In general, joints that normally have more restricted motion are more severely injured when dislocated. For example, the shoulder has very few restrictions in motion. Dislocations of the shoulder are common, but long-term complications, including damage to nerves or blood vessels, are not common. On the other hand, the knee is more restricted in its motion. When it is dislocated, significant injury to surrounding nerves and vessels is more likely.

The cause of a dislocation is usually an outside force. (Dislocations of the kneecap may be an exception to this rule.) As in joint injury, dislocation can result from too much force or from force in an abnormal direction. Once a dislocation has occurred, the joint may remain displaced. If the dislocation spontaneously reduces (goes back into place), it is difficult to be sure what happened unless the dislocation was documented by x-ray or other examination. Sometimes dislocations are accompanied by avulsion fractures similar to those seen with sprains. Such fractures indicate what occurred during the injury. The athlete is usually aware that something has been "out of place" and can often show the position of the extremity or joint when it was dislocated. He may even be able to tell how the dislocation was reduced.

A dislocation is treated initially by reduction. This is usually best left to a physician because further damage can occur if the reduction is not done properly. Treatment following reduction depends upon the joint involved. Dislocations of fingers are treated by immobilization in a position of function, and they rarely recur. On the other hand, dislocations of the shoulder, particularly in the young athlete, often recur. Dislocations of most major joints result in enough disability that the individual is often lost for the season.

OVERUSE SYNDROMES

Overuse syndromes are those conditions that result from overuse, or from inappropriate use, of some part of the body. There are two types of overuse. One merely involves excessive repetition of an activity, resulting in a bone cracking (stress fracture) or a tendon starting to fray or pull loose from its bony attachment. The second kind of overuse might better be termed improper use, for example, continued use following minor injury. In tennis elbow, a normal structure is overused and injured; in tendinitis of the Achilles tendon, an already injured structure is overused.

The following is a list of common overuse problems, most of which are discussed in subsequent chapters.

1. Jumper's knee: inflammation of the tendon(s) at the attachment to the patella (kneecap). This is usually the result of small tears in the tendon that have not healed properly. The condition is most common in basketball players and high jumpers but can occur in any running and jumping short.
2. Osgood-Schlatter disease (Chapter 19): a condition seen in growing children in which the fibers of the patellar tendon (the tendon between the kneecap and shin bone) pull off small bits of immature bone from the tibia (shin bone). The result is a painful, tender, swollen area just below the kneecap. Once the area becomes swollen, it is easily reinjured by falling on it or by other direct trauma, thus aggravating the problem.
3. Stress fracture (Chapter 13): minute cracks that can be found in nearly any bone that has been stressed repetitively in an unaccustomed manner. The bone becomes painful on activity and usually tender to the touch. This condition cannot be visualized on x-ray until two or three weeks after the injury. Ignoring the pain and continuing the activity can result in an overt break in the bone.

4. "Little League" elbow or shoulder (Chapter 19): pain in the elbow or shoulder resulting from too much throwing. The condition might be likened to Osgood-Schlatter disease or, in its more severe forms, may even result in destruction of the joint surface.

SUMMARY

A fracture is a broken bone. A sprain is an injury to a ligament. A strain is an injury to a muscle or tendon. Dislocation is the displacement of a bone at a joint. It is important to be able to recognize significant injury (Fig. 12–1). A player should not return to activity that would result in further damage. Immediate treatment for most athletic injuries includes ice, compression, rest, and elevation.

STUDY QUESTIONS

1. List several ways in which athletic injuries differ from injuries sustained under other circumstances.

2. What three questions must be answered before an injured athlete is allowed to return to participation?

3. What are the nine general criteria used in determining whether or not an athlete has been injured?

4. What initial treatment is appropriate for most athletic injuries?

5. Characterize the signs and symptoms usually accompanying a fracture.

6. What is a sprain? How are sprains classified, and why is the classification important?

7. What is a strain? How are strains classified?

FURTHER READINGS

O'Donoghue, D. H.: *Treatment of Injuries to Athletes*. Philadelphia, W. B. Saunders Company, 1976.

13

COMMON MUSCULOSKELETAL PROBLEMS

THOMAS B. QUIGLEY, M.D.

In this chapter, 30 injuries commonly associated with sports are described. The discussion of each includes mechanisms of injury, methods of diagnosis, choice of treatment, usual time of healing, and expected functional results.

The kinetic energy that results in these injuries is no greater than that of two running bodies in collision. Kinetic energy (E) is equal to one half the product of the mass (m) involved and the square of the velocity (v):

$$E = \tfrac{1}{2}mv^2$$

Kinetic energy is considerably higher in activities such as Alpine skiing and motorcycle racing; the injuries that result from these activities are more complex, severe, and difficult to treat. Such injuries are not included in this chapter.

As discussed in the two preceding chapters, four types of trauma are particularly common in sports: contusion, sprain, strain, and fracture. Often a combination of these injuries is present. The majority of athletic injuries occur between the ages of 15 and 25 years, on the playing fields of high schools and colleges. Fortunately, healing is rapid in this age range. Most tissue that is severely damaged is replaced by scar. In contrast, damaged bone is replaced by new bone.

SHOULDER

Acromioclavicular Joint Injury (Shoulder Separation)

The acromioclavicular joint (Fig. 13–1A) is the point of contact between the acromion of the scapula (shoulder blade) and the clavicle (collarbone). A ligament bridges this joint to stabilize it and is aided by another ligament, which runs from the coracoid process of the scapula to the clavicle. One or both of these ligaments is sprained in a "shoulder separation" (acromioclavicular joint injury).

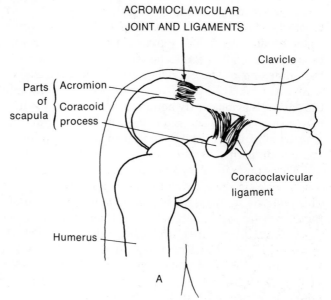

ACROMIOCLAVICULAR
JOINT AND LIGAMENTS

Clavicle

Parts
of
scapula

Acromion

Coracoid
process

Coracoclavicular
ligament

Humerus

A

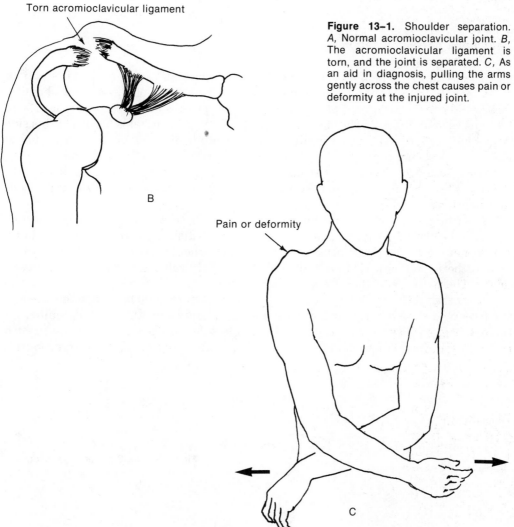

Torn acromioclavicular ligament

B

Figure 13–1. Shoulder separation. *A,* Normal acromioclavicular joint. *B,* The acromioclavicular ligament is torn, and the joint is separated. *C,* As an aid in diagnosis, pulling the arms gently across the chest causes pain or deformity at the injured joint.

Pain or deformity

C

Injury occurs when, in a fall, the shoulder strikes the ground while rotated forward — typically in a football player who is running with the ball held against his abdomen and chest. The player cannot break the fall by extending his arm. There is immediate pain and tenderness over the acromioclavicular joint, and in severe injury, the outer end of the clavicle may be elevated above the normal level (Fig. 13–1*B*). X-rays are essential to rule out fractures. A useful maneuver in examination is to pull the patient's arms gently across his chest (Fig. 13–1*C*). On the injured side, the clavicle may rise above the acromion. Like many other diagnostic maneuvers in evaluation of joint trauma, this is best done within minutes of injury, before spasm, edema, and pain make it difficult.

Three degrees of injury are possible. First-degree injury involves only the acromioclavicular ligament, and there is no deformity even on diagnostic manipulation. Third-degree injury amounts to complete rupture of both the acromioclavicular and the coracoclavicular ligaments, and deformity is marked.

Treatment for first and second-degree injury consists of protection and appropriate strapping. Players can often return to even heavy sports within a week. Complete rupture of acromioclavicular and coracoclavicular ligaments requires surgery within a few days of injury. Return to full activity with relatively little disability should be expected in three or four months.

Dislocation and Subluxation

When the arm is forced backward beyond normal limits of the position of throwing, the upper end of the humerus can be forced out of the shallow shoulder socket and can lie dislocated beneath the coracoid process of the scapula (Fig. 13–2). Diagnosis is not difficult. The shoulder hurts, and the patient holds his arm at his side to prevent movement. The normally rounded contour of the shoulder is lost and is reduced almost to a right angle by the abnormal prominence of the acromion. Except in very muscular individuals, the displacement of the humerus can usually be felt. X-rays are essential to rule out fracture, although it is unusual in high school and college athletes.

A doctor should make the final diagnosis, with careful evaluation of possible injury to the nerves of the arm, and should reduce the dislocation (put it back in place). The sooner this is done, the better. Most dislocated shoulders can be reduced without an anesthetic and with relatively little discomfort if evaluated within 20 minutes of injury. Thereafter, anesthesia may be necessary.

After the first dislocation in a young person, the arm should be held to the side and the forearm held against the thorax by a sling. Shoulder motion is thus limited for three weeks to allow the torn capsule of the joint to heal. There is little point in such postreduction immobilization after the second, or certainly after the third or fourth,

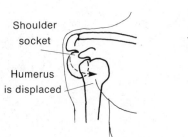
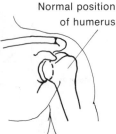

Shoulder socket

Humerus is displaced

Normal position of humerus

Figure 13–2. Dislocation of shoulder.

dislocation. Further dislocation with decreasing provocation is inevitable. Reconstructive surgery is indicated and is remarkably effective. Four to six months after operation, athletes can resume any sport with a chance of further dislocation of only 2 to 3 per cent and almost no limitation of motion in the joint.

Subluxation (momentary or incomplete dislocation) is treated in the same way, although the diagnosis can be more difficult because no displacement is seen. However, the condition can be suspected strongly from the athlete's history. Special x-ray studies, as well as real apprehension on the part of the patient when the upper extremity is moved backward to the throwing position, are important in confirming the diagnosis.

ELBOW

Hyperextension

When the elbow is forced beyond its normal full extension (straightening), its anterior capsule and ligaments, as well as the muscles that cross the front of the joint, can be sprained and strained. Diagnosis is not difficult. Gentle hyperextension produces pain at the front of the elbow, and tenderness is often present. There is no loss of function of the muscles of the forearm, wrist, or hand, nor is there any neurological deficit. X-rays show no bone abnormality. Primary treatment is the same as that for any soft tissue injury: cold, rest (in a sling), and gentle compression for a few days, followed by active motion and protection with a figure-of-eight bandage limiting the last few degrees of extension for a few weeks.

Dislocation

Extreme hyperextension can produce dislocation of the elbow (Fig. 13–3). The ulna is forced backward. Diagnosis is usually simple. The projecting end of the elbow (ulna) produces a gross deformity, and any motion causes pain. X-rays confirm the diagnosis and sometimes show a small fracture of the ulna. Fortunately, nearby arteries and nerves are not usually damaged, although other soft tissues are. Treatment, as in dislocation of the shoulder, is prompt reduction by a doctor. The sooner after injury this is done, the less often a general anesthetic will be necessary.

After reduction, the joint should be splinted for no more than a few days. Immobilization for six weeks, which was orthopedic dogma only a few years ago, all too often resulted in severe permanent limitation of motion. Early active motion should

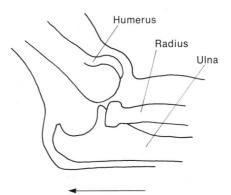

Figure 13–3. Dislocation of elbow.

result in restoration of full mobility in three to four weeks. After any severe elbow injury, a few degrees of extension are often permanently lost, but this is rarely disabling even for sports because the only human activity that requires a completely straight elbow is cleaning leaves out of a gutter spout.

A worrisome complication of elbow injuries such as dislocation is the transformation of injured muscle into bone. This is called *myositis ossificans traumatica* (see page 213). It also occurs in contusion of thigh muscles.

Tennis Elbow

Repetitive motion of the hand, wrist, and forearm, such as occurs in racket games, can produce annoying pain on the outside of the elbow that can be disabling enough to interfere with shaking hands or turning a doorknob (Fig. 13–4). This pain, as well as tenderness, occurs where the muscles that extend the wrist attach to the humerus. Thus, the backhand tennis stroke causes pain at this location. The elbow is otherwise normal, and x-rays almost never disclose any bone abnormality.

This condition has been studied by a number of orthopedic surgeons who are themselves good tennis players. Three stages of treatment have evolved:

1. A trial of pain-relieving medication (e.g., aspirin); rest in a sling for all but essential activities for a week to 10 days; and reevaluation of playing techniques. These simple measures will relieve at least one third of patients.
2. Injection into the painful area of a mixture of cortisone or related substance together with a local anesthetic. This usually produces immediate relief, but the pain unfortu-

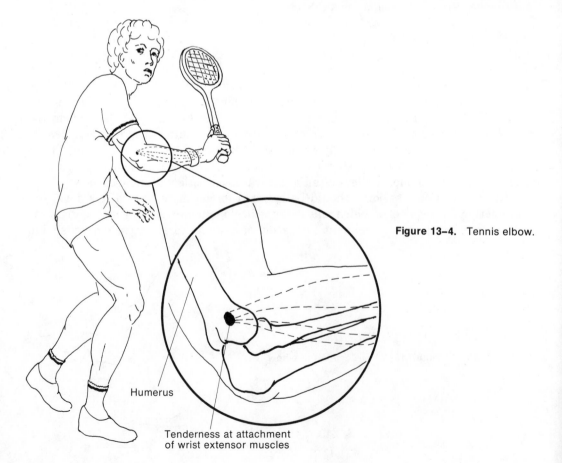

Figure 13–4. Tennis elbow.

Humerus

Tenderness at attachment
of wrist extensor muscles

nately can return within hours or days. Such an injection can be repeated at intervals of about two weeks on three occasions.

3. If symptoms and signs persist after the third injection, surgery can be considered. The essential part of all operations is release of the attachment of the extensor muscles on the humerus. Most patients are relieved following surgery and can return to tennis or whatever activity produced the injury.

WRIST

Fractures

The most important injury to the wrist in young athletes is fracture of the scaphoid (navicular) bone (Fig. 13–5). This boat-shaped bone lies on the thumb side of the joint and, in the years between 15 and 40, is the weak link when the hand and wrist are forced backward (hyperextended). There is pain at the extremes of motion of the wrist with tenderness at the base of the thumb.

Quite often x-rays, even multiple views, taken on the day of injury show no fracture line whatever. Herein lies a serious trap for the unwary. Sprain of the wrist is a diagnosis made only by exclusion. The young athlete who gives a characteristic history of injury by hyperextension and presents tenderness at the base of the thumb should have the wrist immobilized in a cast for at least two weeks, even if x-rays on the day of injury show no fracture line. Very often when this primary cast is removed and another set of x-rays is taken, the fracture line will be visible and the cast can be reapplied. This cast need not immobilize the entire thumb or interfere with writing, an activity of great importance to the usual young person with this fracture. It should be changed and further x-rays taken every four to six weeks. Unfortunately, this is one of the slowest fractures to heal, and immobilization for four to six months is often necessary.

If this pattern of evaluation is not followed and if no x-rays are taken, or if the x-rays taken on the day of injury are regarded as definitive in showing no fracture and the injury is dismissed as a sprain of the wrist, nonunion (lack of healing) and painful degeneration of the fractured scaphoid bone can occur. The treatment of such a

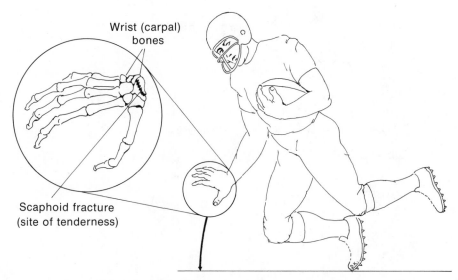

Wrist (carpal) bones

Scaphoid fracture (site of tenderness)

Figure 13–5. Fracture of scaphoid bone of wrist.

nonunion is by bone graft, which, if carefully done, usually achieves union of the fracture. Nonunion is completely avoidable, a fact that cannot be emphasized too strongly.

HAND

Fractures

When the fist is driven against an object such as another person's jaw, a good deal of energy can be transmitted directly along the shaft of the thumb metacarpal, and a fracture at its proximal end can occur (Fig. 13–6). This injury is known universally as Bennett's fracture after the surgeon who first described it. It is manifested by immediate pain, swelling, and tenderness at the proximal end of the thumb metacarpal, and its pattern is clearly visualized in x-rays. Stability is lost, and the powerful muscles of the thumb pull the entire metacarpal proximally, sometimes as much as a full centimeter. This fracture must be treated by surgery and fixation with small metal pins if serious disability is to be avoided. When this is done, a very good functional result is usually obtained, and return to sports is possible eight to 10 weeks after the operation. If the fracture is not diagnosed, eventual degenerative change and limitation of motion are inevitable and will require careful reconstructive surgery which relieves pain more reliably than it restores motion.

Helical (oblique) fractures of the mid-shaft of the middle and fourth metacarpals (Fig. 13–6) rarely become significantly displaced because of the presence of intact metacarpals on either side. The fracture fragments, however, do tend to override, producing shortening of the metacarpal and a deformity known as "dropped knuckle." Surgery is rarely required to restore length. Healing is usually complete in a matter of four to six weeks, and little more than splinting of the forearm, wrist, and palm for

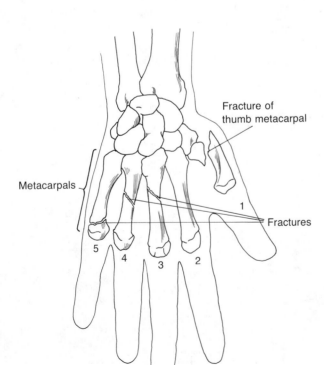

Figure 13–6. Common fractures of hand.

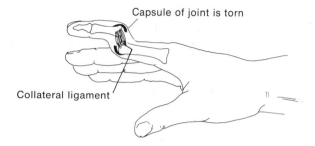

Figure 13–7. Dislocation of finger.

comfort is required. The "dropped knuckle" deformity is rarely disabling, even for playing a musical instrument.

The distal end of the fifth metacarpal can be the site of fracture in athletes (Fig. 13–6), causing angulation of the bone and inability to extend fully the fifth finger. If the angulation of the bone is less than 20°, the bone does not need to be straightened out. If the deformity is greater than 20°, it should be corrected by manipulation or surgery. In four to six weeks, function should be adequate for participation in sports.

Dislocations

Dislocations of the fingers (Fig. 13–7) are common in sports. It is almost instinctive for the player to seize the finger beyond the dislocation and pull it into normal alignment. However, the player still should see a doctor. X-rays are advisable to determine whether associated "chip" fractures are present. If full flexion and extension of the joint are possible, there is probably no soft tissue trapped within it. If the sides of the joint are stable, the collateral ligaments are probably intact. Simple splinting for a few days for comfort, such as taping the affected finger to an adjacent finger, is adequate treatment, and the player can resume almost any game immediately. If, however, full motion is not present or if the joint is unstable on lateral manipulation, prompt surgical correction is indicated.

A common ligament injury that often escapes recognition occurs particularly in skiers during a fall because of stress on the thumb from the loop of the ski pole. There is pain and swelling at the base of the thumb, and on manipulation there is instability between the thumb and its metacarpal. Prompt surgical repair of this collateral ligament rupture or avulsion is indicated. Even late reconstruction, weeks or months after injury, produces very good results.

Baseball (Mallet) Finger

When the hand is in position to catch a rapidly moving ball and a slight miscalculation occurs, the ball may strike the tip of the third or fourth finger, and the distal joint can be forced violently into flexion (Fig. 13–8). This can severely stretch or even

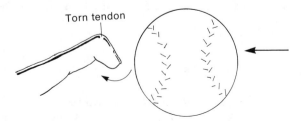

Figure 13–8. Baseball finger.

completely rupture the flat tendon that extends the distal joint. When the fingertip droops limply and no amount of muscular effort can make it straighten, the tendon is completely ruptured. The preferred treatment is surgical repair and immobilization by impaling the distal and middle phalanges (finger bones) on a pin across the joint until healing has occurred. X-rays at times show a chip of bone pulled off with the tendon, and unless this can be accurately reduced by manipulation, the same surgical treatment is indicated.

If the tendon is stretched and not ruptured and if the player can actively straighten his finger, the treatment is a specially molded cast with the distal joint in extension and the proximal joint of the finger in flexion.

Subungual Hematoma (Blood Under Nail)

A blow on the fingernail can occur in any number of sports and cause a rapid accumulation of blood beneath the nail. This produces purple discoloration visible through the nail and, at times, an extraordinary degree of pain. Blood is released by applying the end of a red-hot, partly straightened paper clip to the nail, preferably within the first 24 hours. This produces a small sterile hole through which blood immediately wells forth. The nail is then depressed for a couple of weeks with a band-aid. Very few surgical procedures produce as much relief from pain as this.

LOWER BACK

Most low back pain in athletes between the ages of 15 and 25 years is the result of either direct injury producing a fracture of a transverse process of a lumbar vertebra or inherent weakness due to a congenital defect known as spondylolisthesis.

Fracture of Transverse Process of Vertebra

Traverse processes are short ribs that extend outward from the vertebrae in the lumbar region below the rib cage (Fig. 13–9). They are encased in powerful muscle. When the flank (lower back and sides) is the site of a severe blow such as that from the helmet of a football player, or when the heavy back musculature is suddenly stressed, severe pain can occur. The muscles immediately become tight, and motion of the back is limited. There is usually marked tenderness just to the side of the spine, and x-rays will show fracture of one of the transverse processes.

Treatment consists simply of rest, occasionally in bed for a few days, followed by the wearing of a well-fitted corset with stiff steel braces. When properly protected, a few athletes can return to collision sports in 10 to 14 days. More often, recovery requires three to four weeks. Permanent disability does not occur from this injury.

Occasionally, the adjacent kidney is bruised. This produces blood in the urine, which may be obvious or which may not be apparent unless the urine is examined with a microscope. Such an examination should always be done when this fracture occurs.

Spondylolisthesis

The most frequently encountered developmental or congenital defect producing pain in the low back in young athletes is known as spondylolisthesis (a slipping

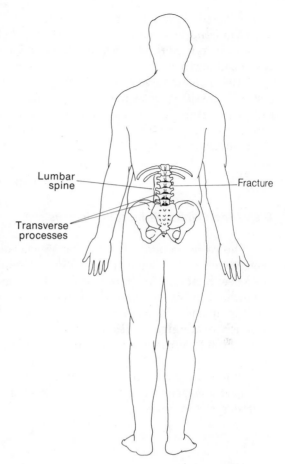

Figure 13–9. Fracture of transverse process of vertebra.

forward of the spine — Fig. 13–10). It results from a defect in the bony ring that holds a vertebra in place. The involved vertebra slips forward on the one beneath it. The reason for this abnormality is not clear. In some cases it appears to be inherited, since about 40 per cent of all Eskimos have it. It also may be the result of a fracture that failed to heal.

An interesting observation was made by a physician attending a large Midwestern university's football team. Football players of considerable ability and promise who had no previous back pain seemed to develop it during their sophomore year at about 18 years of age. X-rays disclosed the abnormality, and their careers in football were ended. A policy of taking x-rays on all athletes recruited from high schools was

Figure 13–10. Spondylolisthesis. The lowest vertebra has slipped forward, carrying with it the vertebral column.

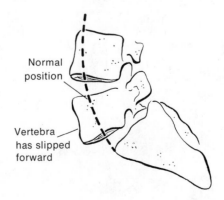

then adopted, whether or not the player complained of back pain. Those who showed spondylolisthesis were not offered athletic scholarships. They were followed at the other universities they chose to attend and, as predicted, in the sophomore year they developed low back pain.

Treatment involves the following: reducing the stress on the back; putting it at rest with a stiff corset when acutely painful; building up the musculature that holds the back upright (the paravertebral, abdominal, and gluteal muscles); and, when pain becomes truly disabling, operating and surgically uniting the involved vertebra with those adjacent to it by a bone graft.

HIP

Displaced Capital Femoral Epiphysis

The rather chubby 13-, 14-, or 15-year-old boy who is a little delayed in sexual development may have a limp due to pain apparently on the inner thigh above the knee. Examination, however, will show no abnormality at the knee but will reveal abnormal limitation of motion at the hip. X-rays disclose a displacement of the growth plate (epiphysis) of the femur near the hip joint (Fig. 13–11). This is potentially a very seriously disabling condition. If this displacement is neglected, poor alignment of the neck of the femur is inevitable, and painful degeneration of the hip joint is sure to follow.

When the condition is recognized, treatment is usually prompt surgery by an orthopedic surgeon skilled in growth problems. Such surgery often results in excellent function within a few years.

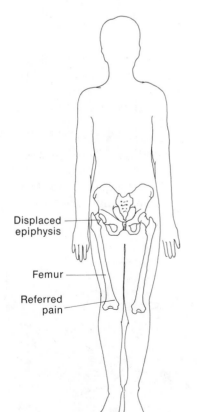

Displaced epiphysis

Femur

Referred pain

Figure 13–11. Displaced capital femoral epiphysis.

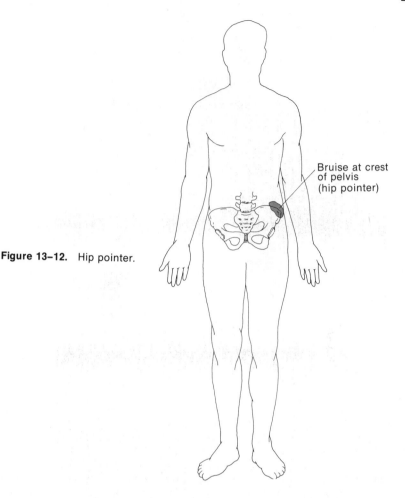

Bruise at crest
of pelvis
(hip pointer)

Figure 13–12. Hip pointer.

Hip Pointer (Bruise)

In all collision sports, appropriate energy-absorbing pads should be worn over the two sides of the pelvis. However, these pads can slip out of place or can be old and inadequate, and bruises of the upper edge of the pelvis (iliac crest) can occur (Fig. 13–12). The disability produced by these bruises is out of proportion to the degree of injury because the abdominal and lateral hip muscles attach at that site, and any motion of these muscles aggravates the pain. This injury is well known to trainers as a "hip pointer." Its treatment is the same as that for any contusion: cold, compression, and rest. In addition, since this is one of the few conditions in which pain is considerably out of proportion to the degree of actual tissue damage, the area is sometimes injected with cortisone or a related substance, diluted in a local anesthetic, to diminish the body's reaction to the injury and thereby reduce pain.

Groin Pull

The "groin pull" is common in all athletic activities involving running, particularly in those requiring sudden bursts of speed. Immediate groin pain is present as a result of strain, usually of the iliopsoas muscle (Fig. 13–13). This muscle arises at the back of the abdomen and inserts on the femur. Its function is to pull the leg forward

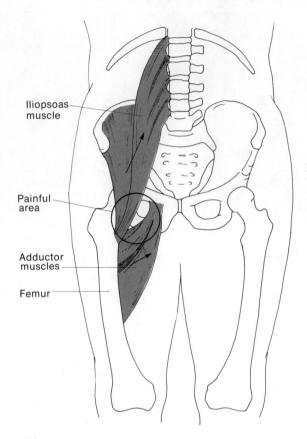

Figure 13–13. Groin pull (strain of ilio-psoas muscle).

and upward. For purposes of diagnosis, the pain can be reproduced if the patient lies on his back and lifts the leg directly upward with the knee straight and the leg externally rotated. Strain of the adductor muscles of the leg (Fig. 13–13) is also called a groin pull.

Treatment involves no more than restriction of activity that produces pain and protection on return to participation in sports. Return is usually possible within 10 to 14 days. There is not much point in applying cold or heat because the iliopsoas muscle is so deeply situated. Protection is achieved by a bandage wrapped around the pelvis and the thigh. If skillfully applied, the wrap limits motion to some extent but not enough to interfere with adequate function on the playing field.

If symptoms persist beyond 10 to 14 days, x-rays should be taken to rule out possible avulsion of the muscle's attachment to the femur. Treatment of avulsion is the same, but full function does not return for three or four months.

THIGH

The two most frequent injuries in the thigh in athletes involve the largest muscles in the body, the quadriceps and the hamstrings (Fig. 13–14).

Contusions of the Quadriceps

The quadriceps muscle is at the front of the thigh. Contusion of this muscle occurs primarily in collision sports and is the reason that thigh pads are worn. The anterior and

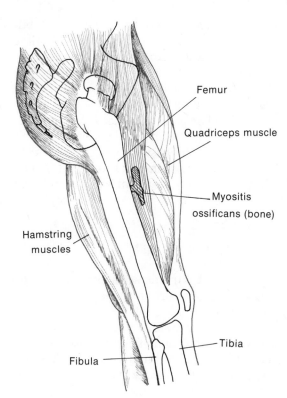

Figure 13–14. Thigh muscles. Myositis ossificans can develop from a muscle bruise.

Femur

Quadriceps muscle

Myositis ossificans (bone)

Hamstring muscles

Tibia

Fibula

lateral aspects of the quadriceps muscle are the most vulnerable to a direct blow. The bruised area is swollen, painful, and tender. Contusion results in a limp caused by swelling, accumulation of blood, and consequent loss of elasticity of the muscle. The limp produces what athletes have long called a "charley horse." The origin of this quaint term goes back to the Brooklyn Dodgers baseball team at the turn of the century. The mowing machines for the outfield were pulled by a horse that limped. When a player sustained a blow on the thigh that made him limp, the other players said, "You are walking like Charley the horse."

Treatment consists of simple measures to assist nature: rest, by use of crutches if necessary; cold applied intermittently for 24 to 48 hours, followed by heat, often in the form of a whirlpool bath; and a gradual increase in active motion. Massage aggravates the condition and can double the period of disability. Forcing motion beyond the limit of pain is equally inadvisable.

Myositis Ossificans. A small percentage of contusions of the quadriceps fail to resolve in the usual 10 to 14 days. Swelling persists, and limitation of motion of the knee, and sometimes hip, develops. A mass that can be felt gradually appears, and starting at about three weeks, x-rays will show the beginning of new bone formation within the muscle (Fig. 13–14). This is known as *myositis* (muscle inflammation) *ossificans* (bone formation) *traumatica* (from trauma). Slowly, over many weeks or even months, the new bone develops and matures like any other bone to form a cortex, a medulla, and a marrow, which can and does contribute to the elements of blood.

The origin of this process is a mystery. It seems to be associated with vigorous muscular activity in youth. However, it is common in the totally paralyzed muscles of paraplegics.

Treatment is the same as for the original contusion — primarily rest. The temptation to manipulate and to massage must be vigorously avoided because the result is simply prolongation of the period of disability. The new bone, in its final form some months after the original contusion, is almost never sufficiently disabling to require surgical removal. Any surgery carried out before the new bone is mature only aggravates the condition and delays final resolution.

This peculiar bone formation response to injury has important implications for research. A great advance would be made if a substance that changes the basic fibroblast of scar into the basic cell of bone, the osteoblast, could be isolated. If this substance could be injected or otherwise applied at the site of fractures, nonunion would be a thing of the past. In addition, when bone marrow is destroyed, as by excessive radiation, the new marrow in an island of myositis ossificans might be able to take over. There is considerable promise that we are close to isolating this substance. At the time of writing, it has been reduced to a complex polypeptide.

Hamstring Pull

The hamstring muscles form a large group on the back of the thigh (Fig. 13–14). Their tendons insert on the leg bones below the knee, and their action is to bend the knee.

Hamstring muscle "pull" is the bane of the runner, particularly the sprinter and hurdler. Contraction of the hamstrings in sudden takeoffs can cause a strain that is immediately painful and makes further running almost impossible. The diagnosis is clear; there is tenderness at the point of separation of muscle fibers. Complete rupture of the muscle is exceedingly rare, and surgery, therefore, is almost never indicated.

Treatment is the same as for contusion: immediate cold, rest, and gentle compression; and after a day or so, heat and guided motion. The injured muscle fibers are replaced by scar tissue that is not elastic and does not contribute to function of the muscle. Thus, in the final stages of treatment, resistance exercises, involving progressively greater forces, are used to increase the bulk and power of the remaining muscle. Unfortunately, the end result may be poor. About half of the athletes who suffer a severe hamstring pull never can perform quite as well as before the injury.

KNEE

Upon first considering the knee, the student may be reminded of the legendary definition of a camel as "a horse designed by a committee." However, with further study, the knee's structural and functional beauty become apparent. It is, of course, not perfect. Man has been walking on two legs for only a moment in evolutionary time, and a half million years hence (if man does not become an endangered species) the knee will undoubtedly be different and probably better.

The knee is basically a hinge between the biggest and strongest long bones in the body, the femur and the tibia (Fig. 13–15). Two washers (cartilages or menisci) lie between these bones, which are held together by tough ligaments both inside and outside the joint. Tendons of the great thigh and lower leg muscles cross the joint and make it move.

Injury in athletes can occur from rotational wrenching, a direct blow, or both together. Rotational stress alone, as in a sudden change in direction with a foot fixed to the ground (the "cutting" of a football back running with the ball), can tear the menisci but is unlikely to injure ligaments severely. Rotational forces combined with a direct blow, particularly when the blow is unexpected, as in the "clip" in football, can produce both meniscus injury and severe ligament stretch, rupture, or avulsion from bony attachment. The first defense against such injuries is the power and bulk of the muscles.

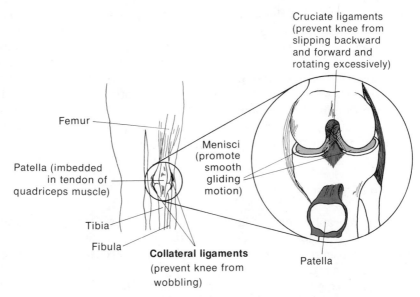

Figure 13–15. Normal left knee. In the enlarged view, the knee is somewhat bent in order to show the cruciate ligaments and menisci within.

Only when muscles have been overcome do ligaments and cartilages become vulnerable. Exercises, notably progressive resistance exercises, are ideal for increasing muscle bulk and power.

Bones in young athletes are very strong and resilient. They are rarely fractured or otherwise injured by the forces of sports in the period between achievement of full growth and middle age.

Ligament Injury

Partial tear of a knee ligament is treated as are other sprains: immediate application of ice, compression, rest, and elevation. Subsequently, crutches may be required for temporary immobilization of the joint. Complete rupture of a knee ligament requires surgery, as described in the example below.

Let us follow the management, under the best circumstances, of a severe injury to the knee sustained in high school or college football today. The injury is observed by the doctor in attendance, who proceeds directly to the playing field where the injured player is lying. A few words with the player and a brief examination are all that is needed to determine that the injury is potentially severe. The player is then transported from the field on a stretcher. To ask him to walk, even with assistance, might aggravate the injury or turn a mild injury into a severe one. Within minutes, the injured player is lying on an examining table in a warm room with his clothing removed. The doctor can examine the knee, compare it with the other knee, and carry out gentle diagnostic manipulation. If such examination is delayed for even an hour, pain and swelling, as well as spasm of the muscles that cross the knee, will prevent accurate evaluation. Then, diagnostic manipulation under anesthesia may be required to determine the extent of injury.

In this example, the following diagnoses are made: (1) rupture of the medial collateral ligament, (2) rupture of the anterior cruciate ligament and (3) probable tear of the medial meniscus. The knee is placed in a comfortable splint, the parents of the player are advised of the situation, and arrangements are made for surgical repair of ligaments and possible removal of the torn meniscus within the next few days.

Prompt surgical repair is the accepted treatment for ruptured or avulsed ligaments of the knee. The results of immediate surgery are much better than those of later reconstructive surgery and are infinitely superior to those achieved with immobilization of the knee in plaster. When surgery is promptly done, return to full participation in sports within four to six months is the rule rather than the exception. Unfortunately, this ideal scenario is not always followed, and the injured athlete may reach the surgeon weeks or even months after the original injury.

Aids to Diagnosis

Arthrography ("arthro" indicates joint) is a type of x-ray procedure in which a small quantity of harmless substance is injected into the knee and coats the menisci, making them visible on the x-ray films. This technique is accurate in detecting tears of menisci in about 90 per cent of cases.

Arthroscopy consists of the introduction of a small (5 mm) diameter tube into the knee through which the internal ligaments and the menisci can be viewed directly. The information provided by these two diagnostic aids overlaps in certain areas. When both are used, very accurate preoperative information can be obtained.

Meniscus Injury

Torn menisci far outnumber ligament ruptures or avulsions at the knee. Most commonly, the medial meniscus is torn (Fig. 13–16). That part of the meniscus that has torn loose sometimes gets caught in the joint and prevents motion, causing the joint to "lock."

The following points strongly suggest a torn meniscus: (1) a history of rotational stress, (2) tenderness at the joint line on either side of the knee, (3) the presence of fluid in the joint, or (4) inability to extend the joint fully (locking). If inability to extend the joint was present from the moment of injury, the chances are very good that the block is caused by a torn meniscus rather than by spasm of the hamstring muscles holding the knee in a comfortable position of flexion. Sometimes mechanical block due to a torn meniscus is difficult to differentiate from a sprain.

A torn meniscus that causes mechanical block should be removed surgically. The entire meniscus must be removed. If this is done, a new meniscus grows. That is, fibroblasts make a scar of very much the same shape and size as the meniscus; as time passes, the new tissue becomes microscopically indistinguishable from the original

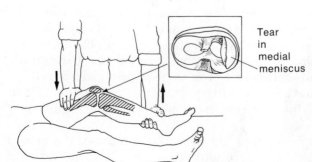

Tear in medial meniscus

Figure 13–16. A torn meniscus ("cartilage") sometimes causes locking of the knee so that extension is limited.

cartilage. Convalescence after removal of a torn meniscus should be rapid. Splinting of the knee is generally required for only a matter of days for immediate postoperative comfort. Crutches can be discarded when active motion is from 180° (straight) to 90°. Full participation in sports with no restrictions can be permitted when the thigh muscles have been built up to normal and when the meniscus has completely regenerated —from three to four months after operation.

There is no nonoperative treatment for torn menisci in the knee for the simple reason that the torn meniscus does not heal. Nourished only by the joint fluid, it has no blood supply to allow scar formation.

Dislocation of the Patella

Dislocation of the patella (kneecap) occurs more often in women than in men and is usually associated with a moderate misalignment of the patella with its associated structures. The patella always dislocates laterally. The injury, therefore, involves considerable tearing of the soft tissues on the medial side of the patella.

Treatment for the first dislocation is immobilization for two to three weeks to allow the torn soft tissues to heal. Recurrence of dislocation is frequent but can be corrected by surgery, which reconstructs the entire anterior aspect of the soft tissues of the knee, realigning the quadriceps, the patella, and the patellar tendon. The results are very satisfactory, and 3 to 4 months after operation an athlete should be able to resume any sport without disability.

LOWER LEG

Shin Splints

The bane of the runner is pain on the inner aspects of both tibiae (shin splints —Fig. 13–17). This condition is associated with running or even jogging. The onset is usually subtle, and although discomfort can be severe, the condition does not always interfere with performance. An athlete may wince while settling into the starting blocks, run a hundred yards in 10 seconds, and limp back to the locker room. Usually, tenderness is present on the inside (posteromedial) surface of the tibia throughout most of its length (Fig. 13–17). This is the attachment of the posterior tibial muscle, the large tendon of which supports the arch of the foot as a sling.

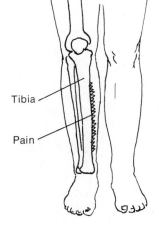

Figure 13–17. Shin splints.   Tibia

Pain

The mechanism of injury is unknown but may be repeated microtrauma (tiny tears) where the posterior tibial muscle attaches to the tibia. However, we have no information from direct observation — autopsies are not done. X-rays show no abnormality unless a stress fracture is found, which is quite different and is somewhat unusual in the tibia.

The only real cure is rest, that is, to stop or decrease running for a number of days. Running on a softer surface may be helpful. Shoes should be of good quality. Shin splints are sometimes relieved by decreasing stress on the arch of the foot through taping or with arch supports. Heat, massage, and aspirin are of some help. There is no permanent disability.

Achilles Tendon

Tendinitis. The heel by which the infant Achilles was held as he was dipped in the River Styx to make him almost invulnerable became the site of his eventually fatal wound. The Achilles tendon (Fig. 13–18) is a point of weakness (fortunately never fatal) in modern sports as well. This tendon of the powerful gastrocnemius and soleus muscles is surrounded by a loose sheath, which provides lubrication as the tendon slides up and down to move the ankle and foot. For reasons that are not clear, repetitive motion, as in long distance running, can apparently exhaust the lubricating function of the sheath so that the sheath and tendon do not glide well; they become irritated and painful. The condition is called tendinitis.

On examination, the sheath is often larger than the normal one on the opposite leg, is usually tender, and can be painful enough to cause a limp. Sometimes, as the foot and ankle are moved, crackling of the roughened surfaces of the sheath and tendon can be felt or heard, a phenomenon known as crepitation.

There is no sure cure. Heat and rest are always effective in time, but a week to 10 days may be required before the athlete can resume full active running. In severe tendinitis that causes a limp, crutches may be worthwhile.

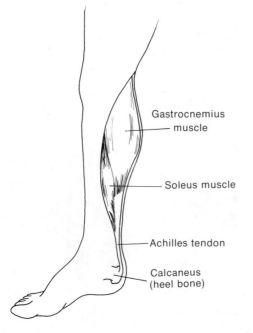

Gastrocnemius muscle

Soleus muscle

Achilles tendon

Calcaneus (heel bone)

Figure 13–18. Achilles tendinitis. Pain, tenderness, and often crepitation are present over the Achilles tendon.

Rupture. Rupture of the Achilles tendon is usually seen in the middle-aged athlete, such as in the aging tennis player who makes an extra effort to get a difficult shot. It can also occur in athletes at the college level. The victim is more conscious of a snapping sensation than of pain. Many describe this sensation as similar to being struck above the heel by a ball or stick. There is immediate disability and loss of almost all "push-off" power in the foot and ankle. It is not possible for the patient to rise up on his toes on the involved side. Surprisingly, the diagnosis is missed fairly often not only by those suffering the injury but also by their family doctors, who simply do not think of it and are led astray by the fact that other less powerful muscles, such as those that move the great toe, are able to make the foot and ankle move as well. The following test proves the rupture has occurred. The patient kneels on a chair, and the belly of the gastrocnemius muscle is compressed by grasping it. If the Achilles tendon is intact, the foot will move a few degrees. Otherwise, the foot will not move.

Treatment requires surgery within a week to 10 days, and results are good. Most athletes can return to their sports in four to five months with little disability. Ballet dancers, however, can never perform quite as well as before rupture. Treatment by immobilization and cast must be condemned, since surgery to reconstruct tendons that heal with abnormal length is often necessary.

The "Ruptured Plantaris"

The official in football or the middle-aged commuter running for a train may feel a sudden snap over the gastrocnemius muscle (Fig. 13–18), as if the site were struck by a thrown stone. There is immediate pain. The muscle and Achilles tendon are intact, but there is tenderness over the gastrocnemius. This sequence of events has long been attributed to a rupture of the plantaris, a small muscle and long tendon under the gastrocnemius. Actually, it is usually a small portion of the gastrocnemius muscle that is torn.

Treatment consists of resting the limb with the use of crutches, followed by gradual resumption of walking with an elevated heel to relax the gastrocnemius muscle. An elastic stocking is helpful both for giving a sense of support and for helping the muscles of the lower leg return blood to the heart. Full function is usually restored in four to six weeks.

ANKLE

The interdependence of form and function is especially demonstrated in the ankle. Even in the most sedentary person, the ankle supports and pushes forward the full weight of the body several thousand times a day, and its durability can withstand all but the most violent stresses produced by sports.

The framework of the ankle consists of three bones (Fig. 13–19A). The heavy tibia bears most of the weight; the graceful, thin fibula forms a resilient lateral buttress, and into the slot between these bones fits the talus, which can move to form a hinge joint.

Firm ligaments stabilize the ankle and limit its motion. Injury to a ligament is called a sprain. When a ligament is stressed beyond its limit, it may be partially torn, ruptured completely (Fig. 13–19B), or avulsed from its insertion on bone, with an accompanying fracture.

Ligament ruptures can occur without fracture, and fractures can occur without ligament rupture. Since ligaments cannot be seen on x-rays, possible rupture must be

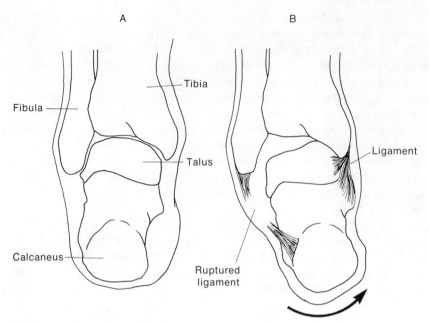

Figure 13–19. Left ankle, viewed from behind. *A*, Normal position. *B*, A sprain results when the foot turns inward.

suspected during evaluation. X-ray evaluation is essential for all but the most minor sprains. There is no other way to determine with certainty the presence or absence of fracture. Ligament rupture without fracture, which almost always occurs on the lateral side of the joint, can be determined by diagnostic manipulation within a few moments of injury. Later, arthrography can be a very useful tool.

Sprains can be graded according to severity, with grade 1 being the least possible injury (tear) to the ligament and grade 3 being complete rupture. Most sprains are grade 2. Immediate treatment, as for other soft tissue injuries, is cold, compression, and rest. A donut of foam rubber held in place with an elastic bandage produces compression. The hole in the donut avoids excessive pressure on the bony protrusion (malleolus) of the ankle. Rest can be achieved either by use of crutches or, in severe sprains, by a temporary plaster of paris splint, extending from the toes to the upper calf. Motion in all sprains except rupture of ligaments should begin promptly within two to three days. The usual grade 2 sprain in an athlete so treated will improve sufficiently in a week to 10 days to allow return to full participation in any sport as long as there is tape protection. Tape should never be used as primary treatment of a sprain lest the encircling tape impede the return of blood to the heart and strangle the swollen soft tissues. However, until the scar in the healed ligament injury has finally matured (which takes months), the ligament will be weaker than normal, and protection with tape is almost always advisable to prevent a second sprain.

Ligament rupture should be promptly repaired by surgery. Unfortunately, too many ligament ruptures are dismissed as minor sprains, and months or years pass before the true diagnosis is recognized. A history of an original severe sprain followed by an increasing frequency of recurrent sprain with decreasing provocation strongly suggests old ligament ruptures. The diagnosis usually can be confirmed by manipulation and by recording abnormal mobility of the ankle joint by x-rays. Reconstruction of ligaments at the ankle is very satisfactory. Most athletes can return to full participation in any sport in three to four months.

Fracture

Fractures must be very carefully analyzed. If the fragments of bone cannot be restored by manipulation to almost perfect alignment, surgery and fixation of bone with appropriate screws, bolts, plates, or pins is often indicated. The injured ankle of an athlete does not tolerate irregularity of the bones that make up its framework.

FOOT

Considering that the foot bears the entire weight of the body 1500 times while walking a mile, it is indeed a wonder that people get about at all, let alone participate in marathons.

Deformities of the foot are, at times, greatly overemphasized. This is not to say that corns and calluses, which are the body's reaction to repetitive pressure, do not need attention when they become painful. Such attention can be most helpful. It should be directed not only toward the corn or callus itself but also, by changing the athlete's shoes, toward relief of the pressure that caused the problem. A sound general rule is to disregard foot deformities in athletes unless they are symptomatic.

The following are three conditions that occur frequently and, when analyzed and treated carefully, that can be relieved almost invariably.

Stress Fracture

When a piece of tempered steel is put through repetitive bending, it will eventually crack and break. The modules of iron become crystallized and lose their original elasticity. A similar phenomenon occurs in bone. Stress fracture has been reported in all weight-bearing bones but is most frequently encountered in the fibula (Fig. 13–20), where marked twisting is produced by the ankle joint during running.

Another common stress fracture occurs in the second metatarsal (Fig. 13–20). Here it is sometimes called a "march" fracture because of its frequency in sedentary military recruits who are suddenly required to march several miles a day. Pain at the site of fracture, and indeed all through the forefoot, occurs on weight-bearing. The pain is often severe enough to cause a limp, and there is tenderness at the site of the fracture. Unfortunately, x-rays taken shortly after the onset of pain rarely show the fracture line. Proof of the fracture can come only after two to three weeks, when callus (healing bone) is visible on the x-ray.

The treatment is rest. If a limp is present, crutches are well worthwhile. A stiff shoe is more comfortable than a moccasin. A plaster of paris boot is rarely worth the trouble and nuisance it causes. With sufficient rest, most runners can return to full participation without disability six to eight weeks after the occurrence of the fracture.

Intermetatarsal Neuroma

Nerve fibers carrying sensation to the brain arise in the skin on the sides of the toes (Fig. 13–21). These join to form larger nerves that travel between the metatarsals. At the point of junction, neuromas can form (Fig. 13–21). These consist of masses of nerve fibers that have become jumbled from repetitive trauma and grow together to form a small ball. This little ball, which need be no more than a millimeter or two in diameter, can be exquisitely tender. It is thought that neuromas arise because the Y-shaped nerve

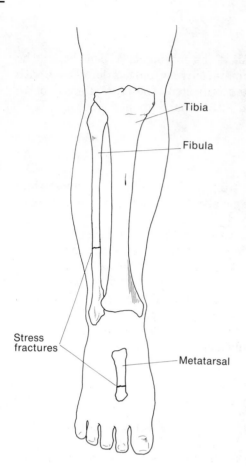

Figure 13–20. Common stress fractures.

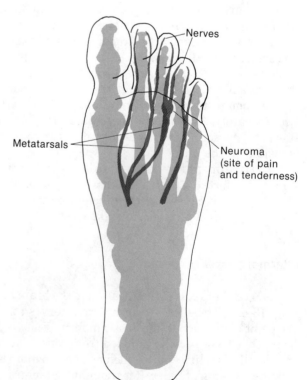

Figure 13–21. Neuroma within foot as seen from beneath.

junction is repeatedly compressed. The continuing compression against the raw, jumbled nerve junction becomes very painful.

In addition to tenderness on examination, diminished sensitivity to pinprick along one side of each involved toe, usually the third or fourth, is very suggestive of neuroma. This diagnosis can be confirmed by the injection of a little anesthetic into the neuroma, which should relieve pain completely.

Treatment is primarily aimed at relieving compression in the forefoot by providing adequate shoes and a pad beneath the distal metatarsal arch. If this fails, surgical removal of the neuroma is satisfactory, producing permanent anesthesia of the opposing sides of the affected toes. This anesthesia is almost always preferable to pain.

Calcaneal Bursitis

A bursa is a normally collapsed, saclike structure that aids motion in various parts of the body by the lubricated movement of its walls, one against the other. Bursitis is inflammation of a bursa.

On the weight-bearing surface of the heel, between the calcaneus and the energy-absorbing pad of soft tissue, lies a bursa (Fig. 13–22). Like other bursas in the body, it is susceptible to painful reaction when, for one reason or another, it fails to produce enough fluid to lubricate its surfaces. Then there is tenderness at the point of pain, and x-rays often show a bony spur. This spur is not the primary cause of the bursitis, but when it is present, it can be an aggravating factor. In middle-aged patients — those who are joggers, for example — gout should be suspected and ruled out by a determination of blood uric acid level.

Local treatment consists of rest and relief of pressure by a horseshoe-shaped pad placed around the tender ares. This pad should be made of firm, clean felt at least one-half inch thick. Pads made of foam rubber do not hold up well under compression, and cotton quickly becomes moist and wadded. Felt, in contrast, retains its resiliency for a long time.

The second line of attack in treatment is injection of the tender bursa, which is done in treating bursitis elsewhere in the body, with a local anesthetic and cortisone preparation. Very rarely, an operation may be indicated, but it should not be carried out until all other methods of treatment have been exhausted and the patient cannot walk but must rely on crutches completely.

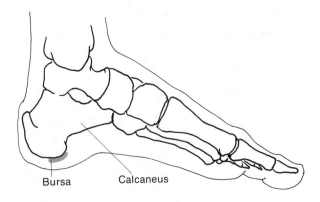

Figure 13–22. Calcaneal bursa.

Bursa   Calcaneus

SUMMARY

A number of musculoskeletal injuries common to athletes are discussed. The immediate diagnosis and treatment of each is outlined, as well as the degree of disability to be expected.

STUDY QUESTIONS

1. What is the typical mechanism that results in "shoulder separation" (acromioclavicular joint injury)?

2. How soon should a dislocated shoulder be reduced, and by whom?

3. What is the treatment for hyperextension of the elbow?

4. Describe the deformity associated with the usual dislocation of the elbow.

5. What is the usual site of tenderness in tennis elbow? What is the initial treatment?

6. In a fracture of the scaphoid bone of the wrist, how is nonunion avoided?

7. Fracture of which metacarpal often requires surgical reconstruction?

8. A player dislocates his finger and immediately puts it back into place by himself. What, if any, further care is advisable?

9. What is spondylolisthesis?

10. What is the immediate treatment for a "hip pointer" (contusion of the iliac crest)?

11. Of what use is the wrapping of a "groin pull" when the player first returns to participation after a number of days of rest?

12. From what does myositis ossificans traumatica usually develop? What is the treatment?

13. What is the main function of the collateral ligaments of the knee?

14. What is the treatment for a mild sprain of a collateral ligament of the knee?

15. Give several signs or symptoms of a torn meniscus of the knee.

16. In dislocation of the patella, what soft tissue is usually injured?

17. Give several possible treatments for shin splints.

18. What are the signs and symptoms of Achilles tendinitis?

19. When is x-ray evaluation unnecessary in a suspected ankle sprain?

20. How soon after occurrence does a "march" fracture become visible on an x-ray?

21. What is the initial treatment for calcaneal bursitis?

FURTHER READINGS

GENERAL

American Academy of Orthopaedic Surgeons: *Bibliography of Sports Medicine,* 1970.
O'Donoghue, D. H.: *Treatment of Injuries to Athletes.* Philadelphia, W. B. Saunders Company, 1976.
Quigley, T. B.: Sports injuries symposium. Am. J. Surg. *98*:1–516, 1959.
Quigley, T. B.: Fractures, dislocations and sprains. *In* Warren, R.: *Textbook of Surgery.* Philadelphia, W. B. Saunders Company, 1963.
Thorndike, A.: *Athletic Injuries,* Philadelphia, Lea and Febiger, 1956.

DISLOCATION OF SHOULDER

Quigley, T. B., and Freedman, P. A.: Recurrent dislocation of the shoulder. Am. J. Surg. *128*:595–599, 1974.

DISLOCATION OF ELBOW

Meyn, M. A., and Quigley, T. B.: Posterior dislocation of the elbow. Clin. Orthop. *103*:106–108, 1974.

TENNIS ELBOW

Ryan, A. (ed.): Special portfolio on tennis elbow. *In The Physician and Sports Medicine.* New York, McGraw-Hill Book Company, 1976.

WRIST AND HAND

Quigley T. B.: Injuries of the hand, wrist, forearm and elbow sustained in organized college athletics. American Academy of Orthopaedic Surgery, Instructional Course Lectures, 368–376, 1960.
Ruby, L. K., and Quigley, T. B.: Primary treatment of hand injuries. Med. Times *105* (8):96–103, 1977.

BACK

Belkin, S., and Quigley, T. B.: Finding the cause of back pain. Med. Times *105*(7):59–63, 1977.

KNEE

Bierbaum, B. E.: Double contrast knee arthrography. J. Trauma *8*:165–173, 1968.
Cascells, S. W.: Arthroscopy of the knee joint. J. Bone Joint Surg. *53*:287–298, 1971.
Hughston, J. C.: Acute knee injuries in athletes. Clin. Orthop. *23*:114–133, 1962.
Hughston, J. C.: Subluxation of the patella. J. Bone Joint Surg. *50*:1003–1026, 1968.
Quigley, T. B.: Management of knee injuries incurred in college football. Surg. Gynecol. Obstet. *87*:569–575, 1948.
Slocum, D. B., and Larson, R. L.: Rotatory instability of the knee. J. Bone Joint Surg. *50*:211–225, 1968.
Smillie, I. S.: *Injuries to the Knee Joint.* Baltimore, The Williams and Wilkins Company, 1946.

ACHILLES TENDON

Quigley, T. B.: Can rupture of the Achilles tendon be treated without surgery? Mod. Med., Jan. 12, 1970, p. 85.

ANKLE

Quigley, T. B.: Analysis and treatment of ankle injuries produced by rotatory, abduction, and adduction forces. American Academy of Orthopaedic Surgeons, Instructional Course Lectures *19*:172–182, 1970.

14

REHABILITATION OF THE INJURED ATHLETE

ARTHUR L. BOLAND, JR., M.D.

Rehabilitation is an important, and often neglected, aspect of sports medicine. Careful questioning and examination indicate that many previously injured athletes fail to regain full strength, range of motion, and endurance before returning to competition.[1] The result is not only a substandard athletic performance but also a high incidence of reinjury with risk of permanent disability. Coaches, trainers, and team physicians must understand the principles and benefits of rehabilitation and insist upon full functional recovery of the players to insure safe and effective performances.

The importance of rehabilitation was appreciated by the ancient Greeks nearly 2500 years ago. During the Age of Pericles, athletic contests, military drills, and calisthenics were an integral part of the educational program of young men and women. Fear of invasion by neighboring tribes required citizens to be physically prepared to defend their shores and cities. The individuals responsible for training these young people also supervised their rehabilitation following injury. One such "physician-trainer" was Herodicus, whose fame spread throughout Greece.[2] Hippocrates, the acknowledged father of modern medicine, studied under him, adopting and modifying his principles of rehabilitation.

In modern times, these concepts of rehabilitation have been accepted and improved. In the 1940's, DeLorme advanced the role of progressive resistance exercises.[3] Bender stressed the value of isometric programs.[4] More recently, Nautilus and Cybex units, which utilize the theory of isokinetic exercises, have been introduced. In addition to these strengthening techniques, the importance of flexibility exercises has been emphasized at coaches' clinics throughout the country. Trainers and team physicians must understand the principles of these various techniques in order to prescribe a safe, effective rehabilitation program for their injured athletes. Finally, the extent of rehabilitation and the duration of disability may vary between two patients who have similar injuries but who are involved in different sports. Allman has referred to this concept as the SAID principle, Specific Adaptation to Imposed Demands.[5] In summary, as much thought and care should be expended in prescribing and supervising the rehabilitation of injuries as is given to the initial diagnosis. Errors at either end of the treatment spectrum will have the same unfortunate results: residual disability, loss of function, and inadequate performance.

PRESEASON REHABILITATION

The preseason physical examination is an important means of identifying conditions that may require rehabilitation before competition is allowed. A history of fractures, dislocations, recurrent sprains, muscle "pulls," backaches, and surgical procedures should be noted. Careful questioning is essential, since eager young athletes often minimize the significance of their previous injuries. Back pain should alert one to the possibility of a congenital or developmental deformity of the spine, such as scoliosis (curvature) or spondylolisthesis (slippage). These patients often exhibit loss of lumbar spine flexibility and tightness of their hamstring muscles. After careful assessment by examination and appropriate x-rays, a program of abdominal strengthening and hamstring-stretching exercises may be necessary to prevent recurrent pain.

Fractures can lead to leg length discrepancies, restricted joint motion, or residual muscle weakness. Careful muscle and joint examinations will identify these potential problems so that appropriate rehabilitation measures can be initiated.

Injuries such as recurrent ankle sprains and shoulder dislocations may result in permanent ligamentous laxity, instability, and secondary degenerative joint damage. Although strengthening exercises are less effective in these cases, protective taping or bracing may be indicated to prevent further injury.

Candidates for contact sports should also be screened and classified according to body habitus, overall strength, and joint laxity. Although more information is needed on this subject, Nicholas pointed out the vulnerability of loose-jointed people to significant ligamentous injury.[6] Muscle-strengthening programs should be proposed for these individuals to help reduce the risk of injury.

Preseason determination of fitness, a function of cardiopulmonary reserve, is important for all candidates for strenuous sports. Sustained muscular activity produces metabolic waste products, which must be cleared by the blood stream. The ability of the heart and lungs to keep up with the oxygen consumption required for these physiological processes is essential. Thorndike described a "step-test," standardized by Forbes at Harvard's Fatigue Laboratory and utilized to determine quantitatively the condition of Harvard athletes.[7] Cooper outlined programs of aerobic exercises that allow one to estimate levels of fitness.[8] A popular method is the measurement of the distance run over a fixed period of time. An athlete in good condition should be able to run a minimum of 1½ miles in 12 minutes. By determining fitness before formal practice sessions begin, coaches and trainers can identify those individuals who may not be able to withstand the stress of strenuous activity. These players can be conditioned more slowly to avoid exhaustion and injury.

Finally, individuals who are candidates for a sport with which they have had no previous experience should be identified. Although most athletes pursue activities that are familiar to them, some young people, male and female, attempt sports about which they have little knowledge of the physical demands involved. Soccer, cross-country skiing, lacrosse, and crew are examples of strenuous activities that cannot be safely or effectively performed without adequate strength and endurance. Novices should be carefully screened and special attention given to their conditioning to avoid excessive fatigue, injuries, and the discouragement that inevitably follows.

In summary, individualized rehabilitation and conditioning programs may be required for those athletes who, during the preseason physical examination, have been found to have had previous injuries, underlying orthopedic problems, poor physical fitness, or lack of experience in their chosen sports.

REHABILITATION FOLLOWING ACUTE
INJURY

Rehabilitation begins with the initial diagnosis and treatment of acute injuries. Nothing is more important to successful rehabilitation and return to competition than prompt, accurate diagnosis. Delay in treatment leads to prolonged disability caused by excessive swelling, pain, joint stiffness, and muscle atrophy.

The ideal place to examine athletes is in the training room, where the uniform and protective equipment can be removed for thorough assessment of the injury. Evaluation on the playing field should be directed toward determining the severity of the injury and ascertaining which means of conveyance is most appropriate to transport the patient to the training or medical room. An exception to this rule is the unconscious patient with a life-threatening head or neck injury. This individual must be more fully assessed and often treated on the field. When there is doubt about how to move the patient, a stretcher, which is the safest and most comfortable method of evacuation from the field, should be employed. Hauling a player to the sidelines, suspended between two burly trainers, is unnecessary, painful, and potentially harmful. Such a technique may be expedient, but it allows an injured lower extremity to swing like a pendulum, causing discomfort and risking further damage to bones, ligaments, nerves, and muscles. Splints and crutches should be utilized until complete examination and x-rays can be obtained.

Common contusions, ligament sprains, and muscle strains are best treated initially with ice, compression, elevation, and immobilization.[9, 10] Crushed ice, placed in a towel and wrapped around the involved area, is an effective method of simultaneously cooling and compressing the injured tissues. Duration of treatment should be 20 to 30 minutes, repeated three to four times per day for the first 48 hours. Ice applied directly to the skin for longer than 20 to 30 minutes is painful and may cause damage to the skin. The use of synthetic cold packs is a convenient, but often less effective, way of providing uniform cooling and compression. Ethylchloride sprays lower skin temperature, but the effect is of insufficient duration. In addition, damage to skin from freezing may occur if these sprays are improperly applied.

Cooling results in reduced metabolic activity and in vasoconstriction, which diminishes bleeding and leakage of fluid into the soft tissues. Compressive dressings, such as elastic wraps, applied between ice treatments also diminish swelling and help to immobilize the injured part. Occasionally a severe joint injury will require a splint for more rigid immobilization.

Elevation during the initial phase of treatment aids venous and lymphatic return, thus decreasing potentially disabling swelling. Either a non-weight-bearing or a minimal weight-bearing gait with crutches should be encouraged when lower extremity injuries are involved. Unprotected walking with ankle and knee injuries is painful and may cause further damage to the swollen tissues. When the progression of swelling and pain has been controlled by these methods, usually within 48 to 72 hours, one can proceed to the next stage of treatment and rehabilitation: heat and physical therapy.

Heat produces vasodilatation and increases blood flow and metabolic activity. Circulating white blood cells engulf the by-products of injury, thus reducing soft tissue swelling. Many modalities of heat are available, including whirlpool baths, hydrocollator packs, moist towels, heating pads, and lamps. Elevation of the involved limb is suggested during treatments to further assist venous and lymphatic drainage. Whirlpool baths necessitate a dependent position but have the added advantages of supplying uniform distribution of heat and gentle massage. Water temperatures should be approximately 110 to 115° F, and treatments should last for 15 to 20 minutes. Hydrocollator packs contain a chemical, which, after heating, continues to give off warmth for several minutes. These packs should be wrapped in a towel and applied to the injured areas. Care should be taken not to lie on them, or burning may occur. Hydrocollator packs are safe and effective, and require a minimum of supervision by the trainer.

Heat can also be effectively supplied by lamps. Standard tungsten bulbs emit infrared rays capable of penetrating the subcutaneous layers. A gooseneck lamp is a convenient means of directing the source toward the involved part. Draping the surrounding area with towels will help to reduce heat loss. The therapist must keep a close check on the position of the lamp to avoid burns. The distance between the light source and the subject should be at least 1 foot.

Short-wave and microwave diathermy machines are also methods of applying heat to injured areas. These devices produce heat by conversion of the electromagnetic radiation produced by high-frequency currents. The heat is dissipated by absorption into tissues of high water content such as muscle and subcutaneous tissue. Depths of 1 to 2 inches can be penetrated. An experienced therapist is essential, since excessive heat can damage deeper tissues without producing the superficial warning signs of redness of the skin and pain.

Ultrasound machines generate mechanical vibrations, which are transmitted by an applicator through a coupling agent such as water or oil. The therapist must keep the applicator moving and avoid direct contact with the skin. The heat generated by this device is absorbed in tissues of low water content such as bone. This device should not be applied to the head, face, areas over large nerves, or growing epiphyses. Ultrasound is potentially dangerous if used improperly. It requires an experienced therapist and offers no real advantage over the simpler, less expensive, and safer forms of heat application mentioned previously.

As swelling and pain recede, gentle active motion is encouraged. Passive stretching or active motion in a painful arc is not advised, since this can cause tearing of edematous soft tissues, resulting in further hemorrhage and swelling. Early, active joint motion helps to prevent adhesions, joint fibrosis, and stiffness. If motion is allowed within the painless arc, no harm will result. Compressive dressings, continued until swelling is significantly reduced, permit activity within this limited range and restrict excessive motion, thus avoiding further damage.

Progressive, protected weight-bearing with crutches is encouraged as pain and swelling subside and joint motion improves. A normal heel-toe gait, within the limits of pain, will help restore joint and muscle function and prevent stiffness. Crutches should not be discontinued until the patient can walk comfortably without a limp.

Massage has been utilized for many years as an adjunct to rehabilitation. When performed properly, it is both soothing and beneficial. However, it should be avoided during the first few days following injury, when further damage can result from manipulation of soft tissues. Light, stroking massage from a distal to proximal direction assists venous and lymphatic return. Kneading and percussion techniques are used for injuries to the deep muscle layers. The disadvantage of massage is that it is time-consuming for a busy athletic trainer.

The treatment program for athletic injuries just outlined is directed at reducing swelling and pain; minimizing soft tissue adhesion (sticking together) and joint stiffness; and restoring function as quickly as possible. This requires an understanding of the purpose and importance of each step in management, and the experience to know when to proceed to the next level of care. This knowledge can be acquired only by careful observation and daily participation in the treatment of these injuries.

REHABILITATION OF STRENGTH AND ENDURANCE

When the preceding measures have been carried out, with reduction in swelling and return of satisfactory joint motion, one can consider the next step in rehabilitation, the restoration of strength and endurance. It should be kept in mind that inactivity leads to atrophy and weakness. Often a program to minimize loss of strength in the uninvolved extremities can be initiated during the period of treatment of an acute injury. Trunk, upper extremity, or contralateral (opposite) leg-strengthening exercises may be continued if they do not cause pain or stress to the involved limb. This program may help to reduce the period of total disability and bolster the sagging spirits of the ;sidelined athlete. Similarly, shoulder motion can be encouraged for patients immobilized in a sling because of elbow, forearm, or wrist injuries.

Muscles function to support and move the skeletal frame. To recondition muscles weakened by injury or inactivity, a variety of exercise techniques are available, including isometric, isotonic, and isokinetic exercise. An isometric activity is a muscle contraction without simultaneous joint motion. This can often be prescribed early in the rehabilitation program. For example, isometric quadriceps exercises are frequently suggested almost immediately following knee injuries or surgery. They can be carried out while the injured part is in a splint or cast, without risk of further injury. Since painful motion of the joint is avoided, this is an effective early method of preventing excessive atrophy.

When a muscle contracts isometrically, only a portion of the fibers do so. Therefore, as rehabilitation proceeds and motion improves, it is important to vary the position of the limb to strengthen more of the muscle fibers. Although isometric exercises are an excellent method of improving strength, they are less effective than other techniques for developing endurance.

With the return of a pain-free range of motion, isotonic (constant load) exercises can be utilized. For safety, joint motion must not be so great that it causes pain or unnecessary stretching. If it is initiated too soon, hemorrhage and swelling may ensue, delaying return of function. During rehabilitation, the exercise program can be altered to develop both strength and endurance.[11, 12] Frequent repetitions of lifting and lowering light weights produce endurance, whereas fewer repetitions using heavier weights increase strength more effectively.

Although isotonic exercises may ideally move a joint through a full range of motion, the amount of tension placed on the various muscle fibers is not equal throughout that range. Because a fixed weight is used, resistance changes as the speed of flexion or extension increases and stress on the muscle fibers is altered. Consequently, not all muscle fibers are strengthened maximally.

The isokinetic machines, such as the Cybex and Nautilus units, are designed to provide a uniform speed throughout a full range of motion so that contraction can be maximized voluntarily. The theoretical advantage of this method is that a maximum number of muscle fibers are strengthened with each repetition. Trainers and team physicians must be aware of the advantages of and indications for the available techniques. Each one can be utilized effectively for specific problems during certain phases of the rehabilitation period. Care must be taken to introduce each technique at the proper time to avoid unnecessary harm.

Two additional aspects of rehabilitation must be considered: the flexibility and the strength of adjacent muscle groups. Following knee injuries, weakness and contractures regularly occur in muscle groups proximal and distal to the injury. For example, tight hamstring and adductor (groin) muscles are the rule with immobilization or crutch walking after knee injury. Heel cord contractures can also occur after inactivity

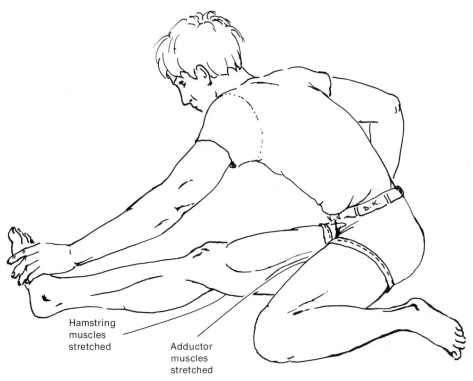

Hamstring
muscles
stretched

Adductor
muscles
stretched

Figure 14–1. Flexibility is improved by simultaneously stretching the hamstring (back of thigh) and adductor (groin) muscles of opposite legs. The "hurdler's" position is shown.

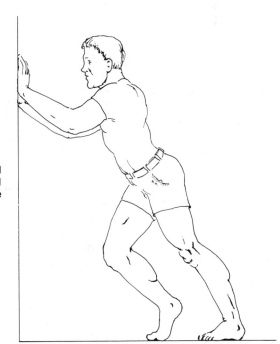

Figure 14–2. Heel cord stretching is performed by leaning forward while keeping the affected foot flat on the floor and perpendicular to the wall.

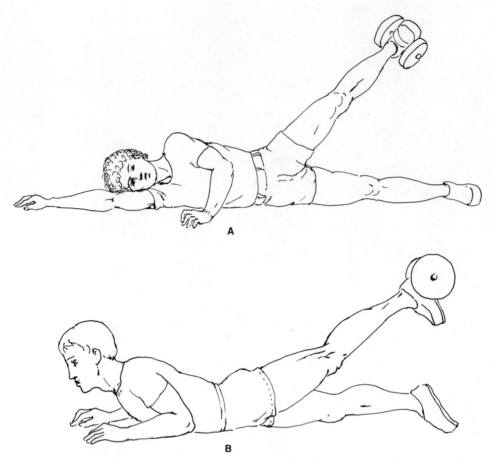

Figure 14–3. Hip abductor (A) and extensor (B) muscles can be strengthened by lifting weights.

resulting from a knee injury. These contractures must be anticipated and thus prevented by including stretching exercises in the general rehabilitation program (Figs. 14–1 and 14–2).

Athletes sometimes "pull" muscles after their return to participation. Appropriate exercises can reduce the incidence of this complication. Similarly, hip abductor muscles (which spread the legs) and hip extensor muscles are weakened during recuperation from a lower extremity injury. These muscle groups must be stretched and strengthened as conscientiously as the quadriceps and hamstrings (Fig. 14–3).

In summary, several strengthening techniques are available and can be used effectively. The rehabilitation schedule must be individualized and modified according to the nature of the injury and the degree of recovery. These decisions must be made by the team physician and trainer jointly. Finally, weakness and contractures routinely occur in areas other than the site of injury. These must be anticipated, recognized, and corrected before participation is resumed.

RETRAINING

The final stage of rehabilitation is performed on the practice field. After flexibility, strength, and endurance have improved, the athlete is allowed to resume training for his specific sport. Certain injuries, such as joint sprains, may require protective taping or bracing. These devices should be worn for both practice and competition. The returning player and the coach must be informed of restrictions. Jogging and stretching often are the initial activities. Sudden acceleration, cutting, and pivoting movements are discouraged in lower extremity injuries. The athlete is advised to work by himself, striding, running figure-eight patterns, back pedalling, and moving laterally until he has confidence in his ability to perform these maneuvers. Often, after the initial vigorous workout, the athlete may experience some discomfort or stiffness the following day. Immediate application of ice and compression after the practice will frequently counteract symptoms produced by the initial activity.

As speed, strength, endurance, and confidence are gradually regained, the player must refine the specific techniques necessary for participation. Throwing, kicking, and jumping are essential in many sports and require coordination and timing. These skills return only with repeated practice either individually or with members of the team. Allman stressed the necessity for team physicians and trainers to comprehend the specific demands placed on athletes by their sport.[5] A baseball pitcher with a shoulder injury, for example, will require more rehabilitation and retraining to be fit for competition than a similarly injured athlete in a nonthrowing sport. A soccer player with an ankle sprain may be able to run effectively but not kick satisfactorily. Those individuals supervising injured athletes must be aware of all the demands placed on their patients and never return them to participation until they are physically able to meet the requirements. A safe general rule is to require *absence of pain, full range of motion,* and *normal strength* in the injured part. Only then can one hope to avoid the physical and psychological disasters that beset athletes who become reinjured, disappointed, and discouraged.

SUMMARY

The rehabilitation of injured athletes begins with prompt, effective treatment to limit swelling and pain. Ice, compression, immobilization, and elevation are followed by heat, gentle motion, and protection from excessive activity. An individualized program to regain strength, endurance, and flexibility is instituted when pain and swelling subside and joint motion improves. Finally, carefully supervised reconditioning on the field, with attention to the demands of the player's specific athletic activity, must be completed before the athlete can safely and confidently return to participation.

STUDY QUESTIONS

1. What conditions requiring rehabilitation may be detected in the preseason history and physical examination?

2. How does delay in treatment of acute injuries complicate rehabilitation?

3. Which treatment measures facilitate venous return and reduction in swelling?

4. When is it generally safe to discontinue use of crutches?

5. Ultrasound treatment should not be used in injuries to which areas?

6. Why is early joint motion within the limits of pain helpful in rehabilitation?

7. List two functions of compressive dressings.

8. When should massage be avoided?

9. How do isometric and isotonic exercises differ?

10. Compare the rehabilitation program for strength with that for endurance.

11. What type of exercise can be initiated promptly and safely after injury? Why?

12. What is the theoretical advantage of isokinetic exercise?

13. Why is it important to examine the muscles and joints proximal and distal to the injured areas?

14. List the criteria for return to participation following injury.

15. Explain the SAID principle.

REFERENCES

1. Abbott, H. G., and Kress, J. B.: Preconditioning in the prevention of knee injuries. Arch. Phys. Med. Rehabil. *50*:326–333, 1969.
2. Allbutt, C.: *Greek Medicine in Rome.* New York, Macmillan & Company, 1921, p. 328.
3. DeLorme, T. L.: Restoration of muscle power by heavy-resistance exercises. J. Bone Joint Surg. *27*:645–667, 1945.
4. Bender, J.: *Isometrics in Athletics.* Carbondale, Ill., University of Southern Illinois, 1962.
5. Ryan, A. J., and Allman, F. L., Jr.: *Sports Medicine.* New York, Academic Press, 1974.
6. Nicholas, J. A.: Injuries to knee ligaments. Relationship to looseness and tightness in football players. J.A.M.A. *212*:2236–2239, 1970.
7. Thorndike, A.: *Athletic Injuries, Prevention, Diagnosis and Treatment.* Philadelphia, Lea & Febiger, 1948.
8. Cooper, K. H.: *The New Aerobics.* New York, M. Evans & Co., 1970.
9. Ferguson, A. B., Jr.: *The ABC's of Athletic Injuries and Conditioning.* Baltimore, The Williams & Wilkins Company, 1964.
10. Ryan, A. J.: *Medical Care of the Athlete.* New York, McGraw-Hill Book Company, 1962.
11. DeLorme, T. L., and Watkins, A.: *Progressive Resistance Exercises.* New York, Appleton-Century-Crofts, 1951.
12. Ferguson, A. B., Jr.: Exercises for the athlete. J. Bone Joint Surg. *44*A:1177–1182, 1962.

15

LIFE-THREATENING CONDITIONS

JOSEPH S. TORG, M. D.

Life-threatening situations in competitive and recreational athletics are by no means epidemic; however, they can and do occur. In 1976, 28 deaths in the United States resulted either directly or indirectly from playing football. In recent years, the number of deaths in football has ranged from 25 to 35 per year — about 2 deaths per 100,000 participants. Although mortality rates for the numerous other athletic activities are not available, deaths nonetheless occur. Thus, the team physician, trainer, and coach must realize that there is the possibility that death may result from athletics, even though the probability is low. Anyone involved in sports medicine and responsible for the care of athletes should be able to recognize and deal effectively with the various life-threatening conditions.

Basically, there are seven immediate threats to the life of an athlete: airway obstruction, respiratory failure, cardiac arrest, heat injury, craniocerebral (head) injury, cervical spine injury, and hemorrhagic shock.[1]

AIRWAY OBSTRUCTION

Obstruction by the Tongue

When an athlete is unconscious, especially when lying on his back, the tongue may fall against the back of the throat and block air flow. Immediate action is required. Simply support the neck with one hand and tilt the head back with the other hand (Fig. 15–1). This maneuver pulls the relaxed tongue forward and opens the airway. If this does not work, the next step is to grasp the lower jaw firmly and pull it forward, again with the head tilted backward. However, when a neck injury is suspected, care should be taken not to manipulate the cervical spine forcibly. An oral airway (tube) can be placed in the mouth by an experienced individual and is very effective.

Obstruction by a Foreign Object

The victim choking on a foreign object is unable to speak or breathe, becomes panic-stricken, turns pale and then blue, and collapses. If effective measures are not

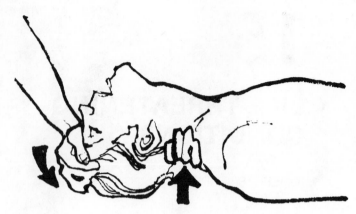

Figure 15–1. Head-tilt method of opening airways. (From *Standards for Cardiopulmonary Resuscitation (CPR) and Emergency Cardiac Care (ECC).* Reprinted from the Supplement to Journal of the American Medical Association, February 18, 1974. Copyright 1974, the American Medical Association. Reprinted with permission from the American Heart Association.)

performed, death will occur within four to five minutes. Heimlich[2] recently described an effective method for dislodging objects obstructing the throat, larynx, or trachea. The *Heimlich maneuver* is a first-aid procedure that can be performed by an informed layman without specialized instruments or equipment.

Airway obstruction occurs when a foreign object is sucked against or into the larynx during inspiration Thus, at the time of obstruction, the lungs are expanded. The Heimlich maneuver produces pressure on the upper abdomen, which is transmitted upward to the lungs. Heimlich states, "Sudden elevation of the diaphragm compresses the lungs within the confines of the rib cage, increasing the air pressure within the tracheobronchial tree. This pressure is forced out through the trachea and will eject food or other objects that are occluding the airway. The action can be simulated by inserting a cork in the mouth of an inflated balloon or compressible plastic bottle, then

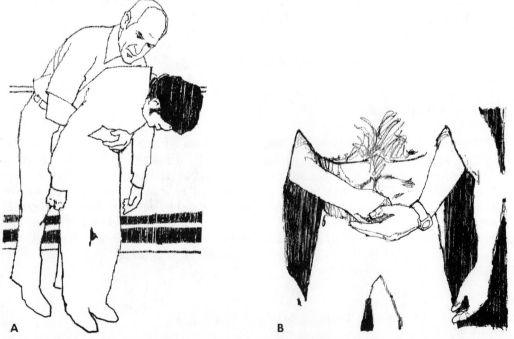

A   **B**

Figure 15–2. *A,* Application of Heimlich maneuver when the victim is standing. *B,* Position of rescuer's hands. (From Heimlich, H. J.: The Heimlich maneuver to prevent food choking. JAMA *234*:399, 1975. Copyright 1975, American Medical Association.)

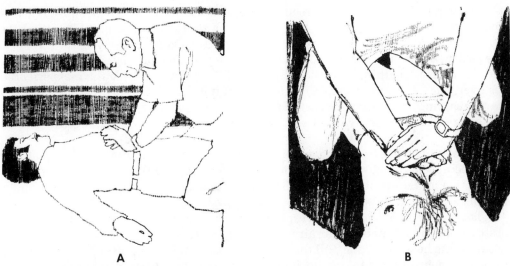

A   B

Figure 15–3. *A,* Application of Heimlich maneuver when the victim is lying on back. *B,* Position of rescuer's hands. (From Heimlich, H. J.: The Heimlich maneuver to prevent food choking. JAMA *234*:400, 1975. Copyright 1975, American Medical Association.)

squeezing the balloon or bottle suddenly. The cork flies out due to the increased pressure, similar to the forceful 'pop' of a champagne cork."[2] In the emergency situation, the maneuver can be performed with the victim standing, sitting, or supine.

Rescuer Standing. The rescuer should stand behind the victim and wrap his arms around the victim's waist (Fig. 15–2*A*). The rescuer then grasps his fist with his other hand and places the thumb side of his fist against the victim's abdomen, slightly above the navel and below the rib cage (Fig. 15–2*B*). The rescuer presses his fist into the victim's abdomen with a quick upward thrust. This should be repeated several times if necessary. When the victim is sitting, the rescuer stands behind the victim's chair and performs the maneuver in the same manner.

Rescuer Kneeling. A variation of the maneuver can be performed when the victim has collapsed or the rescuer is unable to lift him. The victim is lying on his back (Fig. 15–3*A*). Facing the victim, the rescuer should kneel astride his hips. With one of his hands on top of the other, the rescuer places the heel of his bottom hand on the abdomen slightly above the navel and below the rib cage (Fig. 15–3*B*). The rescuer then presses into the victim's abdomen with a quick upward thrust. This thrust should be repeated several times if necessary. Should the victim vomit, the rescuer should quickly place him on his side and wipe out his mouth to prevent aspiration (inhalation of foreign material).

On very rare occasions, obstruction can result from a blow to the larynx that fractures or deforms it. This type of obstruction is not cleared by the Heimlich maneuver. A physician may choose to create an air passage into the larynx by putting a tube or large needle through the cricothyroid membrane of the larynx. An emergency tracheostomy (incision into the trachea) is not generally done because it usually creates more problems than it solves.

RESPIRATORY FAILURE

Respiratory failure occurs in several situations, the most common being simple syncope (fainting) with apnea (cessation of breathing). (See also page 259.) This usually occurs in the training room or physician's office when the husky, body-conscious athlete is threatened by a diagnostic or therapeutic procedure such as removal of fluid from a joint. Anxiety or mild pain triggers a physiological response. The patient's blood pressure falls, and he becomes pale and nauseated, loses consciousness, and stops breathing. Occasionally, convulsions also occur. To the inexperienced observer, such an episode can be quite frightening. However, such patients usually start breathing again in a few seconds. If they do not, simply pull the jaw forward to make sure that the airway is not obstructed and, if necessary, initiate rescue breathing.

A player who has been rendered unconscious by a head injury may stop breathing either because of impaired function of the brain or, as mentioned earlier, because of obstruction of the upper airway by the relaxed tongue. Also, breathing may stop for reasons other than those that have been discussed.

The initial management of respiratory failure is the same as that for airway obstruction. First, establish an airway. As already described, carefully support the neck, tilt the head back, and pull the lower jaw forward. If spontaneous breathing fails to occur, mouth-to-mouth rescue breathing should be initiated (see page 418 for technique). A plastic oropharyngeal (oral) airway should be available to maintain the airway once it has been established in an unconscious patient. Equipment for artificial ventilation (an Ambu bag) should also be available in the event that respiration must be supported for a prolonged period.

A basic rule in dealing with an unconscious football player is not to remove the helmet. Head injuries are frequently associated with injuries to the cervical spine. Therefore, assume that the victim has a broken neck until he regains consciousness or until an x-ray proves otherwise. Forced manipulation of the cervical spine to remove the helmet may, in the injured patient, cause irreversible damage to the spinal cord, including paralysis. It is recommended that when respiratory problems occur in the unconscious football player, the face mask be removed with a No. 1 bolt cutter, leaving the helmet in place.

CARDIOPULMONARY RESUSCITATION

Cardiac arrest (cessation of heartbeat) can result from cardiovascular collapse, ventricular fibrillation, or ventricular standstill. When cardiac arrest occurs on the playing field, a precise diagnosis is immaterial. Regardless of the cause, if the heart has stopped, as determined by the absence of the carotid (main artery of the neck) pulse, cardiopulmonary resuscitation should be initiated immediately. A working knowledge of cardiopulmonary resuscitation is a must for every physician, trainer, and coach. Such knowledge can be obtained only through supervised training. A review of the essential principles of cardiopulmonary resuscitation is given in Appendix C (p. 418).

INTRACRANIAL INJURY

Injuries that occur within the skull, or cranium (intracranial injuries), may damage the brain, the skull, or the blood vessels lying between the brain and skull.

Concussion

Concussion of the brain (cerebral concussion) is characterized by a temporary disturbance in the function of the brain without structural damage. The electrophysiology of the brain is altered as a result of impact. Schneider[3] classifies cerebral concussion as first-, second-, and third-degree.

In first-degree (mild) concussion, there is no loss of consciousness. There may be slight mental confusion and possibly memory loss, dizziness, and tinnitus (ringing of the ears). There is no unsteadiness or lack of coordination. Recovery generally occurs within a few minutes. The point to remember is that even though an individual is not knocked unconscious, he may suffer a concussion. Postconcussion symptoms — headaches, aversion to light, and inability to concentrate — may persist for one or two weeks.

In second-degree (moderate) concussion, there is a loss of consciousness for up to three or four minutes, followed by transient mental confusion and mild retrograde amnesia (loss of memory for events leading up to the injury). Moderate tinnitus, dizziness, and unsteadiness also occur. Individuals with second-degree concussion generally recover quickly but may have symptoms for several weeks.

In third-degree (severe) concussion, there is prolonged loss of consciousness (over five minutes), followed by mental confusion, prolonged retrograde amnesia, severe tinnitus and dizziness, and marked unsteadiness. Recovery is slow and characterized by the presence of postconcussion symptoms.

When can an individual who suffers a concussion return to play? That depends on the sport and the level at which it is played. In high school football, the player who sustains any degree of concussion should not be allowed to play for the remainder of the game. In college or professional football, the situation is different. When an experienced team physician can evaluate the player and keep a close watch on him, a player with a mild concussion can return to the game.* As far as moderate concussion is concerned, if there is *any* loss of consciousness, a player should not return to the game — whether he is in high school or college. In professional football, however, there is no general rule. A player with third-degree concussion should be taken to the hospital where he can be evaluated adequately, no matter what the level of play.

Skull Fracture

In any situation in which a player receives a severe blow to the unprotected head, a skull fracture should be suspected and x-rays should be taken. Skull fractures may be so subtle that they are difficult to detect even on x-ray. A piece of the skull may be depressed so that it presses on the brain. The formation of a hematoma (blood-filled swelling), however, may prevent the examiner from detecting a depressed skull fracture by looking at or feeling the injury. A fracture of the base of the skull, on the other hand, may produce more obvious signs, since it can cause blood to leak from an ear canal or clear cerebrospinal fluid to drip from the nose.

Danger Signs

Several signs indicate brain malfunction that is getting worse and that thus requires emergency action. These signs are: (1) increasing headache; (2) nausea and vomiting; (3) unequal pupil size; (4) disorientation; (5) progressive impairment of consciousness; (6) a gradual rise in blood pressure; and, finally, (7) a decrease in pulse rate. Any of these signs means that the individual has a serious problem and should be taken to a hospital immediately.

---

*Editor's note: In some universities, the player with even mild concussion is not allowed to return to the game.

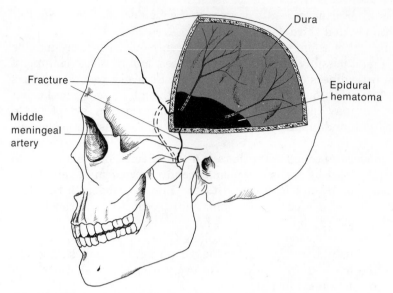

Figure 15–4. Skull fracture tears middle meningeal artery, causing epidural hematoma.

Epidural Hematoma

The dura is a relatively thick membrane that lies between the skull and the brain (Fig. 15–4). Following injury, blood can accumulate on either side of the dura and may put pressure on the brain, causing it to function improperly. Occasionally, a skull fracture at either temple will tear the middle meningeal artery, which runs in a groove on the inner surface of the skull. Blood then accumulates rapidly between the skull and dura to form an epidural hematoma (Fig. 15–4). This sequence is rapid because arterial blood is under high pressure. For example, a batter is struck in the head by a pitched ball. He may (or may not) be unconscious for a moment but then seems to be all right. However, 10 to 20 minutes later he begins to demonstrate the danger signs just described. He needs immediate surgery to remove the hematoma.

Subdural Hematoma

Veins run from the brain to the dura, across a space that is filled with cerebrospinal fluid. A blow to one side of the head can stretch and tear the veins on the opposite side as the skull is moved away from the brain. Venous bleeding is low-pressure, so blood collects slowly and damage may not become apparent for several weeks. However, many victims show signs of the problem within six hours. Neurosurgery is required to remove the blood. It is therefore extremely important to be suspicious of a blow to the head and to observe the victim closely.

In addition to the head injuries just described, the brain itself can be bruised or otherwise injured, causing one or more danger signs or death.

Cervical Spine Injuries

Injury to the cervical spine is potentially the most disastrous traumatic insult that can happen to the athlete.[4] Irreversible spinal cord damage can result in paralysis

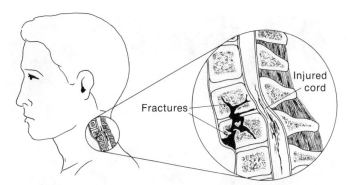

Figure 15–5. Fracture of cervical vertebrae with dislocation. The spinal cord is injured.

(paraplegia, quadriplegia) or death. Damage may be the result of fracture, dislocation, or fracture-dislocation of the cervical vertebrae (Fig. 15–5). When such an injury occurs or is suspected, it is imperative that the individual responsible for the safety of the players protect the victim from further damage to the nervous system. A lesion without neurological involvement must not be converted to one with irreversible cord or peripheral nerve damage by ill-advised examination or manipulation in transportation.

Head and neck injuries can occur together; thus, every athlete who is unconscious because of trauma should be assumed to have a neck injury. Neck trauma precautions (see the next section) should be taken with those who have severe neck pain, with or without paralysis, following injury. Anyone suspected of having a cervical spine injury who cannot actively perform the full range of cervical spine motion, free from pain or spasm, should be withdrawn from competition and have appropriate x-rays taken. If x-rays and the neurological examination are normal, the individual should not return to activity until his neck stops hurting —that is, until he has full, active range of motion of the cervical spine without pain or spasm.

Transportation

The basic principle in moving an unconscious player, or one suspected of having a cervical spine injury, is that he or she be "moved like a log" (Figs. 15–6 to 15–12). One person must assume command of the situation and instruct four assistants to transfer

Figure 15–6. Figures 15–6 through 15–12 show the proper way to move a player who has a suspected cervical spine injury. First, determine whether the unconscious player is breathing and has a pulse. Next, consider the possibility of an associated neck injury. Head and neck injuries frequently occur together. Care must be taken so as not to complicate further an existing cervical spine fracture or dislocation. The injured athlete should be transported on a fracture board when the possibility of cervical spine injury exists. The basic principle is "move him like a log." (Courtesy of William Newell, R. P. T., Purdue University.)

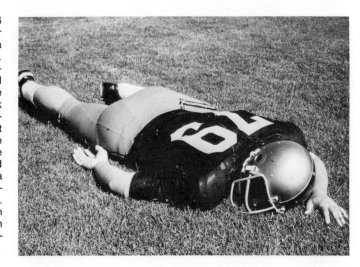

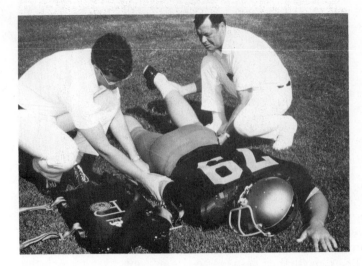

Figure 15–7. First, the extremities should be carefully placed in axial alignment with the torso. (Courtesy of William Newell, R. P. T., Purdue University.)

Figure 15–8. Rolling the injured individual requires a team of five persons. The "captain" of the team is responsible for protecting the head and neck during transfer to the stretcher. Care must be taken to prevent the neck from being flexed, extended, bent laterally, or rotated. (Courtesy of William Newell, R. P. T., Purdue University.)

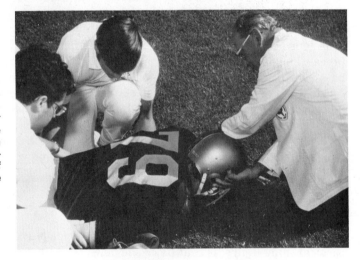

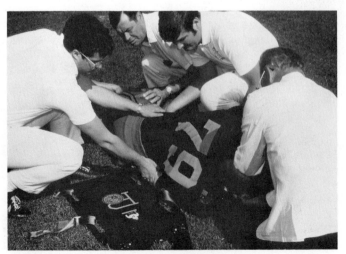

Figure 15–9. On the command of the team leader, the patient is carefully rolled onto the fracture board with the head and neck protected at all times. (Courtesy of William Newell, R. P. T., Purdue University.)

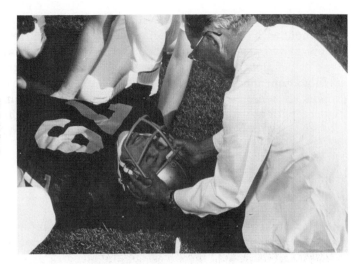

Figure 15–10. After the patient has been rolled onto the fracture board, the head and neck must still be protected. (Courtesy of William Newell, R. P. T., Purdue University.)

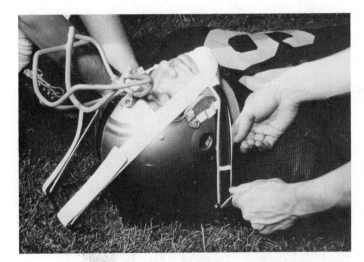

Figure 15–11. *Do not remove the helmet.* If it is necessary to get to the face, as for resuscitation, the face mask should be removed from the helmet. The Purdue fracture board is fitted with an outrigger and buckles for a four-tailed chin strap. Other methods of spine immobilization may be used when such an apparatus is not available. The head and neck may be supported with sandbags, wet towels, adhesive tape, or simply by having someone hold the head. (Courtesy of William Newell, R. P. T., Purdue University.)

Figure 15–12. Evacuation proceeds with the head and spine immobilized, thus avoiding the possibility of compounding an existing injury. Constant attention must be given to the maintenance of a clear airway. (Courtesy of William Newell, R. P. T., Purdue University.)

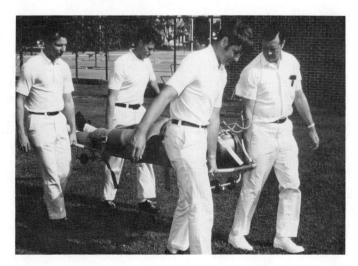

the player to a fracture board so that the head and neck remain in straight, loglike alignment with the rest of the spine. The football helmet should never be removed, and a pillow should never be used. Once on the fracture board, the head and neck must be kept in position by sandbags, tape, wet towels, or outrigger traction. Absolute immobilization must be maintained until appropriate x-rays are taken. Although the canvas stretcher is commonplace and suitable for evacuation of the vast majority of injured patients, a fracture board is necessary when spine injury is suspected.

HEMORRHAGE AND SHOCK

Hemorrhage

Hemorrhage may be external and obvious or internal with blood loss into a body cavity or soft tissue planes. When hemorrhage is caused by laceration of skin, soft tissues, and associated blood vessels, the bleeding should be controlled by application of *direct pressure* to the injury site — preferably with a sterile pad. Generally, direct pressure will control bleeding from veins as well as from small- and medium-sized arteries. However, when hemorrhage cannot otherwise be controlled, a tourniquet may be applied to an arm or leg. Proper application of the tourniquet is essential. It should be at least 2 inches wide to avoid damaging the tissue under it and should be placed near the injury on the side closer to the heart. It must be applied firmly and tightened to occlude both venous and arterial flow. A tourniquet that is loosely or improperly applied can increase blood loss by permitting arterial outflow but preventing the low-pressure venous return of blood to the heart.

Internal bleeding may occur as a result of a fracture, crush injury, or ruptured organ. For example, rupture of the spleen resulting from blunt trauma to the abdomen is seen occasionally in contact sports. In these situations, the loss of blood from the cardiovascular system may not be recognized immediately unless it is looked for. Depending on the nature of the internal laceration and the rate of bleeding, the signs and symptoms of blood loss may appear rapidly or be delayed for several days or even weeks. In either case, loss of blood from the cardiovascular system presents a threat to life.

Shock

Hemorrhagic shock occurs when excessive blood loss leaves too little blood in the cardiovascular system to circulate effectively. Death can result if bleeding is not stopped and the blood volume restored.

When bleeding is external, the recognition of impending or actual shock should not be difficult. However, shock associated with internal hemorrhage may not be as obvious. In the latter situation, the early clinical manifestations of shock must be recognized. They are: (1) cold, pale, clammy skin; (2) collapse of superficial veins; (3) pale or blue mucous membranes; (4) restlessness; (5) increased pulse rate and decreased blood pressure; (6) nausea; and (7) decreased urine output.

When shock is suspected, the victim should be placed on his back on a stretcher with his legs elevated. The victim should be kept warm, but not overheated, and he should be evacuated to a hospital. The sideline, locker room, or school dispensary is no place to observe the individual. When internal hemorrhage is suspected, the judgment of an experienced surgeon and the facilities of a hospital are necessary.

HEAT INJURIES*

Heat injuries include three separate entities: heat cramps, heat exhaustion, and heat stroke. Only the last two are life-threatening. Signs of heat injury include muscle cramps; excessive fatigue or weakness, or both; loss of coordination; a slowing of reaction time; headache; decreased comprehension; nausea and vomiting; and dizziness.

Heat cramps occur most frequently in calf muscles when an individual sweats excessively and does not adequately replace the lost water and, sometimes, salt. To treat heat cramps, first stretch the involved muscles. Then have the player rest and drink water or a commercial electrolyte solution.

Heat fatigue, or heat exhaustion, occurs when an individual is exposed to a high environmental temperature and sweats excessively without fluid replacement. Insufficient circulating blood volume causes fatigue and collapse. Lay the player in a cool, shaded spot, remove clothing, and provide fluids. If he does not improve promptly, evacuate him to a hospital *immediately*. Death may result if heat exhaustion is not recognized and treated promptly.

Heat stroke occurs particularly in unacclimatized individuals who are exposed to high environmental temperatures. The thermal regulatory mechanism fails, sweating stops, and body temperature rises. Above 107° F, brain damage occurs and death follows if vigorous measures are not instituted. This is a real medical emergency. The clue to diagnosis of heat stroke is the high body temperature in the absence of sweating. The athlete with these signs should be packed in ice and evacuated to a hospital immediately. Note that heat cramps and heat exhaustion are not necessarily a prelude to heat stroke — but they can be.

Prevention. The athlete who has just returned from vacation should be allowed a period of acclimatization of 14 to 21 days before being placed in a competitive situation in which he must perform regardless of temperature. Try to arrange the initial practice time for the cooler hours of the day — early morning, late afternoon, or early evening rather than high noon. Make sure that practice clothing permits moisture to evaporate. Above all, make sure that the players get adequate fluid replacement. Weight charts are a good way to monitor the daily fluid loss. One quart of water weighs about 2 pounds. It is not unusual for an athlete to lose 8 pounds (1 gallon of fluid) in several hours. Provide unlimited fluid before, during, and after practice and games. To condition by dehydration is not only antiquated, but currently can almost be considered criminal. Salt can be replaced by the liberal use of table salt at mealtimes. The use of commercial electrolyte solutions is optional.

SUMMARY

In the unconscious individual, relaxed muscles of the tongue and upper airway may obstruct airflow. Tilting the head back usually opens the airway. However, when a player has been knocked unconscious, the neck may also be injured; do not manipulate the head forcibly. Pull the jaw forward or insert an oral airway. If breathing does not resume spontaneously, start rescue breathing; if the heart has stopped, perform cardiac resuscitation as well. If an individual chokes on a foreign object, try to clear the airway with a quick thrust against the upper abdomen (Heimlich maneuver).

Concussion is a transient impairment of brain function without structural damage. The player may be unconscious briefly or merely confused, but he should be

---

*This topic is covered in greater detail in Chapter 21.

observed for further damage. Danger signs indicating serious head injury include headache, confusion, nausea, unequal pupils, loss of consciousness, and increased blood pressure. Anyone with such signs should be taken to a hospital immediately. Brain damage can result from a skull fracture, epidural hematoma, subdural hematoma, or other injury.

Cervical spine injury can cause paralysis. Persons with suspected serious neck injuries must be "moved like a log" so that additional damage is not done. The player's helmet should be left on.

External hemorrhage usually can be stopped by direct pressure on the wound. Internal hemorrhage is less obvious. Signs of shock include pale, damp skin; restlessness; nausea; and decreased blood pressure. The victim is placed on his back with legs elevated and taken to a hospital immediately.

Heat stroke, a condition marked by high body temperature and absence of sweating, is a medical emergency because the high body temperature can cause brain damage and death within a few minutes. Immediately cool the victim by packing him in ice or immersing him in cold water; then evacuate him to a hospital.

STUDY QUESTIONS

1. Describe the appearance of an individual with upper airway obstruction due to a foreign body.

2. Describe the Heimlich maneuver.

3. Describe the appearance of an individual who experiences syncopal apnea.

4. Describe the emergency management of syncopal apnea.

5. Should the helmet be removed from an unconscious football player? Why?

6. Classify cerebral concussions, and state guidelines for emergency management.

7. List signs requiring emergency action in instances of head injury.

8. Explain what is meant when an individual with a cervical spine injury is "moved like a log."

9. Describe the appearance of an individual experiencing hemorrhagic shock from internal bleeding.

10. Give the signs and symptoms of heat injury.

11. Describe the appearance of an individual with heat stroke, and give principles of emergency management.

For Those Trained in Cardiopulmonary Resuscitation.

12. Describe the steps in establishing an airway and initiating rescue breathing.

13. How is adequate ventilation insured on each breath by the rescuer?

14. State the indications for external cardiac compression and describe the accepted technique.

REFERENCES

1. Torg, J. S., Quendenfeld, T. C., and Newell, W.: When the athlete's life is threatened. Physician and Sports Medicine 3:54–60, 1975.
2. Heimlich, H. J.: A life-saving maneuver to prevent food-choking. J. A. M. A. 234:398–401, 1975.
3. Schneider, R.: *Head and Neck Injuries in Football*. Baltimore, The Williams and Wilkins Company, 1973.
4. Torg, J. S., Quendenfeld, J. C., Moyer, R. A., Truex, R., Spealman, A. D., and Nichols, C. E.: Severe and catastrophic neck injuries resulting from tackle football. J. Am. Coll. Health Assoc. 25:224–226, 1977.

16

NONTRAUMATIC
MEDICAL PROBLEMS*

RICHARD H. STRAUSS, M.D.

A small number of medical problems, other than injuries (trauma), are common among athletes and account for a large portion of their visits to doctors. Many diseases will impair performance if not recognized and treated at the start, and some are made worse by athletics. This chapter encourages the reader to prevent illness whenever possible or to recognize problems early so that simple ones can be treated by the athlete himself. The physician's treatment, if necessary, is outlined; and finally, possible effects of the disease on sports participation are given.

Microorganisms (germs) can infect the body and cause disease.† Viruses cause the common cold, cold sores, and many other problems. They are the simplest microorganisms, reproduce only within the cells that they attack, and are unaffected by antibiotics. Bacteria (Fig. 16–1) come in various shapes and can reproduce outside other cells. They cause common skin, throat, and other infections, which generally can be treated effectively with antibiotics. Fungi cause skin infections such as athlete's foot. They grow outside cells, more slowly than bacteria. Antibiotics are helpful in fighting these microorganisms.

SKIN

"Staph" Infection

Occasionally an infection will get started where there has been a small break in the skin, such as a scrape on the leg. Staphylococcal bacteria are frequently the cause, but not always.

Prevention. The best way to prevent infection is to wash the wound well with ordinary soap and water soon after the injury, such as in showering after practice. There is no evidence to show that iodine, Merthiolate, or other solutions are helpful.

For the first few hours, a small amount of blood and clear yellow serum may leak

---

*This chapter is written for the *reader-athlete* and points out certain treatments that the athlete may elect for himself. The prudent coach or other nonmedical person generally avoids suggesting specific medical treatments to others. The coach is often helpful in recognizing medical problems and referring them to the appropriate health professional.

†See Chapter 10, Principles of Infection, for a more complete discussion of this topic.

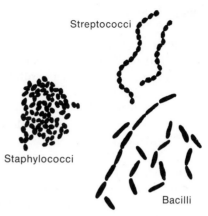

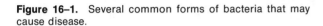

Figure 16–1. Several common forms of bacteria that may cause disease.

from the wound. During this time the wound can be covered with a Band-Aid or sterile gauze. Thereafter, the wound should be left uncovered as much as possible in order to air-dry. Bandages tend to promote growth of bacteria through retention of moisture, heat, and debris. With normal healing, the wound will be a little red and sore. If infection sets in, the wound, after a day or so, will not dry up with scab formation; instead, pus will form and leak from the wound. Then medical attention should be sought.

Treatment. The infection usually can be halted at this point by washing the wound well three times a day with pHisoHex (Rx)* or Betadine Skin Cleanser (non-Rx). An antibiotic ointment such as Bacitracin (non-Rx) may be applied. Watch out for danger signs of spreading infection, such as enlargement of the red area around the wound; red streaks running up the arm or leg, indicating inflamed lymph channels; enlarged, sore lymph nodes (lymph glands) in the groin, armpit, or elsewhere; or fever. These are serious signs, and it is imperative at this point to see a physician for treatment with an appropriate antibiotic. The affected part should be rested, and the athlete may be out of action for several days. Serious signs may appear even though an original injury was never noticed.

Impetigo

Impetigo is an infection caused by streptococcal or staphylococcal bacteria. It is highly contagious and is transmitted, for example, among wrestlers by direct contact or by contact with the mat or infected towels. It usually appears on the face or upper body as sores with honey-colored crusts.

Prevention. The infected individual should not wrestle or have other personal contact until the crusts are gone (healed) because the crusts are infectious. Use of common towels to wipe off sweat should be avoided.

Treatment. This problem must be seen by a physician because it requires treatment with an antibiotic. If the infection is not treated, it occasionally leads to serious kidney disease (glomerulonephritis) at a later time. When antibiotic pills are prescribed, they must be taken for the entire period designated—usually 10 days—in order to eliminate the bacteria. The infected area is kept clean with an antimicrobial soap such as Dial (non-Rx) or pHisoHex. Between cleansings, the wound is kept dry.

---

*A number of medications are discussed. "Rx" indicates those that require a prescription; "non-Rx" indicates those that are sold without prescription.

Athlete's Foot

This extremely common problem is caused by a fungus that exists almost every-where but needs a warm, moist environment in order to grow. Some people seem to have a natural immunity, while others get the infection repeatedly.

Prevention. Wear clean socks each day. Wash and dry well between the toes after each practice. Those with a tendency to get the infection can dust Tinactin (non-Rx) or Desenex (non-Rx) powder between toes after drying.

Treatment. Itching and peeling skin between toes is usually the first sign. Stop the problem at this point so it doesn't cause more trouble. In addition to following the hygienic procedure described in the preceding paragraph, get Tinactin (non-Rx) solution or cream from the trainer or drugstore. Rub only a small amount into the affected areas after washing (at least twice a day). Certain other antifungal creams are also effective, but powders do not penetrate the skin well enough. The infection will usually start to get better after a few days, but it is necessary to continue this treatment for at least two weeks. Treatment for several months is sometimes necessary in order to get rid of hidden fungus.

A later stage of athlete's foot is cracking of the skin, which can then become infected with bacteria. This leads to pain, swelling, and redness, which can make walking difficult. If this occurs or if the disease persists after initial treatment, see a doctor.

Jock Itch (Tinea Cruris)

This is a fungal infection of the groin similar to athlete's foot. It appears as an itching, red rash and is more frequent among men than women. The treatment is the same as for athlete's foot: keep the area clean and dry and apply an antifungal solution or cream (e.g., Tinactin) twice daily after bathing. See a physician if it does not improve in a few days. Wearing cotton boxer shorts rather than tight-fitting under-wear will speed recovery.

Cold Sores (Herpes Simplex, Fever Blisters)

This viral infection often occurs at the edge of the lips but may appear anywhere on the body. It is contagious when the sore is present but can live quietly for years in some people until activated by sunburn, fever, irritation, or other stimuli. The first evidence of the infection is the appearance of a blister, which breaks and later becomes crusted.

Treatment. Healing of a cold sore generally takes two weeks and is hard to speed up because viruses are not affected by antibiotics. The infected area should be kept clean by washing gently with soap (e.g., Dial, pHisoHex) twice daily and should remain exposed to air for drying. Since there is no sure treatment, many remedies of marginal value exist. Application of a drying agent such as alcohol or Campho-Phenique (non-Rx) twice a day may help. New drugs that are under investigation may be effective. Direct contact, as in wrestling, should not be allowed until crusts are gone.

Canker Sore

A canker sore is a small, painful ulcer within the mouth that generally appears for no apparent reason. The cause is unknown.

Treatment. The canker sore heals by itself in about two weeks, and treatment helps only a little. A protective paste containing hydrocortisone [Orabase HCA (Rx)] when dabbed onto the ulcer may ease the discomfort. Certain foods such as citrus fruits make the ulcer feel worse.

Warts

Common warts are caused by a virus and are slightly contagious. They can appear almost anywhere, sometimes disappear for no apparent reason, and are generally treated only if they cause problems. If they are located where rubbing occurs, they may become irritated or infected.

Treatment. Physicians use a number of methods for removing warts, including freezing, applying chemicals, and cutting them off. Still, they often come back. Salicylic acid plasters, which can be purchased in a drugstore (non-Rx), work occasionally.

Plantar warts are those that are located on the bottom of the foot. They are painful for the same reason that a stone in the shoe is painful. It is best to have them removed while small, but not usually during the competitive season because removal often makes walking difficult for a number of days. During the season, the plantar wart can be pared down periodically to keep walking comfortable. A donut-shaped pad can help to keep pressure off the wart.

Acne

Changes in hormonal balance during maturation result, in some people, in an overproduction of oils and fatty acids by the skin. These accumulate to form blackheads and promote infection (pimples), especially on the face and shoulders. Sports can make the situation worse because of sweating and increased oil production associated with exercise, especially in warm environments. Football is particularly stressful.

Treatment. The treatment consists of keeping the skin clean and removing excess oil. First, make sure the affected skin is washed with soap each morning, after practice, and at bedtime. If this doesn't work, use a drying agent such as Fostex (non-Rx). Wiping the face with a Stri-dex (non-Rx) pad, which contains a drying liquid, during a break in practice may also help. Acne is sometimes a severe problem that requires the long-term care of a physician.

Poison Ivy and Poison Oak

Oils from these plants in contact with the skin can cause eruptions with intense itching. One or two days after contact, red bumps or lines appear and usually proceed to develop many small blisters, which ooze clear fluid.

Prevention. Avoid touching any part of the plant. If shoes or clothing have brushed against the plant, wash them thoroughly. The oil can be carried on the fur of pets or in smoke from burning plants. If your skin has touched poison ivy or poison oak, washing it thoroughly with soap and water for several minutes may prevent a reaction if done soon enough — preferably within one hour. Persons who have never before reacted to poison ivy can suddenly become "allergic" to it.

Treatment. See a physician, who may prescribe a "steroid" ointment for the rash. Such corticosteroid medications (related to cortisone) do not cure the problem but decrease the inflammation and itching. If the rash is widespread, steroid pills such as prednisone may be prescribed. Such steroids have possible serious side effects and should be taken only as directed. Moderate cases of poison ivy take about two or three weeks to heal. The old standard treatment, calamine lotion, is temporarily soothing but not otherwise helpful. Scratching should be avoided because it can lead to infection.

Mild cases of poison ivy need not interfere with sports participation. After the plant oil has been washed off the skin, the rash is not contagious and does not spread, although new areas may continue to appear for several days. Bad cases, because of oozing, itching, and irritation by friction, may prevent participation temporarily.

Contact Dermatitis (Irritation from Equipment, Chemicals)

The ending "-itis" on a word is widely used in medicine to indicate inflammation: redness, swelling, and heat from increased blood flow. Thus, dermatitis means inflammation, or rash, of the skin. Sometimes players develop severe rashes under equipment such as hockey gloves or running shoes. Chemicals from leather or dye in clothing may be the cause, in which case switching to a different brand may solve the problem. Sweat, when trapped under a hockey glove, can cause irritation in some people. This may be prevented by wearing a cotton glove underneath to absorb the sweat and by changing it when it becomes damp.

Treatment.   Eliminate the irritating material. Treatment by the physician is similar to that for poison ivy.

Sunburn

Our society views a tan as a sign of health and vigor; this is incorrect. Exposure to ultraviolet rays of the sun damages skin so that the rate of aging is increased. Extreme exposure, as in farmers and sailors, leads to a higher incidence of skin cancer. If you get a suntan, avoid burning by increasing exposure gradually.

Prevention.   The sun is strongest between 10 a.m. and 3 p.m., so restrict the first exposure of any surface to a few minutes if it occurs during this period. Increase exposure time gradually. Three classes of sun lotions (non-Rx) are sold: (1) the "dark tanning" lotions are simply oils and do not block ultraviolet rays or protect against sunburn. (2) "Sun screen" lotions generally contain a benzoate, which partly absorbs ultraviolet light. These permit tanning and longer exposure to sun before burning occurs. (3) "Sun blocking" lotions (Presun, Pabafilm) usually contain PABA (para-aminobenzoic acid) and block ultraviolet light as much as possible.

Treatment.   After the redness and pain of sunburn have appeared, the damage is done, and it is just a matter of waiting for healing to take place. Aspirin (non-Rx) helps to relieve the pain. So do surface anesthetics such as Solarcaine (non-Rx); but they may cause an allergic reaction, so stop using them if the burn seems to be getting worse even though sun is avoided. Cold, moist applications can be soothing.

Sun-damaged skin may peel after a few days. Application of oil to the skin can temporarily prevent peeling, but eventually the dead skin will come off, and with it the tan. If blisters appear, you have a more serious burn and should see a doctor.

Bee Sting

If the stinger is still present, remove it immediately with tweezers. The pain and swelling of a bee or wasp sting can be relieved by applying ice for twenty minutes or by putting Adolph's Meat Tenderizer on it. Some people are allergic to stings and within a few minutes may have difficulty breathing and go into shock. This is a life-threatening emergency that requires immediate medical treatment.

EARS

Swimmer's Ear (Infected Canal, Otitis Externa)

In warm weather or when people swim a great deal, the ear canal (Fig. 16–2) tends to remain damp. This allows infection to occur, usually from bacteria. The result is an itching or painful ear, which feels worse if the outer cartilage of the ear (the pinna) is tugged on. Sometimes fluid drains from the ear.

Prevention. Those swimmers who tend to get this infection can generally prevent it by using any of a number of ear drops that dry the canal. A cheap and effective solution is rubbing alcohol (70 per cent isopropyl or ethyl alcohol). Using a dropper, fill the ear canal with alcohol after swimming. Then turn your head and let the alcohol run out, carrying the water with it. There are more expensive, commercial preparations that are similar but have a little acetic or boric acid added. Some people find alcohol too drying or irritating and should not use it. As an alternative, Domeboro solution (Rx) can be used.

Infection of the canal can also be caused by inserting foreign objects, including cotton swabs, into the canal. As the pediatricians say, "never put anything smaller than your elbow into your ear." Wax falls out normally. If it accumulates so that it blocks the canal and impairs hearing, wax can be washed out or otherwise removed at a medical facility.

Treatment. Any painful ear should be seen by a physician. The infected canal is usually treated with antibiotic ear drops. Healing is probably faster if the patient stops swimming, but competitive swimmers do not always take that advice.

Middle Ear Infection (Otitis Media)

The eardrum creates a seal between the canal and the middle ear (Fig. 16–2). The middle ear normally contains air and is connected to the back of the pharynx (throat) by the eustachian tube. The middle ear may become infected following colds that cause swelling and blockage of the eustachian tube. The major symptoms are deep ear pain with a full feeling and decreased hearing. Sometimes there is fever. If the infection is

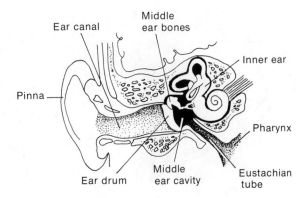

Figure 16–2. Anatomy of the ear.

allowed to progress, the eardrum may burst and drain infected material from the ear. Also, the delicate bones of the middle ear, which conduct sound, may be damaged.

Treatment. See a physician. Treatment usually includes antibiotics by mouth for 10 days, often with a decongestant. There is no particular way to prevent this infection.

EYES

Because vision is so important and the eyes are so easily damaged, almost every eye problem should be seen by a physician. This is especially true for pain in an eye, decreased vision, or double vision, all of which indicate that something serious may be happening.

Foreign Body (Dirt in Eye)

An occasional exception to the rule just given is the speck of dirt that drifts into the eye from the air. The feeling of irritation that results causes tear production, which often washes out the foreign body. Do not rub the eye because this may cause the clear cornea (Fig. 16–3) to be scratched. When tears do not wash the speck out, go to a water fountain or faucet where there is *clean,* cool water and let it flow gently, opening the eye underwater several times. If this does not work, see someone who is medically trained. Sometimes the foreign body has been washed out but still feels present because it has scratched the cornea. In such cases, antibiotic drops are often used. Glass or metal in the eye require the immediate attention of a physician (ophthalmologist).

Infection (Pink Eye, Conjunctivitis)

Infection of the eye by bacteria is easily spread by sharing towels or by rubbing the eye. The eye feels irritated and looks red (bloodshot) because the tiny blood vessels of the conjunctiva (Fig. 16–3) have dilated to help fight infection. Pus appears at the corner of the eye. In the morning the eye is usually crusted and difficult to open.

Treatment. The physician may prescribe antibiotic drops or ointment. The athlete should stay out of practice until symptoms are gone — usually a day or

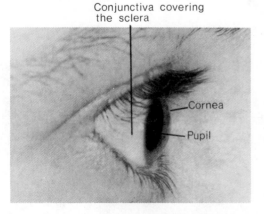

Conjunctiva covering
the sclera

Cornea

Pupil

Figure 16–3. The clear cornea of the eye transmits light rays. The conjunctiva is the thin, usually invisible, membrane that contains blood vessels and covers the white portion of the eye (sclera). (From Scheie, H. G., and Albert, D. M.: *Textbook of Ophthalmology,* 9th ed., p. 4. Philadelphia, W. B. Saunders Company, 1977.)

two—for his own comfort and to avoid spreading the disease. He should continue using the medication for an additional two days to prevent a relapse.

Sty

A sty is an infection of a gland in the eyelid, which then causes the tissues of the lid to swell. It is difficult to reach the infection with antibiotics. The physician will generally prescribe hot compresses and antibiotic eye drops to prevent spread of infection to the conjunctiva. Often the infection will come to a head and release pus, after which the eyelid quickly returns to normal. This problem may prevent sports participation for several days.

Irritation (from Swimming, Snow Blindness)

Swimming can lead to eye irritation, especially if water in the pool is not carefully controlled for its pH (acidity) and chlorine concentration. Even with ideal water conditions, many competitive swimmers wear goggles. Irritation and redness can appear during swimming or soon afterward. Eye drops such as Murine (non-Rx) or Visine (non-Rx) may soothe temporarily, but the irritation will go away by itself in a few hours and is better avoided than treated.

Snow blindness comes from sunburn of the cornea during skiing, hiking, or climbing on snow. The same problem can occur during other sun exposure, as in sailing, or from the burning rays of sun lamps. Several hours after exposure, the eyes become very irritated and the victim cannot stand bright light. In general, healing takes place within 12 hours. If not, a physician should examine the eyes. The problem can be prevented by wearing dark glasses or goggles.

THE RESPIRATORY SYSTEM

Common Cold

In this annoying disease, a virus infects the lining of the respiratory tract, where it causes swelling and secretion of fluid. As everyone has experienced, symptoms may include runny nose, sneezing, stopped-up ears, sore throat, hoarseness, and cough. Victims often feel weak but have little fever.

Prevention.   The disease is transmitted from person to person by infected secretions in the form of droplets in the air, which are then inhaled; by the sharing of items such as drinking glasses; or by direct personal contact. Avoiding communal water cups and towels will help to decrease transmission. An individual becomes immune to the particular virus that infected him, but because there are several hundred different viruses that cause the common cold, he is not immune to colds in general. Vitamin C does not prevent or cure colds, according to most available evidence.

Treatment.   There is no cure for the common cold. Antibiotics, such as penicillin, do not work because they do not affect viruses and may result in more harm than good by allowing growth of bacteria that are resistant to the drug. Colds tend to last about a week, and the *symptoms* can be treated, although not always effectively. Some age-old advice may well be the best treatment: get plenty of rest, especially if you feel tired; drink fluids to insure normal hydration (chicken soup is fine); and take aspirin every four hours for headache, sore throat, or fever.

There are a number of medications available without prescription that may help a little. For a runny nose, most "cold tablets" such as Coricidin D or Contac contain a decongestant to decrease nasal stuffiness and an antihistamine. Antihistamines help to relieve allergies but probably not colds. They often cause drowsiness. A good decongestant is Sudafed. Nasal sprays, such as Neo-Synephrine, act as decongestants for a few hours. They should be used for only two or three days because their effectiveness decreases with use; and when the drug is overused, a "rebound" effect may cause worse congestion. Throat lozenges or sprays (Cepacol, Chloraseptic), which are surface anesthetics, alleviate a sore throat.

Cough is often helped by placing a vaporizer in the room. Available cough syrups (e.g., Robitussin [non-Rx]) help to liquefy secretions so they can be coughed up more easily. They are, at best, moderately effective. Benylin Cough Syrup (Rx) contains an antihistamine, so if taken before bedtime it can promote sleep. When a cough at night prevents sleep, it is best to see a physician, who may prescribe a cough medication containing a narcotic in order to suppress the cough somewhat. The cough that follows a cold can linger for a few weeks. Occasionally a cold may be followed by a bacterial infection of the bronchi, ears, or sinuses that requires treatment with an antibiotic.

A number of viral illnesses, such as measles, may start like a cold but go on to cause other problems. See a physician if fever is high or persistant, if cough is severe, or if symptoms are other than those of the common cold.

Sports Participation.   Many people ignore a mild cold. The athlete should not participate when he has a fever or significant cough, or when he feels tired or achy. People may recover sooner if they rest when they feel sick rather than exercising.

Because antihistamines such as those in cold remedies often cause drowsiness, they may decrease athletic performance. Decongestant pills and sprays are stimulants related to epinephrine and, where drug testing is done, may disqualify the participant, as will narcotics such as those in cough-suppressant medications (see Chapter 27).

Influenza

Influenza is another viral infection of the respiratory tract ("stomach flu" is a different disease). It feels like a bad cold but with so much weakness and achy feeling all over that the victim often can hardly move. Also, fever and chills are usually present.

Prevention.   Influenza usually occurs in epidemics in the fall and winter. Vaccination against a specific type of influenza is usually, but not always, effective because the strain of virus varies from year to year and must be predicted correctly to allow for manufacture of the right vaccine. The vaccine is recommended for persons with severe heart and lung diseases because they may die from complications of influenza. Normal individuals get sick but rarely die and are not generally vaccinated. Some teams prefer to receive the vaccine in order to avoid the illness during their competitive season. The vaccine itself may cause mild influenzalike symptoms.

Treatment.   There is no cure, and symptoms are treated like those of a severe cold.

Sports Participation.   There is little question of competing during the illness because the victim feels terrible. After all symptoms are gone, the athlete should gradually increase workouts over a number of days until reaching his normal level.

Strep Throat

Another cause of sore throat is the streptococcus bacterium, which can infect the throat and tonsils. Infection by one particular type (group A beta-hemolytic streptococccus) is potentially dangerous because it can lead to rheumatic fever and heart damage at a later time. These complications may be prevented if the sore throat is treated early with antibiotics. The victim usually has a sore throat, especially when swallowing, swollen lymph nodes in the neck, fever, headache, and weakness. Sometimes a bright red rash covers much of the skin, in which case the name "scarlet fever" is used. It is still, basically, strep throat. Other diseases such as colds and mononucleosis can begin as a sore throat. A throat culture can determine whether the streptococcus germ is present. Results of the culture are known in about one day.

Treatment. Penicillin is the usual treatment, either as pills or by injection. The victim generally feels cured after a few days. However, it is important to take the pills as prescribed, for the full 10 days or more, in order to wipe out the infection completely and decrease the chances of later heart damage. When feeling ill, the patient should rest in bed and take fluids and aspirin for the fever. Gargling with warm salt water (½ teaspoon of salt in a cup of water) can ease the throat pain.

Prevention. Transmission is by droplets in the air or on infected materials, or by direct contact. If you have been near someone with strep throat, be alert for symptoms in yourself.

Sports Participation. Do not participate until you feel completely recovered.

Collapsed Lung (Pneumothorax)

Occasionally a healthy person's lung will suddenly collapse for no apparent reason. This occurs most frequently among college-age males either at rest or during exercise. A bleb, or weak spot, on the surface of the lung breaks, letting air *(pneumo-)* into the chest cavity *(thorax)*. This air decreases the "vacuum" or negative pressure surrounding one of the two lungs and allows it to collapse, usually only partway (see page 67). The victim feels sudden chest pain and has difficulty breathing.

Treatment. If the air leak has stopped and the collapse is small, bed rest for a few days allows the air to be absorbed and the lung to expand by itself. If air continues to leak or the collapse is nearly complete, a tube is inserted into the chest cavity to remove the air, but this is rarely necessary. After two such collapses, surgery is usually done to prevent further episodes.

Occasionally the air of a pneumothorax will rapidly build up to such a pressure that it seriously interferes with breathing and the return of blood to the heart. The victim may then go into shock and become unconscious. This is a life-threatening emergency that must be treated surgically by immediate removal of the air.

Hyperventilation (Overbreathing)

Sometimes, when people are injured or upset for almost any reason, they unconsciously breath faster and deeper than necessary. This can cause symptoms that make them even more anxious: dizziness; tingling of fingers, toes, and lips; and the feeling of being unable to get their breath. They then breathe even more and can remain in a panic for many minutes. Hyperventilation (overbreathing) results in carbon dioxide being lost from the body more rapidly than it is produced. The lowered levels of carbon dioxide and acidity in the blood cause the symptoms.

Treatment. Getting the patient to calm down is the main concern. Point out, if appropriate, that the problem is minor, that help is being given, and that he is breathing too fast. Advise slow, quiet breathing or intermittent breath-holding. If the victim will cooperate, have him breathe into and out of a paper bag covering his nose and mouth. That way, exhaled carbon dioxide will be rebreathed; and since the system is leaky enough, oxygen is not used up. Stop when the patient is calm.

Hay Fever

Hay fever is not a fever but an allergy to small inhaled particles (allergens) such as pollen, mold, or sheddings from animal fur. It resembles a cold, with runny nose and sneezing, and is often associated with spring and fall pollen. The athlete with this problem can try a number of methods, as they are appropriate or possible. He can: (1) ignore it; (2) avoid performing at times when the allergy is severe or at locations that aggravate it; (3) try hyposensitization (allergy shots) over a number of months; or (4) take medication. There are two main types of medication: antihistamines, which decrease symptoms but cause drowsiness; and decongestants, which are banned where drug testing is done.

Asthma

Asthma can be caused by allergies, infection, or breathing irritating substances. Breathing becomes difficult during an asthma attack because the muscles around small airways in the lung contract, making the bronchi narrower. Also, more mucus is secreted by the bronchi and contributes to wheezing and coughing. In people who have asthma, exercise can trigger an attack, owing to cooling or drying of the airways by the inhaled air. This does not mean that people with asthma should avoid exercise. On the contrary, they can increase their exercise tolerance by gradually increasing their daily exertion. The pace should be determined by the individual. Swimming is an exercise least likely to trigger asthma, probably because it can be done at a nonstrenuous rate as well as because of the warm, humid air surrounding indoor pools.

Exercise-induced asthma also occasionally develops in athletes who have never had asthma before. Immediately after exertion, or sometimes during it, the individual becomes unusually short of breath and sometimes wheezes. Symptoms usually disappear after a rest of 15 minutes or so. This problem can be treated with medication, but certain of the usual asthma remedies should be avoided. Those that contain sedatives such as barbiturates may decrease performance, and the stimulant drugs related to epinephrine are banned where drug testing is performed. Several drugs (including cromolyn sodium [Rx]), however, are allowed by drug control programs.

THE HEART

Heart disease is discussed in Chapter 26. Only problems related to the basically healthy heart are presented here.

Functional Heart Murmur

A number of normal young persons have a very soft heart murmur detected at some time during a physical examination. It may be heard one day and gone the next and is called a "functional" (innocent) heart murmur because no structural cause for the murmur can be found. It does not indicate a heart problem and should be ignored.

Premature Ventricular Contractions
(Premature Beats)

Occasionally, the ventricle of the heart may contract prematurely and cause an irregularity in rhythm. Usually this is detected only during a physical examination. In the normal heart, exercise causes these irregularities to disappear.

Viral Infection

Some viral illnesses can affect the heart muscle, which is one reason that people are advised not to exercise when they feel sick or have a fever. On very rare occasions, apparently healthy athletes have died during a game or practice. This is usually attributed to ventricular fibrillation, in which the contractions of heart muscle fibers suddenly become uncoordinated and blood is not pumped. A few such cases have been associated with viral illness.

Fainting (Passing Out, Syncope)

There are a number of reasons why otherwise healthy people may lose consciousness, including a blow to the head or blood loss (see Chapter 15). However, psychological stimuli can also cause loss of consciousness, as for example, when a large football player is approached by a small nurse carrying a hypodermic needle with which to draw blood from his vein. The individual turns pale, feels weak and sick to his stomach, and suddenly passes out. The mechanism behind this response (vasovagal syncope) is that anxiety or pain in some people can cause the blood vessels of the body to dilate. Blood then drains to the lowest parts of the body —away from the brain if the person is standing or sitting. The brain loses consciousness within a few seconds after its blood supply has decreased.

Treatment. Catch the person as he falls so he does not hit his head. Then immediately lay him flat on his back on the ground. You may note during the next few seconds that the victim almost appears dead. That is, breathing is shallow and hard to detect, the pulse is slow and hard to find, and the skin is pale. This situation will generally improve in a few more seconds as blood flow returns to the brain with the help of gravity. Lifting the victim's heels a foot or so off the ground will help blood drain from the legs toward the heart and brain.

A mistake commonly made by onlookers is to support the collapsing or unconscious person in an upright position. This is absolutely the *wrong* move and can lead to brain damage. The injured player sitting on the bench who says, "I feel like I'm going to pass out," should be helped to lie down on the spot and will probably begin to feel better immediately.

THE DIGESTIVE SYSTEM

Nausea, vomiting, and diarrhea can result from a number of causes that are sometimes hard to differentiate.

Viral Gastroenteritis ("Stomach Flu")

Several viruses tend to disturb the normal function of the stomach and intestines. (The influenza virus is not one of them. It infects the respiratory system.) Symptoms of this common disease include loss of appetite, nausea, vomiting, diarrhea, cramping abdominal pain, and a generally achy feeling. They usually last about two days and, as with all viruses, there is no cure.

Treatment.   Simply stay in bed and, as appetite returns, start drinking liquids and progress to a regular diet. When symptoms are severe, the physician may prescribe medication such as Lomotil (Rx) or paregoric (Rx) (both narcotics) to calm the intestine, or antinausea drugs. Persistent vomiting for more than one day can lead to serious dehydration and should be reported to a doctor.

Prevention is difficult. The disease spreads easily by inhalation of the virus from droplets in the air and may pass rapidly among many persons in a team or school.

Food Poisoning (Staphylococcal Food Poisoning)

The most common cause of food poisoning is contamination by the staphyloccus bacterium, especially in warm weather. Dairy products such as cream fillings or meats may become contaminated from the infected skin or respiratory tract of a food handler. If the food is not kept refrigerated, the bacteria can multiply over a few hours and produce a toxin (poison) that causes severe vomiting and diarrhea a few hours after being eaten. These unpleasant effects usually last less than 12 hours. The bacteria do not multiply inside the digestive system, so it's simply a matter of getting rid of the poison. (Other bacteria can cause more severe food poisoning.)

Treatment.   Medicines to reduce the vomiting and diarrhea are not usually given. Occasionally, treatment of severe dehydration may require administration of fluids by vein. The disease is prevented by proper food handling. It can strike large groups eating the same food such as at club picnics.

Travelers' Diarrhea ("Montezuma's Revenge")

People who live in temperate climates such as that of the United States and who travel to warmer nations such as Mexico often get diarrhea a few days after arriving. This is thought to be from infection by a strain of the bacterium *Escherichia coli* that is new to the traveller. *E. Coli* normally lives in the human intestine but the new strain causes diarrhea for a few days before the disease cures itself.

Prevention.   This disease is difficult to prevent, but chances of avoiding it are improved by eating in establishments that are known to prepare food hygienically and by avoiding water of unknown quality. When in doubt, avoid fresh salads, eat only those fruits that you have peeled yourself, eat foods that are served hot, and drink bottled beverages.

Treatment.   Drinking liquids, such as soup, helps to replace lost water and salt and prevent dehydration. Diarrhea can be relieved by Lomotil (Rx) or paregoric (Rx). [Caution: these narcotics can disqualify participants in drug control programs. Kaopectate (non-Rx) or Pepto-Bismol (non-Rx) may alleviate diarrhea and are allowed in such programs.] Antibiotics do no good and possibly prolong the disease. Certain drugs, such as Entero-Vioform, are sold without prescription for treatment of diarrhea in some countries but not in the United States. They can cause damage to the nervous system, may mask serious disease, and thus should not be taken.

Alcoholic or Aspirin Gastritis

The morning after an evening of alcohol consumption, an individual may find that he has an irritated, upset stomach (alcoholic gastritis). Taking an antacid such as Maalox (non-Rx) or Gelusil (non-Rx) may help somewhat. Repeated episodes can cause bleeding from the stomach lining.

Aspirin or certain other drugs that are taken over a number of days for problems such as tendinitis may irritate the stomach or, in rare instances, cause ulcers. Symptoms of abdominal pain or nausea should be reported to the prescribing physician. Taking aspirin with meals or with a full glass of water or milk tends to prevent stomach irritation.

Exertion, Anxiety

Many athletes have observed independently that if they eat and then exercise hard, they vomit. This can be avoided by eating lightly about three hours before the workout (see Chapter 17). Water should be drunk to satiate thirst throughout the practice or game to keep up with loss of water through sweating. Dehydration impairs performance and may result in heat injury (see Chapter 21).

An athlete being interviewed on national television was asked what he did while getting "psyched up" before a race. "I go to the bathroom a lot," he replied. One result of anxiety or tension is the tendency for the intestines to churn more vigorously than usual. Thus, an individual may need to defecate one or more times before competition. Unless diarrhea is severe, this is not a problem that requires medical attention.

Appendicitis

The appendix is a small, dead-end tube connected to the large intestine. When it becomes infected, it is like a boil deep inside the abdomen. The symptoms at first are vague — diffuse abdominal pain and loss of appetite — so it can be confused with many other diseases. Within 12 hours the pain usually settles in the right lower quarter of the abdomen.

Treatment. An infected appendix needs to be removed without delay so that it does not burst and spread infected material into the abdominal cavity. Full recovery following surgery takes a number of weeks, and the time interval before returning to sports depends on the type of activity involved.

Hemorrhoids

The hemorrhoidal veins are those that surround the junction of the rectum and anus. When these veins become abnormally large, they are called hemorrhoids. This occurs particularly in weight lifters, people who row, and others who by straining cause increased pressure in the abdomen. Symptoms can include anal pain or itching and appearance of bright red blood on defecation.

Treatment. Treatment may include stopping exercise for a few days and sitting in a warm bath several times a day. Suppositories such as Anusol (non-Rx) may help. Stool should be kept soft by a diet that includes bulk-forming foods, such as lettuce, apples, or bran; or by taking a laxative such as Metamucil (non-Rx) or milk of magnesia (non-Rx) if necessary. Rarely, in severe cases, surgical removal of the enlarged veins may be required.

THE URINARY SYSTEM

Protein in Urine

The kidney normally filters blood and further processes the resulting liquid to produce urine. Cells and protein molecules, which are large, are kept in the blood, where they belong. Protein in the urine, as revealed by a test, is usually a sign of disease. However, following strenuous exercise, many normal persons have a moderate amount of invisible protein in their urine. Sometimes a few red blood cells leak in also and can be seen under the microscope. This is not a sign of disease, although visible blood in the urine is and should be reported to a physician immediately. What must be remembered is that urine tests should always be done before exercise, not after, or the results may falsely suggest disease.

Urinary Tract Infections

Infections of the urinary system occur more often in females because the urethra (the tube leading out of the bladder) is short and is a less effective barrier against entry of germs than is the urethra of the male. Sometimes such infections are associated with sexual activity ("honeymoon cystitis": bladder infection). Early symptoms are burning or pain at the time of urination and frequent urination. Blood may appear in the urine. As the infection progresses, pain over the kidneys and fever can result. Urinalysis will usually reveal the presence of bacteria and white blood cells.

Treatment.   After the urine is cultured, appropriate antibiotic drugs are taken for 10 days even though symptoms may be gone in a day or two. The athlete can usually return to sports when all symptoms are gone. In order to make sure that the infection has been eliminated, a follow-up urine culture may be done a week or so after the antibiotic treatment is finished.

SEXUALLY TRANSMITTED DISEASES

All sexually transmitted diseases should be treated by a physician as soon as they become evident in order to relieve the individual's discomfort, to prevent possible serious effects later on, and to stop the spread of the disease. *Sexual contact should be avoided until the disease is cured.*

Nongonococcal Urethritis (N.G.U.)

This is a relatively common problem among males and rarely occurs in females. It is thought that there are several types of microorganisms smaller than bacteria (chlamydia and mycoplasma) that can live in the vagina and cause no problem. However, if they start to grow within the male urethra (the tube within the penis), they become irritating and cause a burning sensation, especially during urination. Also, there may be a slight continuous leakage of mucuslike fluid from the end of the penis.

Treatment.   This is not as dangerous a problem as gonorrhea, but it is unpleasant and can be treated effectively with certain antibiotics following tests for other diseases. The sooner it is treated, the easier it is to eliminate. Nongonococcal urethritis is generally transmitted by sexual intercourse. Urination after intercourse helps to wash microorganisms out of the urethra and decrease the chances of getting the infection. Resumption of sexual contact with the same partner will not necessarily lead to recurrence of the problem.

Gonorrhea ("Clap")

When gonococcal bacteria infect the urethra, they usually cause not only burning on urination but also a considerable leakage of yellow pus from the penis ("the drip"). This prompts most males to head for the doctor by the fastest means available. Some males have no symptoms and become carriers. Females may have no symptoms or may tend to overlook a moderate urethral or vaginal discharge of gonorrhea and therefore are more likely to become carriers of the disease. Burning on urination or vaginal discharge should prompt a visit to a medical facility, where gonorrhea can be detected. Gonorrheal infections of the throat and rectum also occur.

Treatment.   The disease is treated with large amounts of penicillin or certain other antibiotics. If gonorrhea is left untreated, the initial symptoms disappear, but the infection can spread and cause serious problems, including sterility and arthritis.

Methods of prevention have not been successful, and the disease is epidemic with an estimated 3 million cases per year in the United States. A vaccine is under investigation and appears promising.

Genital Herpes (Blisters)

A close relative of the virus that causes cold sores produces similar lesions on the penis or female genitals. These sores may be very painful, and medical treatment is designed to relieve pain; but healing still takes about two weeks. In the female, such infections may possibly be associated with an increased chance of cervical cancer at a later time.

Syphilis

Syphilis is caused by a microorganism known as a spirochete. The first sign is a painless ulcer or sore (chancre) on the penis, female genitalia, or other site of sexual contact. Treatment is usually with penicillin.

Frequently the painless ulcer is not noticed by the victim, and it goes away after a couple of weeks. However, the disease may then spread throughout the body and years later can result in permanent damage to the brain, spinal cord, heart, and other organs. For this reason, a blood test for syphilis is usually done whenever any of the sexually transmitted diseases is treated.

Crab Lice (Pediculosis Pubis)

Crab lice, though as small as the head of a pin, are extremely ugly (Fig. 16–4). They live in hairy, pubic areas, where they suck blood and create small red spots that

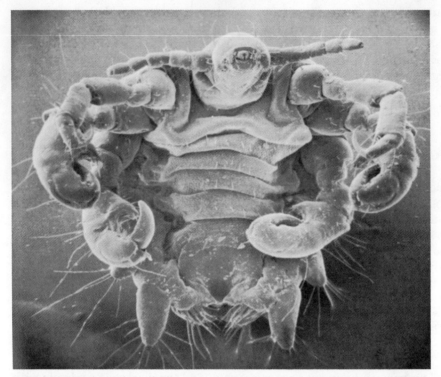

Figure 16–4. A human crab louse, seen from underneath (× 150). The thick legs and large claws are used to grasp hair shafts on the host. (From Kogan, B. A.: *Health — Brief Edition.* New York, Harcourt, Brace Jovanovich, 1976, p. 73.)

itch a great deal. They can, in fact, be caught from toilet seats or clothing, but the more frequent mode of transmission is sexual contact. (Gonorrhea and syphilis are not caught from toilet seats. The germs producing these diseases die when they get dry.)

Treatment. The lice are killed by Kwell (Rx) lotion or shampoo or certain other lotions. Clothes and bedding must be washed well or cleaned when the individual is treated.

Scabies

Scabies is produced by tiny mites that cause problems much like those created by crab lice. These mites differ from crab lice because they may infect not only the pubic area but also the hands and elsewhere. They create small, red, itchy bumps or lines by burrowing into the skin, and they are eliminated by the same medication used for crab lice. Scabies is transmitted by close personal contact, such as by sleeping with another person.

GENERAL PROBLEMS

Mononucleosis

This disease occurs most commonly among young adults. It is caused by a virus that is probably transmitted through respiratory droplets, that is, through the air or close personal contact. Fortunately, it is not very contagious, so other family members or roommates generally do not catch the disease. The incubation period is several weeks.

Mononucleosis generally lasts from two to four weeks. It often begins with a feeling of tiredness for several days; then fever and sore throat follow, and enlarged, tender lymph nodes usually develop, first in the neck. Lymph nodes under the arms and in the groin also frequently become enlarged and tender. Initially, it may be hard for the physician to distinguish mononucleosis from other viral illnesses or from strep throat. A few more days may have to pass before blood tests become helpful.

Treatment.   There is no specific treatment for mononucleosis. The sore throat can be alleviated with salt water gargles and aspirin. Bedrest is appropriate when the victim feels tired or has a fever. Otherwise, moderate activity is permissible. Athletic practice should be avoided, not only because of tiredness and other symptoms but also because the disease can affect heart muscle as well as skeletal muscles. The liver is usually also affected, which may result in an ache or tenderness under the right lower ribs. Blood tests that evaluate liver function may be abnormal for a number of weeks.

The spleen becomes enlarged in about half the victims. It is then more likely to rupture during athletics, especially in contact sports. This causes bleeding into the abdomen and requires immediate surgery to prevent death. Therefore, the athlete should not resume sports until the spleen has returned to normal size, which may take several weeks after the individual feels well. Occasionally, recovery may take two or three months. Following recovery, the individual is immune to the disease.

Viral Hepatitis

Hepatitis is a general term meaning inflammation of the liver. Hepatitis can be caused by microorganisms, alcohol, drugs, or other agents. *Viral hepatitis* is a relatively common disease that is caused by a virus, of which there are two types. Infectious hepatitis (type A) is generally spread by direct contact with an infected individual or by contact with items touched by that individual (fecal-oral contamination). Serum hepatitis (type B) is spread mainly through blood transfusions or use of contaminated needles, but can also be passed by sexual contact or close personal contact.

Infectious hepatitis often begins with tiredness and loss of appetite, sometimes accompanied by flulike symptoms (runny nose, sore throat, cough, and fever). Over several days, the skin and eyes may become yellow (jaundiced) because the liver functions improperly and allows accumulation of certain metabolic products in the blood stream. Often the liver becomes enlarged and causes an abdominal ache under the right ribs. The main treatment is rest. Frequently the individual is isolated until convalescence begins. Infectious hepatitis generally lasts a month or more. The athlete can gradually return to participation when he feels well, has no jaundice, and has a normal-sized liver, and when tests of liver function are nearly normal. Serum hepatitis is a similar disease but is frequently more severe and lasts longer.

Travel

Motion Sickness.   Persons who tend to become nauseated because of motion can take one of the standard nonprescription medications (Bonine, Marezine, Dramamine) one-half to one hour before departure. These pills may also alleviate unexpected motion sickness during travel if the victim is not actively vomiting. Such medications make many people sleepy and should be avoided for several hours before competition.

Diarrhea. (See page 259.)

Ear Pain During Flying (Aerotitis Media). Some people have trouble "popping" their ears (opening the eustachian tube) when planes change altitude, especially when landing. (See also page 346.) A cold or allergy can create this problem. Try chewing gum or swallowing as pressure changes. Decongestant cold tablets or nasal sprays may help when the problem is serious.

Jet Lag. The body has natural daily rhythms, such as sleep, which are called circadian cycles. These cycles may be forced to change when a person travels between time zones. Some people require about one day for each hour of time change in order to readjust their sleep habits. In international travel, competitors should arrive a sufficient number of days ahead of time to allow for adjustment and to permit optimal performance. Temporary use of a mild sleeping medication for a day or two may help. Those travelling only briefly to a new time zone may find it more effective to remain on a schedule according to their home time if possible.

The air in jetliners is dry, and passengers tend to become dehydrated. Therefore, make a point of drinking considerable nonalcoholic liquid. In addition, walk around every half hour or so when not sleeping in order to prevent cramping and problems of decreased circulation in the legs.

Immunizations. Travel to Europe presently requires no special immunizations. Travel to other areas may, in which case appropriate medical advice should be obtained several months ahead of time to permit a series of immunizations if necessary.

Everyone should have completed a basic series of immunizations against tetanus, diphtheria, and poliomyelitis. This is usually done in early childhood. A booster immunization against tetanus should be obtained routinely every 10 years in the general population or at least every five years in athletes because wounds are more likely to occur. Tetanus (lockjaw) is a disease produced by bacteria *(Clostridium tetani)* that normally live in the intestine of humans and animals and in the soil. These bacteria can multiply and produce toxin in deep wounds, such as punctures, where they are not exposed to the oxygen of air. The result is spasms of skeletal muscles and convulsions, with death occurring in half of the unimmunized victims. Immunization against tetanus toxin is highly effective, and thorough cleansing of wounds helps to prevent infection.

SUMMARY

This chapter discussed medical problems, other than injuries, that are common among athletes. The object is to improve health and minimize lost time. Causes, symptoms, and certain treatments were explained so that the athlete can help to prevent these problems or, if they occur, can treat them or know when to see a physician.

STUDY QUESTIONS

1. List several danger signs or symptoms that indicate that infection is spreading from a small lesion on the foot to other parts of the body.

2. A wrestler has an infection on his face that may be impetigo. Of what potential danger is this to the individual and to his teammates?

3. What is the appropriate treatment for a small abrasion (scrape) on the arm acquired during a game?

4. Give the treatment for a mild case of athlete's foot.

5. Two days after jogging in the woods, an individual noticed red, itchy bumps and streaks on his legs, face, and chest, even though he had been wearing a shirt. What, if anything, should be done with his running clothes and shoes?

6. It is your first day at the beach for the summer. What precautions should you take?

7. Why should penicillin or other antibiotics not be used for treatment of the common cold?

8. Should an individual with a fever exercise vigorously? Why?

9. You are participating in a world championship where randomly chosen competitors must undergo testing for "doping." You have a cold. Is it wise to take a standard cold tablet (containing an antihistamine and a decongestant) the evening before your event?

10. Why bother taking penicillin or other antibiotics for the prescribed 10 days for "strep throat," even though you feel well after two days?

11. A player standing at the sidelines with a possible sprained wrist says that he feels dizzy. What should you do?

12. In the usual cases of food poisoning, why are drugs to stop vomiting and diarrhea used very little?

13. Your tendinitis has been helped greatly during the past week by taking aspirin four times a day. Off and on for the past two days you have had an annoying ache in the upper abdomen. Give one likely cause.

14. Why should routine urine testing be done before, rather than after, a daily practice?

15. List the symptoms of nongonococcal urethritis.

16. Can crab lice be caught from a toilet seat?

17. Is mononucleosis highly contagious?

18. Why are contact sports not permitted when the spleen is enlarged following mononucleosis?

19. Why should tetanus immunization be kept current in participants in sports?

FURTHER READINGS

Thorn, G. W. (ed.): *Harrison's Principles of Internal Medicine*. New York, McGraw-Hill Book Company, 1977.

Krupp, M. A., and Chatton, M. H.: *Current Medical Diagnosis and Treatment*. Los Altos, Calif., Lange Medical Publications, 1978.

Vickery, D. M., and Fries, J. F.: *Take Care of Yourself — A Consumer's Guide to Medical Care*. Reading, Mass., Addison-Wesley, 1976.

SECTION 4

SPECIAL TOPICS IN SPORTS MEDICINE

This section deals with special groups, environments, and problems. The chapters can be read selectively or, for an overview, in total.

17

NUTRITION AND THE ATHLETE

NATHAN J. SMITH, M.D.

Diet is important in determining available energy and body composition, both of which are of concern to the serious athlete. The amount of body fat should be kept to a minimum in contestants of those sports that match participants on the basis of weight (wrestling, lightweight crew) and of those in which the most efficient ratio of strength to body weight is advantageous (gymnastics, distance running, figure skating). Adequate hydration (water in the body) provides an advantage for all athletes in sports that expend a great deal of energy, and muscle glycogen has been shown to be important in contests that involve prolonged periods of aerobic exercise (distance running, cross-country skiing, rowing, middle- and long-distance swimming). The coach, trainer, and team physician can help to optimize the performance of the athlete by providing guidance concerning healthy eating practices. Advice should indicate how diet can best meet the energy demands of a specific sport, how body fatness can be reduced safely, and how healthy gains in weight can be made.

THE ATHLETE'S DIET

The athlete is highly motivated to improve performance and usually recognizes that food intake may have an influence on it. Unfortunately, poor and even dangerous advice is abundantly available, based on myth, superstition, or the tradition of a given sport. Most readily obtainable is "locker room" advice, which generally lacks any factual basis. Sound nutritional counselling usually is well accepted and, in the young student, may initiate a lifelong program of good eating habits.

Day-to-day dietary practices of the active athlete should be centered on regular mealtime eating in an enjoyable setting with pleasant associates. The food selection should be varied, using the "four food group" plan. This plan (Fig. 17–1) requires two servings of high-protein foods (meat, fish, poultry, legumes); two servings of dairy foods (milk, yogurt, cheese, ice cream); four servings of fruits and vegetables; and four servings of cereal and grain foods. Although these 12 servings will provide all the essential nutrients that the athlete needs (except iron for some women), they supply only 1400 to 1500 kilocalories (kcal),* which is insufficient. Second servings and other

*A kilocalorie (abbreviated *kcal*) is the amount of energy required to raise 1 kilogram of water 1 degree Celsius (centigrade). The "calorie" that is commonly used in nutrition (e.g., in the newspaper) is equivalent to one kilocalorie. One apple furnishes about 100 kcal energy.

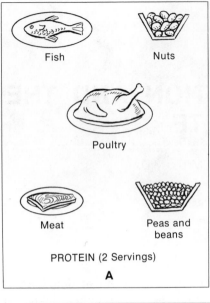

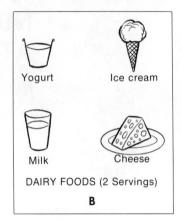

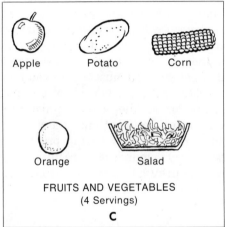

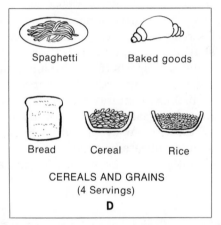

Figure 17–1. The "four food group" plan provides the daily essential nutrients, vitamins, and minerals necessary for an active athlete. Examples of each group are shown. Additional quantities of food are required to provide sufficient calories.

foods such as desserts will provide the necessary additional calories. Some persons, particularly those who are not of northern European origin, do not eat dairy foods because they cannot digest lactose, a sugar found in cow's milk. In such cases, the remaining food groups can furnish sufficient variety for a balanced diet.

Some high-school and college athletes follow a meatless diet consisting of fruits, vegetables, milk, and eggs. Such diets can meet the needs of the athlete if appropriately varied as described in a "six food group" plan for meatless diets. Beans, eggs, nuts, and milk products help to satisfy the large caloric needs of these athletes as well as to provide high-quality protein.

In order to reduce the chances of heart disease later in life, some authorities recommend that male athletes limit fat intake, particularly saturated fats (animal fats). The American Heart Association's "Prudent Diet for American Men" recommends reducing fat to 30 to 35 per cent of total calories, with 10 per cent of the calories contributed by saturated fat. A reduction in customary salt intake is also commonly recommended and is accomplished by avoiding excessive intake of salty foods and by not adding table salt to prepared foods. A reduction of salt intake is thought by some to prevent retention of excess intercellular water and to contribute to the athlete's feeling of fitness.

Selection of an appropriately varied diet following the "four food group" plan is not difficult, considering the typical American food supply. Such a diet will satisfy the needs of the athlete. *Vitamin, mineral, protein, or energy supplements are not necessary.* Although widely used by participants in many sports, such supplements are expensive, useless, and potentially dangerous. Athletes are advised to avoid them.

Among young athletes, there are two factors that commonly interfere with proper diet. These are the cost of a good diet and the lack of a regular meal schedule. The high cost of food necessary for the active adolescent athlete often cannot be met by families with low incomes. At all income levels, young athletes often live with disorganized families or by themselves, where the setting for pleasant and effective mealtime eating does not exist. Irregular and inadequate food intake is commonly encountered in many of these economic or socially compromised circumstances. Even when he receives three good meals a day, the large, growing adolescent in a sport that expends a lot of energy, such as basketball, may need additional midmorning or midafternoon "before practice" snacks to provide for his energy needs. *When an athlete underperforms, find out whether he is getting enough to eat.*

MEETING SPECIFIC ENERGY NEEDS IN VARIOUS SPORTS

Various sports require specific energy sources or combinations of energy sources. The three main sources of energy are phosphocreatine (PC) and ATP in muscle; the anaerobic metabolism of muscle glycogen; and the aerobic metabolism of fat, glucose, and glycogen. Certain activities such as the short sprints, shot-put, high jump, and pole vault require only brief bursts of energy that are provided anaerobically from ATP and PC in muscles. Competitions requiring intense energy expenditure over more prolonged periods, such as crew races, wrestling matches, and middle-distance and long-distance running and swimming races, call upon the aerobic metabolism of muscle glycogen. The length of time that an athlete can maintain a high level of performance in these events is determined in part by the glycogen content of muscles. In endurance events, after anaerobic glycogen metabolism has made its contribution, additional energy comes from the aerobic metabolism of glycogen, glucose, and fat. Attention to certain dietary factors can increase the effectiveness of these three overlapping sources of muscle energy. Optimum performance requires the basic diet described previously, good hydration, and periodic carbohydrate intake during the day of a contest. Sufficient time should be allowed between competing performances for the regeneration of optimum levels of ATP and PC.

Glycogen Loading

The amount of glycogen stored in a muscle can affect the endurance of that muscle. This becomes important in sports that require hard work over a considerable time (i.e., sports in which glycogen is metabolized aerobically over a considerable time). Such sports include cross-country skiing, distance running, and the longer swimming events. Through dietary manipulation, the glycogen stored in muscle can be increased up to three times the normal level (glycogen loading), and endurance can be increased somewhat. To accomplish this, a six-day program is followed.

For the first three days, carbohydrate is severely restricted (100 grams or 400 kcal per day). Proteins and fats provide necessary calories. The muscles involved in the sport are exercised heavily each day in order to help deplete muscle glycogen. During days four through six, the athlete can eat what he wishes but should include 1000 to 1500 kcal of carbohydrate each day. Residue-free carbohydrates are most easily obtained as sugared beverages and candies. A quart of Kool-Aid plus a 12-ounce bag of jelly beans is a readily available source of over 1000 residue-free kcal. Spaghettis, pies, and pastries provide unnecessary bulk. (The pregame meal is discussed later in this chapter.)

A week of dietary preparation should be used very selectively for the serious high-school or college-age competitor before an important competition. In some people, glycogen loading results in a feeling of muscular stiffness. Rarely, if ever, should such dietary preparation be used for the early adolescent or preadolescent athlete.

WATER AND ELECTROLYTE NEEDS OF THE ATHLETE

Water

Water is a nutrient critical to athletic performance and, in certain situations, critical to the athlete's safety. The complex chemical reactions involved in the production of muscular energy take place in water and can be compromised if the body's water content is less than optimal. Essential nutrients and metabolic by-products are transported to and from body tissues in aqueous media. In addition, body water plays a critical role in transporting heat from working muscle cells to the body surface, where it is dissipated — often through the evaporation of sweat.

A young adult male requires about 2.5 liters of water a day when pursuing normal activities in a temperate environment. Strenuous athletic activity increases the water requirement. Younger individuals have a relatively large body surface area for their weight. Thus, the preadolescent "little league" athlete has an even greater requirement for water per unit body weight. Water from the metabolism of food contributes as much as one fifth of the normal water requirement, but the major sources of water are beverages and the water contained in food. In some instances, these two water sources may contribute equally to meeting water needs. Regular mealtimes with proper food and liquid intake help to ensure an optimal level of hydration.

The body's water content is maintained primarily through sensitive control of urine volume and to a lesser degree by the mechanism of thirst. It is important to recognize that thirst is a very insensitive indicator of water need, particularly in the athlete experiencing the tensions and anxieties of competition. Water lack that interferes with performance can develop before thirst is recognized. Scheduled water intakes should be provided during competition to insure adequate hydration. In those sports having day-long or even two- or three-day periods of competition (track, swimming, tennis, wrestling meets), three meals a day should be planned and regular water intakes scheduled. In warm weather when high-energy expenditure is involved, even more frequent consumption of relatively large volumes of water may be required.

Good hydration is necessary to prevent heat stroke. Participants in distance running, bicycle racing, and American football are particularly susceptible to heat disorders resulting from inadequate fluid replacement.

The American College of Sports Medicine has issued a position statement on the prevention of heat injury in distance running (see Appendix B). Athletes participating in distance races (greater than 10 miles or 16 kilometers) should ingest 400 to 500 ml of a dilute aqueous beverage 10 to 15 minutes prior to the start of the race. In addition, there should be drinking stations every 2.0 to 2.5 miles. Certain other conditions have been recommended to assure safety in these events.

Specific recommendations can be made regarding the safe conduct of football games and practices during warm and humid weather. (See also Chapter 21.) For practices early in the season players should wear uniforms of light-colored sleeveless shirts, shorts, and helmets. Water intake should be mandatory every 35 to 45 minutes during practice, and nude weighing before and after each practice is essential. The player who reports for practice with a residual weight loss of more than 2 to 3 per cent of body weight from a preceding practice should not be permitted to participate until adequate fluid intake has corrected his body weight deficit. Scheduled fluid intake and regular meals will replace the large water losses often experienced in football.

Heat stroke is preventable, and the deaths that continue to occur because of heat stroke in sports programs are as needless as they are tragic. A water-deprived athlete, exercising vigorously, cannot effectively transport and dissipate body heat. Heat stroke then becomes a very real possibility, and if it occurs, demands immediate emergency treatment.

Less threatening, but still damaging to the athlete's ability to perform, are the dehydrating practices frequently adopted by athletes attempting to "make weight," as in wrestling, lightweight crew, and junior football. Sweating induced by heat or by exercise in plastic suits, as well as the use of diuretics ("water pills") and cathartics, results in dehydration with varying degrees of water and electrolyte (salt) depletion. With as little as 2 to 3 per cent of body weight lost as body water, endurance and ability to dissipate body heat will be affected adversely. Weight control for competition should not involve any depletion of body water.

Electrolyte Needs

Electrolyte solutions are almost never needed to replace salt lost through sweating. A host of beverages containing salts and sugars have appeared on the market, but the need is more imagined than real. In all but the most exceptional circumstances, salt balance can be maintained optimally by eating regular meals that are salted to individual taste and by drinking adequate amounts of water. The kidneys and sweat glands help to conserve salt, when necessary, by decreasing the amount of salt excreted.

Excessive intake of salt (as occurs with the use of salt pills), combined with limited water intake, results in intracellular dehydration, with all of its handicaps and dangers. Many commercial electrolyte drinks have osmolarities (concentrations) sufficiently high to result in fluid retention within the stomach and small intestine and distress in the upper abdomen. Adequate water and regular food intake are the most effective and safest means of maintain the body's electrolytes.

WEIGHT CONTROL IN SPORTS

For many athletes, attempts to reach and maintain a desired weight for competition can lead to dietary abuses that threaten health and limit ability to compete. In sports in which competitors are matched by weight, athletes sometimes try to reach their lowest possible weight through large weight reductions in a few days. In contrast, participants in contact sports such as football or ice hockey often wish to increase body weight in order to optimize their performance potential.

Gaining Body Weight

The active athlete who desires to increase body weight may seek professional consultation after weeks of unsuccessful effort. Failures are usually due to: (1) lack of appreciation for the amount of food required to create a positive caloric balance in a large, active, young individual; (2) lack of a rigidly structured schedule of food intake; or (3) on occasion, insufficient financial resources to provide the large amount of food required.

Approximately 2500 kcal are required to create 1 pound of lean body tissue. An extra 1000 kcal each day will allow a weight gain of about 2 pounds per week. This is approximately the maximum rate of weight gain of lean body mass that can be expected. The athlete may require anywhere from 4000 to 6000 kcal or even more for weight maintenance with heavy exercise. For an intake of an additional 1000 kcal, diet counselling is required. An example of a high-calorie diet is given in Table 17–1. It is important that only 30 to 35 per cent of the calories be contributed by fat. Most of the fat should be unsaturated (of vegetable origin). High-calorie foods and snacks that include margarines, salad oils, nuts, or peanut butter can be used liberally.

The most commonly encountered factor that frustrates the athlete's efforts to gain

TABLE 17–1.   HIGH-CALORIE DIET FOR GAINING BODY WEIGHT*

Breakfast	Snack
½ cup orange juice 1 cup oatmeal 1 cup low-fat milk 1 scrambled egg 1 slice whole-wheat toast 1½ teaspoons margarine 1 tablespoon jam	1 peanut butter sandwich 1 banana 1 cup grape juice Total: 485 kcal
Total: 665 kcal	
Lunch	**Snack**
5 fish sticks tartar sauce large serving, French fries green salad with avocado and French dressing 1 cup lemon sherbet 2 granola cookies 1 cup low-fat milk	1 cup mixed dried fruit 1½ cups malted milk Total: 660 kcal
Total: 1505 kcal	
Dinner	**Snack**
1 cup cream of mushroom soup 2 pieces oven-baked chicken candied sweet potato 1 dinner roll and margarine 1 cup carrots and peas ½ cup coleslaw 1 piece cherry pie beverage	1 cup cashew nuts 1 cup cocoa Total: 1045 kcal
Total: 1615 kcal	
	Daily Total: 5975 kcal

*Adapted from Smith, N. J.: *Food for Sport.* Palo Alto, Calif., Bull Publishing Company, 1976.

weight is the inability of the active, overcommitted person to eat four to six times a day. Consumption of four or more pleasant, unhurried meals every day is the best way to achieve the necessary caloric intake. Current life styles are often incompatible with such eating patterns.

Any gain in weight should be in the form of lean body mass (muscle). Thus, fatness should be evaluated every two weeks by measuring the thickness of skin-fat folds. Increasing fatness should prompt a reduction in caloric intake and an increase in energy expenditure.

The athlete desiring to gain weight must know that only muscle work will increase muscle mass. No particular food, vitamin, drug, or hormone will increase muscle size in the absence of muscle work. The recommended diet has no specific increase in proteins or vitamins. Most foods that are rich in animal protein (red meats, eggs, dairy products) are also high in saturated animal fats and should not be prominent in the athlete's weight-gaining regimen. The muscle work needed to increase muscle mass should be prescribed by the coach or trainer and usually includes exercise with weights or other resistance devices.

Each year, in an attempt to increase their abilities as football players, hundreds of thousands of high-school boys make themselves overfat on diets rich in animal protein and thus high in saturated fats. These dietary activities, which are often encouraged by coaches and parents, probably constitute the most serious nutrition-related abuses in sports today. On occasion, the health and performance of the athlete are further jeopardized by the unethical use of anabolic steroids (e.g., Dianabol; see Appendix B) and other drugs (e.g., Periactin) that are ineffective and potentially dangerous.

Reducing Body Weight

Many athletes need to achieve an optimal ratio of muscle mass and strength to body weight. This can be accomplished only by reducing body fat to a healthy minimum. In high-school and college wrestlers the minimum amount of body fat that is safe is approximately 5 per cent of body weight. Similar levels of body fatness are desirable in gymnasts, distance runners, lightweight oarsmen, and others. The few limited studies to date suggest that women, as well as men, compete in these sports most effectively when an estimated 5 per cent of their body weight is fat. These estimates of body fat are most commonly made by using a caliper such as the Lange skin fold caliper (Cambridge Scientific Instrument Co., Cambridge, Maryland).

In counselling the athlete regarding weight reduction, body fatness is estimated and the desired amount of fat loss is calculated. The rate of fat loss should be no more than 3 to 4 pounds each week; a 2-pound weekly loss is more desirable. More rapid weight loss often involves the loss of muscle mass and is not compatible with effective training or performance. Thus, the loss of more than a few pounds of body fat demands a significant period of time. The team physician, coach, or trainer is well advised to initiate concern about competing weights and fatness long before the beginning of the competing season.

Fatness is reduced by *increasing energy expenditure and moderately reducing energy intake*. One pound of body fat is equivalent to approximately 3500 kcal of stored energy. Thus, a daily caloric deficit of 1000 kcal will mobilize the energy of 2 pounds of fat each week. Such a caloric deficit is best accomplished by adding an hour each day of active training and by subtracting 500 to 750 kcal from the diet normally required for weight maintenance. Total daily intake should not be less than 2000 kcal for most male athletes or 1600 kcal for most females. Such intakes, selected from the four food groups, can provide all essential nutrients (Table 17-2). More severely restricted caloric intakes may result in loss of muscle mass.

TABLE 17–2. LOW-CALORIE DIET FOR REDUCING BODY WEIGHT*

Breakfast	Snack
½ cup orange juice 1 soft-boiled egg 1 slice whole-wheat toast 2 teaspoons margarine 1 glass skim milk or other beverage	1 banana Total: 100 kcal
Total: 345 kcal	
Lunch	**Snack**

hamburger (3 ounces) on a
  roll with relish
½ sliced tomato
1 glass skim milk
1 medium apple
	1 carton fruit-flavored
	  yogurt
	1 cup grape juice
	
	Total: 385 kcal

Total: 510 kcal	
Dinner	
baked chicken marengo (½ breast) ¾ cup rice 5–6 Brussel sprouts green salad with French dressing 1 small piece gingerbread 1 cup skim milk or other beverage	
Total: 660 kcal	
	Daily Total: 2000 kcal

*Adapted from Smith, N. J.: *Food for Sport.* Palo Alto, Calif., Bull Publishing Company, 1976.

Specific advice for weight reduction includes avoiding foods of high caloric density and keeping records of food intake and training activities.Often, all the athlete must do to have an effective diet is to eat a *single modest serving* of the menu items served at the dormitory or at family mealtime and to *avoid desserts and between-meal snacks.* Raw vegetables, water, or diet colas may be used occasionally as "lifesaving" snacks. Increasing caloric expenditure through increased daily exercise is essential.

Weight reduction programs for athletes must be based on (1) measurements to determine the approximate amount of existing fat and (2) an estimate of desired fatness. Sufficient time for fat reduction must be allowed to permit the intake of a nutritious diet and continued effective participation in training.

As noted earlier, wrestlers and certain other athletes sometimes attempt to lose weight rapidly through sweating. Their methods include exercising in a rubber suit or sitting in a sauna. Weight loss in this manner is exclusively water; it is regained when the individual drinks liquids and returns to normal hydration. No fat is lost through this process. Such dehydration methods are sometimes practiced by wrestlers during the 24 hours before weighing-in as a desperate attempt to reach a lower weight class. Weighing-in is usually done a few hours before competition, and during the intervening time the wrestler attempts to drink sufficient water to return to normal hydration. However, strength and endurance cannot return to normal within this short period, so the individual's performance is impaired.

THE PREGAME MEAL

Food intake prior to competition can be a problem. The uninformed individual experiencing the tensions of competition, armed with myths and superstitions regarding the influence of food on ability to compete, will often respond in one of two ways. Either food and fluid intake will be avoided completely, or they will be excessive. In both instances, the result can be disastrous.

The following guidelines indicate a desirable preparticipation intake of food and liquid:

1. Intake should be sufficient to insure that hunger and weakness due to lack of food do not occur during competition.
2. The type of food and time of eating should be such that the stomach and upper intestine are empty at game time.
3. Food and fluid intake should contribute to an optimal state of hydration.
4. Foods that could transmit disease (e.g., cream pies) should be avoided.
5. The menu should include familiar foods and particularly those foods that the athlete may be convinced will "make him win."

The football team's traditional steak breakfast or a large midday "banquet" for the basketball team fails to satisfy many of these goals. Fat leaves the stomach slowly. If eaten sufficiently early to leave the stomach empty at game time, the large, high-fat steak meal will also leave many players hungry. The large protein intake of such meals may compromise hydration by inducing urinary water loss. Also, after such a large meal the intestinal tract will be burdened with considerable food residue. A good pregame meal is relatively high in carbohydrate; is low in fat, bulk, and salt; and has abundant liquid. An example of such a meal is sandwiches made with lean meat (lean beef, chicken, etc.), jello salad, fruit punch, sherbet, and cookies or angel food cake (Fig. 17–2). The meal should be eaten two to three hours before competition. With some modification it can be provided by the school cafeteria or even "brown-bagged" by a low-budget travelling team.

In recent years, complete liquid meals have become popular with some athletes, particularly those who find their upper gastrointestinal tract the target of preparticipation anxiety. These commercially available products (Ensure-plus, Nutri-1000, etc.) satisfy the requirements of a pregame meal listed above. Home liquid-meal concoctions (instant breakfasts, etc.) are usually less than adequate because of poor flavor, excessive protein and electrolyte contents, and insufficient caloric contribution.

Sherbet

Cookies

Jello salad

Fruit punch

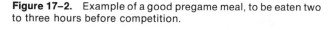

Figure 17–2. Example of a good pregame meal, to be eaten two to three hours before competition.

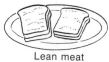
Lean meat
sandwiches

Some athletes like tea and honey before a game. However, after a few cups of tea, caffeine "jitters" can develop in the young athlete who is not accustomed to caffeine-containing beverages, and upper abdominal distress can develop from the osmotically induced fluid accumulation that follows a generous intake of honey. Moderation is the rule in all pregame food intake.

IRON DEFICIENCY

Iron deficiency anemia has long been known to result in decreased ability to do physical work. More recently, studies reveal that iron depletion even without anemia may cause compromised muscle performance and thus may affect athletic performance. Recent surveys have documented iron depletion in as many as 20 per cent of women 12 to 45 years of age in all income groups, and in even greater numbers of teen-age males in poverty populations. Thus, many athletes may be attempting to compete while limited in endurance and muscle function by inadequate sources of available iron.

Women with larger than average losses of iron associated with menstruation do not meet their iron needs even on a well-selected American diet. (This is the only recognized nutritional need not met by a diet selection based on the four food group plan.) These people should be identified and advised to take a daily medicinal supplement providing 15 to 20 mg of elemental iron. Women athletes who use intrauterine devices for contraception are at particular risk of iron depletion resulting from an associated increase in menstrual iron loss. They should take an iron supplement. Teen-age boys on diets inadequate to meet their needs of rapid growth of lean body mass will become iron-deficient. This situation is most frequently encountered in low-income families. In such cases, administration of therapeutic iron is indicated and steps should be taken to increase the availability of food. Iron depletion and even frank iron deficiency anemia are encountered with such frequency that a biochemical assessment of iron status should be included in the preparticipation health evaluation of all female athletes.

SUMMARY

The athlete depends on food to meet the energy requirements of competition. A well-planned, mixed American diet eaten regularly will meet the maintenance needs of the athlete. On occasion, this diet may be varied to optimize energy availability for certain kinds of competition. The athlete should maintain good hydration before and during competition.

Dietary intake often requires modification when an individual wishes to increase or decrease body weight. Reducing body weight (fatness) is accomplished by increasing energy expenditure in training as well as by moderately reducing food intake. Increasing body weight (muscle mass) requires muscular work and a moderate increase in food intake.

An athlete's pregame meal should be well planned in order to avoid overeating as well as hunger, weakness, and poor hydration. When an athlete underperforms, evaluate food intake and be sure that it is adequate to meet the energy needs of training and competition. Vitamin, mineral, and protein supplements have no place in the diet of a healthy athlete.

STUDY QUESTIONS

1. Describe a diet based on the four food groups.

2. Record all the food you eat in a 24-hour period and determine whether the four food groups are appropriately represented.

3. Describe the dietary management of glycogen loading.

4. Describe a desired program of electrolyte replacement during early season football workouts.

5. Describe the role of body water in maintenance of normal body temperature.

6. Describe the essentials of a program to prevent heat stroke in early football season practices.

7. Describe an appropriate weight reduction program for a high-school wrestler.

8. To whom would it be appropriate to prescribe a dietary supplement?

9. List five qualities of a good pregame meal.

10. Why is a pregame meal of steak, broccoli, baked potato, rolls, cake, and ice cream undesirable?

11. List two groups of individuals involved in athletic programs who are at greatest risk for iron deficiency.

FURTHER READINGS

Bergstrom, J., and Hultman, E.: Nutrition for maximal sports performance (glycogen loading). J.A.M.A. *221*:991, 1972.

Blix, G. (ed.): *Nutrition and Physical Activity Symposium of the Swedish Nutrition Foundation.* Uppsala, Sweden, 1967.

Claremont, A. D., Costill, D. L., Fun, W., and Van Haudel, P.: Heat tolerance following diuretic induced dehydration. Med. Sci. Sports *8*:239, 1976.

Frasier, A. D.: Androgens and athletes. Am. J. Dis. Child. *125*:479, 1973.

Lewis, S., and Gretin, B.: Nutrition and endurance. Am. J. Clin. Nutr. *26*:1011–1014, 1973.

Mathews, D. K., and Fox, E. L.: *The Physiological Basis of Physical Education and Athletics,* 2nd ed. Philadelphia, W. B. Saunders Company, 1976.

Smith, N. J.: *Food for Sport.* Palo Alto, Calif., Bull Publishing Company, 1976.

Smith, N. J., and Rios, E.: Iron metabolism and iron deficiency. Adv. Pediatr. *21*:239, 1975.

18

THE YOUNG ATHLETE — AN OVERVIEW

NATHAN J. SMITH, M.D.

THE SOCIAL SETTING

A generation or two ago, the typical adolescent high-school athlete was a boy who participated in two or three of a relatively small number of interscholastic team sports available in his school. He may have played organized baseball in the summer months and, if asked why he took part in sports, he probably would have replied, "For the fun of it!" His high-school student sister did not have an opportunity to participate in interscholastic sports. During elementary or junior high school, the sports experience of both boys and girls was generated with neighborhood children in spontaneous, unsupervised play after school hours and during summer vacation.

How different things are today! Currently there are 32 sports approved for interscholastic competition for boys and 25 for girls, with nearly 6 million high-school students participating. In addition, it is difficult to think of a sport that is not available in a highly organized form for the preadolescent, elementary school-age boy or girl. These programs include a broad spectrum of sports such as baseball, age-group soccer, swimming, gymnastics, and martial arts. The programs are usually community-based, with untrained volunteer coaching and volunteer parent supervision.

The enormous expansion in scholastic and community-based age-group sports has resulted from several contributing forces active in present-day society. First, American economic affluence is able to support the considerable cost of these programs. For example, equipping one 10-year-old participant in a Pop Warner football program may cost more than 150 dollars. Second, opportunities for spontaneous active play by preadolescent boys and girls have become extremely limited in the restrictive environment of urban and suburban residential areas. Active, energy-expending recreation in this setting must be organized, planned, and scheduled. Because such play programs involve significant numbers of children, they become an athletic team experience — a sports program. Also, in poverty-stricken areas, many young people are drawn into intense participation in sports programs at an early age as they or their parents envision the potential for education (a realistic means of overcoming poverty) and wealth through a career as a professional athlete.

The increase in the variety of sports participated in by high-school students reflects a greater desire for sports in which there is less intensity of commitment, more individual competition, and in some instances, the opportunity for lifelong participation. Sports such as distance running, rowing, tennis, and golf attract increasing numbers of participants. They provide excellent alternatives for those girls or boys not prepared physically or emotionally for intense participation in the more traditional programs of football, basketball, or ice hockey.

One can look with satisfaction on the recent expansion of available community sport activities for young people. These programs provide the exercise that vitally contributes to health and fitness. There are additional important needs that a well-managed athletic program can satisfy for the child coming from a single-parent home. (Today, nearly one in five American children live in single-parent homes.) In urban areas, the alternative to such programs is unsupervised play in the streets or in limited play space — an unattractive, high-risk alternative. If active recreation is to be found in community-based sports programs for young children, trained professionals concerned with recreation, child development, health, and safety must be ready to define specific goals and appropriate conduct for these children and work to upgrade the community's athletic activities.

THE UNIQUENESS OF THE YOUNG ATHLETE

Growth is the single quality that is unique to the young athlete. It produces change in body size, proportion, and composition; increase in strength; change in body functions; and, most particularly, maturation of behavior.

The susceptibility of the growing musculoskeletal system to injury is discussed in the following chapter. Strength development in response to training is different for the prepubertal athlete compared with his postpubertal counterpart. The increase in fatness that occurs in 8- to 10-year-old boys should be recognized as a normal antecedent to the upcoming demanding pubertal growth spurt, not an indication of being "out of shape" and in need of a demanding, intense conditioning program. With the onset of pubertal growth, the needs for nutrition and rest increase enormously. These important consequences of normal growth must be considered in the training and competitive behavior of the child athlete.

Two aspects of the young athlete's maturing behavior dominate his relationship to sports particpation.First is the normal evolution of independence that increases as the school experience starts and is finally achieved during adolescence. Independence can be fostered by the relationship with a team, the responsibilities of team membership, the establishment of positive responses to coaching, and winning and losing. Second is the preadolescent's desire and need for acceptance. As he starts school, expands his social contacts, and spends an increasing number of hours away from the accepting environment of home, acceptance must be found among a wide circle of peers or adults. Acceptance by teammates, peers, coaches, and even parents is of utmost importance. The young athlete soon recognizes that athletic excellence is a sure route to highly prized acceptance, and failure on the athletic field can be costly in terms of acceptance. Thus, endless hours of training in the swim program, standing "scared to death" in the batter's box, or "sticking it" to your football opponent may be a high price to pay, but when it results in winning, the rewards are considerable. The young boy or girl athlete should be encouraged to participate in sports but his or her desire for acceptance should not be exploited through adult and parent dominated programs in which fun and development of skills are secondary.

THE PREPARTICIPATION EXAMINATION

The preparticipation evaluation of the young athlete is of particular importance because it may be the first time that his or her health has been evaluated for suitability for an athletic program. Size, maturity, and level of conditioning can be assessed to determine whether the proposed sport is suitable for this particular individual. Such counselling is of particular importance as long as schooling and eligibility for sports participation is based on chronological age. The great variability in rates of maturation places many normal, but late-maturing, individuals at a competing disadvantage and at risk to injury in several sports. On the other hand, the early maturer playing with individuals of similar chronological age may be inappropriately held back from competition with competitors more suited to his level of skill, size, and maturity.

The wide range of ages at which pubertal development begins requires that some documentation of pubertal development be part of the young athlete's preparticipation evaluation. The onset of the menstrual experience is a suitable index for girls. Recording the stage of pubic hair development is a reliable indicator in boys (Fig. 18–1) and is easily accomplished during the health appraisal. Collision, contact sports (football, wrestling, lacrosse, and ice hockey) should not be recommended for boys until they have reached stage 5 development. On the other hand, the highly skilled junior high-school athlete with grade 4 or 5 pubic hair development may be a suitable participant in many high-school programs. Health professionals must continue to urge the matching of young competitors on the basis of maturational age rather than chronological age, as is almost universal at the present time. In a recent study of junior high-school tackle football, it was found that the weights of the players competing on the same two teams of 14-year-olds varied from 83 to 211 pounds. Players at both ends of this wide spectrum were inappropriate participants — at risk to injury or dissatisfied with their roles on the team.

A great advantage in the increasing number of different sports offered in scholastic programs is the availability of a suitable sport for almost every boy and girl. The late maturer can enjoy soccer, swimming, cross country, tennis, and so on, avoiding the injury risks of collision sports. The small, early maturer can excel in wrestling or gymnastics. Thoughtful counsellors can even find rewarding sports experiences for young people with a variety of health handicaps. The student with epilepsy, asthma, diabetes, hemophilia, and so forth can be helped to find a place in most school sports programs.

ADVICE TO PARENTS

The expansion of elaborate programs of organized sports for preadolescent boys and girls is a relatively recent phenomenon and one that many parents may be encountering for the first time. Thus, the parent may seek advice concerning children's participation from physicians, other health professionals, teachers, or school counsellors. The parents may be guided in their decision about participation if they consider questions such as the following: Why does your boy or girl want to become involved in a sport program? Does the young prospective athlete have a realistic appreciation of the time commitment involved and the time that will be taken away from other recreation? Who is in charge of the program? Are the children adequately matched for safe competition? What are the goals of the program and of the coaching staff? Is your son or daughter ready to lose or to be a bench warmer? Are you ready to be parents of a loser or a bench warmer? What if he or she wants to quit? What are the

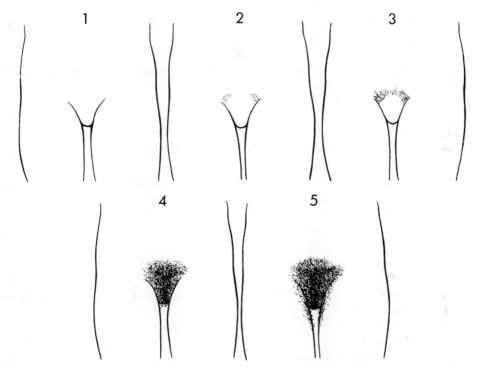

Figure 18–1. Pubic hair development as an indicator of maturational age. *Stage 1.* No pubic hair. *Stage 2.* Sparse growth of long slightly pigmented, downy hair that is straight or slightly curled. *Stage 3.* The hair is considerably darker, coarser, and more curled, spreading sparsely over the pubes. *Stage 4.* The hair is adult in type but covers a smaller area than in the adult. *Stage 5.* The hair is adult in quantity and type and extends down over the inner thighs.

chances of a sports-related injury? How much time will the family have to give to this activity?

The answers to these questions should identify the family with a sincere interest in an age-group sports program and should help them have a realistic idea of what is involved in "going out" for the team. Serious consideration is needed before initiating participation in the preadolescent, community-based sport program.

The risk and severity of sports-related injuries in the preadolescent athlete, even in contact or collision sports, is less than in the high-school or college participant. The frequency and intensity of contact are less in the younger age group. When injuries do occur, most are minor. However, particular guidance should be provided for the very young athlete. Lack of experience precludes making an informed decision about when the intensity of participation should be tempered or when continuing all-out effort is appropriate. When an injury dictates that the serious young athlete drop out of training and competition, the physician, coach, and parents will do well to make sure that the hours and intense interest channelled into athletic activity are not allowed to dissipate into an unhealthy and unhappy void. Special efforts should be made to help the young athlete maintain an active, vigorous commitment to the team or to an appropriate alternative.

RESPONSIBILITIES TO THE ATHLETE

There is increasing concern regarding the safe conduct of sports for young people both in and out of school. In almost all instances there are no requirements for coaches or supervisors of sports programs to have specific training in any aspect of injury prevention, recognition, or management — or in the safe conduct of a sports program.

Health professionals and recreation advisors must become more aggressive in demanding of the community that the five essentials listed below are met without compromise to assure that young athletes will have the opportunity for "healthy and safe" participation in sports programs.

1. Proper conditioning
2. Intelligent coaching
3. The best facilities and equipment possible
4. Capable officiating
5. Competent medical care

SUMMARY

Active, energy-expending recreation is necessary for health and fitness. Increasingly, such recreation is available to youth through rapidly expanding school and community-based sports programs.

Children are unique because they experience the continual changes of a growing body and maturing behavior. Growth changes occur at rates that vary widely within any group of boys or girls. Matching competitors on the basis of maturational age, rather than simply by chronological age, reduces the risk of injury and increases the enjoyment of participation.

Parents should be helped to have a clear understanding of the implications of their children's participation in youth sports programs. Recreation professionals, educators, and health professionals must become more active in demanding that sports programs for young athletes, in and out of school, provide competent coaching, officiating, and medical care.

STUDY QUESTIONS

1. List several ways in which today's sports opportunities for children differ from those of 30 years ago.

2. Give several alternative activities for a young person who is not interested in contact sports.

3. What is the significance of increased fatness among many 8- to 10-year-old boys?

4. Give two emotional factors that dominate a young person's relationship to sports participation.

5. Of what significance is a preparticipation examination?

6. By what criterion can pubertal development be assessed in girls? In boys?

7. Give some questions, with answers, that would suggest that a family is ready for participation in a sports program.

8. Discuss several conditions that help to assure healthy and safe sports programs.

FURTHER READINGS

Magill, R. A., Ash, M. J., and Small, F. L. (eds.): *Children and Youth in Sport*. Champaign, Ill., Human Kinetics Publishers.
Shaffer, T. E.: The adolescent athlete. Pediatr. Clin. North Am. *20*:837–849, 1973.
Shering symposium: the school age athlete. J. Sch. Health, April, 1977, pp. 217–242.
Tutko, T. S., and Bruns, W. I.: *Winning Is Everything and Other American Myths*. New York, Macmillan Publishing Company, 1976.

19

SPORTS INJURIES IN CHILDREN AND ADOLESCENTS

LYLE J. MICHELI, M.D.

THE EPIDEMIOLOGY OF CHILDREN'S INJURIES IN THE SPORTS SETTING

The growth of organized competitive athletics for the preadolescent and adolescent age groups has been a source of controversy in recent years, particularly regarding the risk of injury from organized sports. Unfortunately, sound epidemiological data on the incidence of injury in organized sports versus free play is lacking. Much of the divergent medical opinion is based on personal observation rather than on assessed ratio of injury.[1]

A number of factors contribute to the increasingly organized character of children's sports, including limited recreational facilities, the progressive loss of open space and vacant lots in cities and suburbs, and the decrease in spontaneous neighborhood activities. Organized competitions are more and more common among Americans of all ages and levels of competition, and children have been included in this trend.

The proponents of organized sports argue that organization benefits the child in the following ways: access to trained coaches improves the techniques of play at an early age and results in increasingly skilled participation later on; the development of leagues, playoffs, team uniforms, and separate stadiums increases enjoyment and helps to maintain interest; and, finally, properly supervised games have a lower risk of injury than free play. As noted in the bylaws of the Pop Warner Junior League Football Association, which sponsors community-based football for 10- to 14-year-olds, the specific objectives of the league are "to familiarize all boys with the fundamentals of football and to provide opportunity to play the game in a supervised, organized, and safe manner."[2]

There is no question that properly organized athletic programs for younger children can be highly enjoyable. Unfortunately, poor leadership and the emotional involvement of coaches and parents can, at times, turn organized children's sports into a parody of true sportsmanship. Too often, the adult supervisors place undue emotional stress upon these young athletes without significantly improving either their playing techniques or their enjoyment of the game[3] (Fig. 19–1).

288

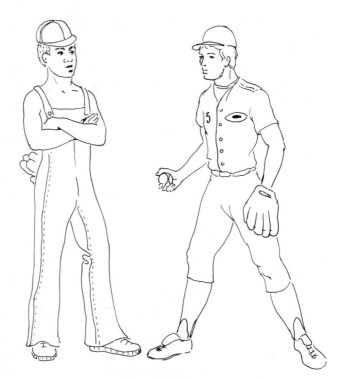

Figure 19–1. Organized sports versus free-play activities for children. Increased organization of children's sports increases the probability of certain injuries. The emotional climate of organized sports may or may not be superior to that in free play, depending on the structure of the sport.

Aside from the question of emotional stress in organized competition, there is concern about injuries to the relatively more vulnerable bones and joints of the child. In the noncontact sports, in which high-velocity trauma is not likely, the recurrent microtrauma of repetitive training (as in throwing practice, gymnastics practice, or distance running) may be harmful. In contact sports (gridiron football, rugby, hockey), the risk of injury, especially irreversible injury to the growth plate of the bones from high-impact trauma, may be greater when the players train seriously and play intensely. The young runner may be hurt by training too hard. The young lineman, because of his training, may be playing too hard.

Fortunately, there is some evidence that the preadolescent athlete, even when engaged in organized football, runs less risk of injury than his counterpart at the high school or college level. Roser and Clawson reviewed the incidence of injury in 2097 participants in the Seattle Junior Football League.[4] They found 2.3 per cent rate of injury* among these players and noted that very few of these injuries were serious. Godshall reviewed the records of the Pop Warner football program in a central Pennsylvania region in which 1700 boys had participated on various teams during a 12-year period.[2] He found only two major injuries (both were fractures of the leg) and a few minor fractures of the wrist, fingers, and foot. He also called attention to the very low insurance rates for teams during the 1973 Junior League football season, with the premiums ranging from 80 to 245 dollars per team for the season. He cited these low rates as evidence that serious injuries were probably a rare occurrence in these age groups. Furthermore, it has been noted by Pop Warner officials that in the first 43 years of their organization's existence, there has not been a single fatality among the more than 1 million participants in the registered football programs.

In contrast, various studies of high-school football have shown injury rates of between 40 and 50 per cent.[5] A study of high-school football injuries in North Carolina from 1969 to 1972 found an overall injury rate of 49 per cent.[6] Garrick and Requa recorded an injury rate in football of 81 per cent in a study of Seattle area high

*Number of injuries per participant per season, multiplied by 100.

schools.[7] Their rate of injury, averaged for all high-school sports, was 39 per cent per season.

The significantly lower rate of injury among preadolescents in contact sports has been ascribed to specific alterations in the rules, such as the prohibition of cross-body blocking, spearing, and so forth, and to the low impact velocity produced by smaller children. Nonetheless, the potential for serious and permanent injury to the growing bones of these younger children remains real, and the risks versus the benefits of a particular sport for a particular child must be carefully weighed by parents and physicians.

TYPES OF INJURY

Since the child is still growing, damage to growth structures, particularly the growing bones and joints of the extremities, is the chief danger in childhood injuries.

Children are susceptible to many of the same injuries as adults, including sprains, strains, and contusions, as well as long bone fractures of their extremities.[8] In addition, four special types of injuries can be sustained by children as a result of musculoskeletal trauma (Fig. 19–2): (1) growth plate injuries; (2) injuries to the epiphysis or end of the bone; (3) avulsions (pulling away) of major musculotendinous insertions from bone; and (4) certain overuse injuries of bones, cartilage, and musculotendinous structures of the upper and lower extremities.

Growth cartilage is the tissue responsible for the growth of the spine and extremities in the child. This cartilage ultimately turns into bone in the adult, but is itself much softer than bone and more susceptible to injury.

Growth Plate Injuries

The growth plate (physis) is a disc of cartilage located near each end of the long bones of the skeleton. The entire growth of the bone occurs from these two sites. The growth plate consists of columns of cartilage cells in various stages of development

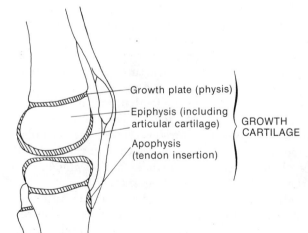

Growth plate (physis)

Epiphysis (including articular cartilage)

Apophysis (tendon insertion)

GROWTH CARTILAGE

Figure 19–2. The knee of the child has three sites of growth cartilage, any of which may be injured.

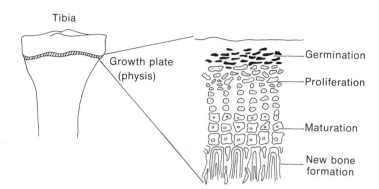

Figure 19–3. Growth plate, showing the four zones of development and maturation.

(Fig. 19–3). The immature cartilage cells at one end subsequently multiply and mature. Young bone cells replace the mature cartilage cells and produce a latticework of solid bone.

The growth plate is sometimes less resistant to deforming forces than either the ligaments of nearby joints or the outer shafts of the long bones (Fig. 19–4). Thus, a heavy blow or twist to an arm or leg of a child can result in disruption or fracture through the substance of the growth plate, with serious consequences. If portions of the germ cell layer are destroyed or if alignment of the growth plate segments is disturbed so that columns of bone form across the plate, subsequent growth or alignment of the

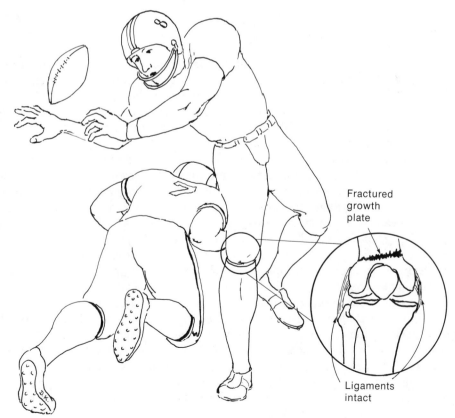

Figure 19–4. The growth plate may be damaged even though ligaments are not.

extremity may be seriously affected. Loss of limb length, angular deformity, or joint incongruity can result from growth plate injury. The potential for development of these three problems depends upon both the extent of the injury and the specific growth plate involved.[9] For example, fractures involving the growth plate of the shoulder rarely result in subsequent joint or growth complications, whereas fractures about the knee have a relatively high incidence of subsequent problems.

An injury about the major joints in a child requires careful evaluation for the possibility of growth plate damage. An injury about the knee or ankle, for instance, must not be dismissed as a sprain of the ligaments until damage to the growth plate is ruled out (Fig. 19–4).

Epidemiology.   Collins and Larsen both felt that significant growth plate injury rarely occurred in organized sports and that organized sports carried no greater risk of these injuries than informal play activities.[10, 11] However, in a review of epiphyseal injuries followed in the Growth Study Clinic of the Boston Children's Hospital from 1965 to 1975, it was found that 26 per cent of the 135 injuries traced had occurred as a result of organized sports activities.[12] The causes of the remaining injuries were almost equally divided between high-velocity or vehicular trauma and free play activities. It was found, after careful review of sports-related growth plate injuries, that the majority of those injuries that occurred about the knee were the result of football activities, usually involving blocking. The majority of injuries about the ankle occurred from participation in baseball — particularly from sliding into base.

As the number of organized sports activities for children increases, careful study must be made of the rate of growth plate injuries in order to insure that increasingly sophisticated techniques of play and higher levels of participation do not result in an increased rate of these most serious injuries.

Articular Cartilage Injuries

The epiphysis is the end of a long bone and forms part of the joint (Fig. 19–3). In the child, the epiphysis is covered with a layer of cartilage, which has a double function. It provides a smooth, gliding surface for the joint. In addition, because the epiphysis must also grow in circumference, the inner cartilage cells are actively replaced by bone as the epiphysis enlarges. This process continues until the child becomes an adult and growth ceases.

During childhood, the articular (joint) surface and the articular cartilage appear to have a special susceptibility to injury that is not present during adulthood. Thus, impact between the ends of two bones, if of sufficient intensity or frequency, can injure the articular cartilage and cause pieces to be knocked free into the joint. Early arthritis can result, or these pieces of articular cartilage ("joint mice"), sometimes with underlying bone attached, can actually roll free in the joint and grow in size until they inhibit joint function. Their growth is supported by the joint fluid. Osteochondritis dissecans is the general term given to this process. It appears to occur more often in certain susceptible individuals, but most authorities feel that trauma, whether recurrent or the result of one distinct blow, plays a significant role.[13]

Joints particularly susceptible to this type of injury include the elbow, knee, hip, and ankle. If detected early, rest or cast immobilization of the extremity is usually sufficient to allow healing to occur. If the fragments are already free in the joint at the time that the process is recognized, surgery is sometimes required to remove them. As with the other forms of growth-related injuries in the child, injury to the articular cartilage always must be suspected if the child complains of persistent pain in a major joint.

Musculotendinous Avulsions (Apophyseal Injuries)

The major muscles of the extremities are attached to the bones by tendons. These major tendinous insertions are at the margins of the joints or on some of the larger bones of the body, such as the scapula or pelvis. The term apophysis is used for these insertion sites when growth cartilage forms part of the attachment.

On occasion, when these musculotendinous units are severely pulled, the apophyses may be partially pulled away (avulsed) from the remainder of the bone, injuring the growth cartilage. In contrast, similar stresses in the adult result in injury to the substance of the muscle belly or tendon; the tendon rarely pulls away from the bone.

These apophyseal avulsions can occur in both the upper and lower extremities in the young athlete.[14] Most frequently, however, they occur in the lower extremity as a result of running or pivoting. Since the pelvis is a site of major musculotendinous insertions, a number of more serious apophyseal avulsions in the young athlete occur about the pelvis. Along the front and side of the pelvis, portions of the iliac apophysis can be pulled off with stress of the lateral abdominal muscles or overstretch of the major muscles that flex and extend the thigh. Avulsions of the apophyseal insertion of the adductor muscles in the groin are frequently seen in hockey players. Avulsions of the hamstring muscle and hip flexors at their apophyseal insertions on the hip and lower pelvis occur relatively often in young track athletes, particularly hurdlers and broad jumpers, and in soccer players[15, 16] (Fig. 19–5).

Apophyseal avulsions of major musculotendinous units about the hip and pelvis can cause such excruciating pain that they are often mistaken for serious fractures or even hip dislocations. On occasion, these avulsions must be repaired by surgery in which the apophysis is reattached to the site of avulsion from the bone. Sometimes, particularly if the torn apophysis remains near the bone, it can heal satisfactorily with rest and immobilization alone.

In addition to the acute separation of an apophysis from a bony insertion as a result of a single traumatic episode, recurrent overstressing of a musculotendinous unit can result in chronic irritation at the apophysis and slow, but progressive, elongation of the apophysis as it pulls away from the bone. Such apophyseal overuse syndromes are most frequently seen about the elbow and knee and will be discussed in the "Sites of Injury" section of this chapter.

Stress Injuries

Stress fractures, or fatigue fractures, are injuries to bone in which there is a slow but progressive loss of bony substance at one particular site. This can result in complete fracture through the bone if the process continues long enough. The stress fracture is due to recurrent submaximal trauma, repeated with such frequency that the body is unable to repair the site of injury adequately. In the young athlete, stress fractures are usually due to the rapid increase of a specific training activity over a short period of time.

Stress fractures may occur at any age or level of activity. The most common stress fracture in the young athlete[17, 18, 19] occurs in association with running activities and involves the tibia below the knee (Fig. 19–6). At first, this stress fracture is often mistaken for shin splints.[20] A typical history is that of a young cross-country runner who begins vigorous training, including hill work, three to four weeks before school begins in preparation for the fall season. Initially, changes in the tibia will not be seen

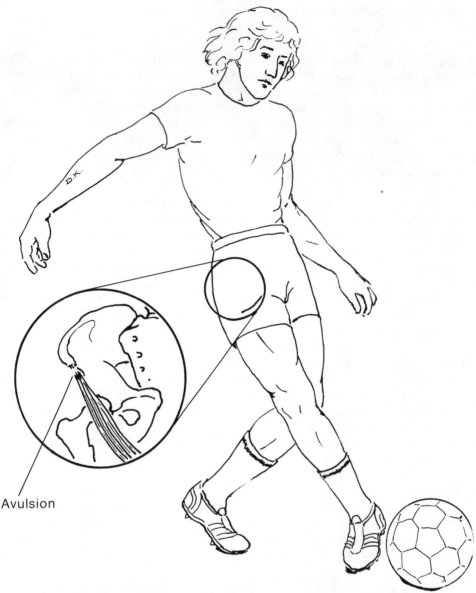

Avulsion

Figure 19–5. Apophyseal avulsion. In this soccer player, the kicking motion has torn the sartorius muscle free from its attachment to the pelvis.

on x-ray despite moderately severe pain while running. After two to three weeks, particularly if the extremity is rested and the bone is allowed to heal, there will be evidence of new bone formation at the site of stress fracture.

The other type of stress fracture frequently occurring in the young athlete is that of the distal fibula (outer leg bone) just above the ankle.[19] This is seen in runners who engage in short turning activities such as those of indoor track, but has also been seen in cross-country skiers and hockey players. Once again, early detection is the key to this diagnosis. Early treatment, including rest and immobilization, can prevent the bone from completely fracturing, which would require prolonged cast treatment or operation.

While stress fractures are more common in the legs, they have been reported in the upper arm (humerus) in conjunction with repeated throwing.[21] Stress fractures can

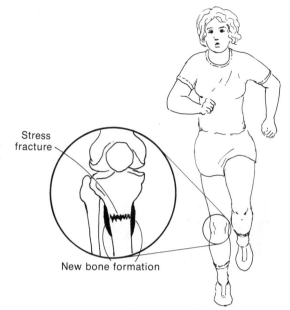

Figure 19–6. Stress fracture of upper tibia. In the young athlete, stress fractures are usually due to the rapid increase of a specific activity over a short period of time.

Stress fracture

New bone formation

also occur in the spine of the young athlete, and can be a source of serious concern.[22] These will be discussed in the following section.

SITES OF INJURY

Elbow

Injuries to the elbow occur relatively often in the young athlete and are of particular concern when associated with repetitive throwing activities in sports.[23, 24, 25, 26] The act of throwing, especially the first part of the delivery, strains the elbow by compressing the outer side and stretching the inner side of the joint (Fig. 19–7). The forces involved are greatest in a sidearm throw (as in pitching a curve ball) and least in a straight overhead throw. In addition to pitchers, javelin-throwers and quarterbacks are the most frequent victims of this type of elbow injury.

Recent rule changes in Little League baseball now limit pitching to six innings per week and have eliminated curve ball throwing. These changes appear to have decreased the incidence of injury, although it is difficult to limit practice throwing. Individual susceptibility to growth cartilage injuries also varies; six innings may be fine for one child and a strain for another.

Suspicion must be maintained regarding complaints of elbow pain in children involved in any sport, particularly the throwing sports. In the early stages of these injuries, pain may be the only symptom, but it is often accompanied by tenderness over the inner side of the elbow. Later, inability to straighten the elbow fully is a sign of serious injury. If the injury is detected in the early stages, symptoms can often be relieved by rest followed by careful physical therapy. Then exercise can be resumed. If neglected, the injury can grow worse and require surgical correction.

The most effective approach to this problem appears to be prevention of prolonged forceful throwing in children and early investigation of a youngster who complains of elbow pain.

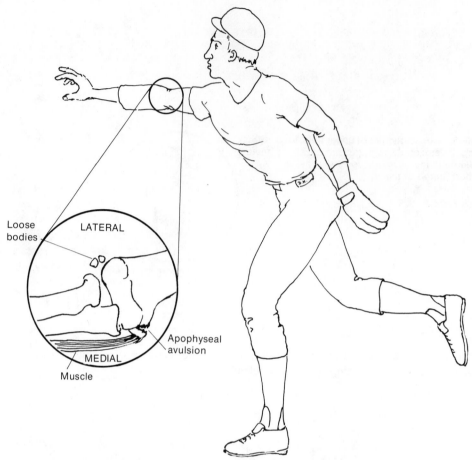

Figure 19–7. Little League elbow is a name for several injuries to the throwing elbow of the child. On the lateral side, impaction can cause the formation of loose bodies (joint mice). On the medial side, traction by muscle can cause avulsion of its attachment (apophysis).

Shoulder

Injuries to the shoulder are relatively frequent in young athletes.[21, 25] Whether the result of macrotrauma or recurrent microtrauma, the site of injury is generally the growth plate located immediately below the shoulder rather than the articular cartilage or musculotendinous insertions. Growth plate fractures at the shoulder resulting from major trauma generally heal rapidly after they have been reduced and immobilized, usually without significant disability.[8]

Repeated forceful throwing that applies torsion (twist) to the shoulder can result in shoulder pain and partial growth plate separation. The results of such microtrauma have been dubbed "Little League shoulder" and should be suspected in any youngster complaining of shoulder pain.[21] Several cases of complete fracture of the proximal humerus at the shoulder have occurred when throwing has been continued despite shoulder pain. Usually, rest alone is sufficient to heal these lesions, and the child is able to throw again after strength has been restored to the shoulder muscles by physical therapy.

Back

Complaints of back pain in the child participating in sports must be evaluated carefully. The child is subject to muscular strains and ligamentous sprains of the back. In addition, several serious conditions may occur in the young spine that is subject to recurrent sports stress.

Spondylolysis and Spondylolisthesis. With repeated impact stress or bending of the spine (as in gymnastics), a stress fracture can occur between the anterior and posterior parts of lower spinal vertebrae (Fig. 19–8).[22, 27] This condition is known as spondylolysis if there has been no slipping forward of the spine. When the upper spine slips forward, the condition is called spondylolisthesis. Athletic trauma, particularly that associated with increased lordosis (swaying of the low back), can result in this injury.

In 1974, McMaster[28] noted an increased occurrence of this condition in football linemen and ascribed this to the greater stress placed on the low back during blocking and tackling. More recently, Jackson[27] observed an increase in this condition in young female gymnasts and attributed it to the extreme extension or swaying of the back in demanding movements such as back flips in the floor exercises and back walkovers on the balance beam. With early detection and treatment, many of these lesions can be healed, and the child can soon return to the balance beam and the uneven bars.

Once again, early recognition of the injury is necessary to prevent a potentially serious problem. If undetected, spondylolisthesis can cause persistent back complaints and a significantly decreased tolerance for vigorous activities in later life.

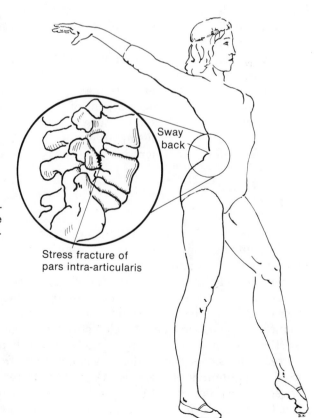

Figure 19–8. Spondylolysis and spondylolisthesis involve a stress fracture of one or more vertebrae at the base of the spine.

Sway back

Stress fracture of pars intra-articularis

Scheuermann's Juvenile Kyphosis.   The other back condition seen with increased frequency in the young athlete is known as Scheuermann's juvenile kyphosis (hunchback).[29, 30] This condition results from an injury to growth cartilage of the vertebral bodies. In it, the growth of the end plates appears to decrease because of recurrent compression of the front of the spine. This disorder is most frequently seen in 12- to 16-year-olds, particularly in boys in contact sports, and usually presents as a nagging low back pain. By the time of detection, there may already be evidence of kyphosis or round back deformity in the spine. X-rays usually confirm the changes in the vertebral bodies, namely, narrowing of the front of the vertebral bodies and tipping forward or rounding of the spine.

Mild cases with minimal bone deformity may be treated with a period of rest followed by specific exercises to correct the deformed posture often associated with this injury. In its later stages, this condition is most successfully treated by the application of specific braces or casts that straighten the spine by taking the pressure off the front of the spinal bodies and allowing growth to resume. If detected early and appropriately treated, complete recovery from this condition can be expected and, after healing has occurred, athletic activities can be resumed without problems.

Hip and Pelvis

The most common injuries of the hip and pelvis in the young athlete are musculotendinous avulsions. These apophyseal avulsions are generally the result of a single traumatic episode and are often extremely painful. They require immediate bed rest, icing of the area, and strong medication for pain. Rarely is surgery required to restore the muscle to its site of insertion; the amount of displacement is generally minimal, and satisfactory healing will occur if proper rest and immobilization of the extremity are provided.[14, 15] If sports participation or exercise is begun too early, particularly when the nature of the injury is not fully realized, healing may not occur or may be significantly delayed. Surgery may then be required to reattach the avulsed muscles and allow proper healing.

Injuries to the articular cartilage can occur at the hip. These are relatively rare, since the hip is a well-protected joint of the ball-and-socket type. Occasionally, very heavy trauma can result in a fracture through the growth plate at the hip or even in complete dislocation of the hip from the socket. This is quite rare but extremely serious. Immediate treatment is necessary to attain optimal results.

Knee

Children are susceptible to many of the same types of knee injuries seen in adult athletes: internal derangements of the meniscal cartilages of the knee; ligamentous injuries to the knee; and injuries to the extensor mechanism of the knee. In addition, all four of the childhood-specific types of injury can be seen about the knee.

The most frequent cause of knee pain in the young athlete is a condition known as Osgood-Schlatter disease.[31] It often occurs among soccer players. This condition is produced by an apophyseal avulsion of the patellar tendon from the tibia at its site of insertion (the apophysis shown in Fig. 19–2).It is usually readily identified by swelling and tenderness over the tendon insertion at the front of the knee and by pain upon forced straightening of the knee. Osgood-Schlatter disease is generally seen in boys between the ages of 10 and 14 years, but it is being noted with increasing frequency in girls. Once identified, this condition is best treated with a period of rest, which may or may not involve cast immobilization, followed by progressive resumption of motion. Physical therapy is used to restore strength and flexibility to the muscles of the leg, which are generally atrophied because the pain of this condition inhibits their use.

Another injury specific to the young athlete is osteochondritis dissecans, an injury to the articular cartilage and underlying bone of the knee. Detected early, this condition generally can be treated successfully by cast immobilization so that there is no pressure on the loose fragment.[13, 29] If detected late, or if the bone and cartilage fragment breaks free in the course of treatment, these fragments can persist and even grow inside the knee and result in intermittent locking of the joint. These free fragments, also known as joint mice, must be removed surgically in order to restore full motion and relieve pain.

Heavy blows (macrotrauma) to the knee, which in older athletes can result in serious ligamentous injuries, can cause growth plate fractures of the distal femur or proximal tibia in the young athlete.[12, 32] These injuries can be detected by tenderness over the growth plate and by x-rays, which often show the displacement at the growth plate. Surgery is sometimes required to realign the growth plate, although it will frequently heal satisfactorily if manipulated into normal position and then held with a cast. Unfortunately, injuries to these particular growth plates can result in a relatively high incidence of growth arrest and shortening of the injured extremity. They do not, however, generally result in significant joint problems because they usually do not enter the joint itself.[11]

Finally, patients with stress fractures of the proximal tibia, occurring often in distance runners, will sometimes present with a complaint of "knee pain." However, careful examination reveals that the site of pain and tenderness is actually just below the knee — over the tibia itself.[17] Again, early detection of these tibial stress fractures and appropriate rest can usually result in complete healing and early resumption of sports activities.

Ankle and Foot

Although children can certainly sustain ligamentous injury (sprain) about the ankle, particularly the outside of the ankle, the possibility of growth cartilage injury is significant. Growth plate fractures of both the tibia and fibula are frequently seen together, although each can occur independently. In particular, growth plate injury of the end of the fibula, on the outside of the ankle, can easily be mistaken for a "sprained ankle" and not treated with proper immobilization. This can result in permanent damage and deformity if the growth of the fibula has been stopped. Osteochondral (bone and cartilage) injuries of the ankle are seen with relative frequency in young athletes and must be suspected when pain and swelling persist in an otherwise stable ankle that has sustained recent injury.

Foot pain in the young athlete can generally be traced to a specific site of tenderness. Complaints are usually the result of musculotendinous strain or avulsion. The most common site of apophyseal avulsion in the child is the outside of the foot where the strong peroneal muscles insert at the base of the fifth metatarsal. In general, early recognition of these musculotendinous injuries and treatment with rest is sufficient for cessation of symptoms and healing, although occasionally, complete avulsion of the apophysis can result in prolonged disability.

Stress fractures can sometimes occur in the foot bones of the child. Persistent complaints of pain over the midfoot may be due to stress fracture of the metatarsals, a diagnosis that must be suspected and evaluated appropriately.

INJURY PREVENTION

It is evident from the preceding discussion that the most important ways of preventing serious injury to the young athlete are early attention to complaints of pain and dysfunction, particularly about the major joints, and maintenance of suspicion for growth cartilage or stress injuries. With proper early attention and appropriate treatment, which usually involves nothing more specific than *rest of the painful extremity,* complete healing and total resumption of activities can be anticipated.

In addition, certain children in certain stages of development appear to be particularly susceptible to injuries in the contact sports. Lichtor has noted that loose-jointed children appear to be particularly susceptible to injuries in contact sports and has recommended that these children participate in noncontact sports such as track and field or rowing.[33] At the opposite extreme, the child with very tight ligaments appears to have an increased risk of injury, particularly to the back and spine, from ballet or gymnastics. Unfortunately, consistent criteria for classification of youngsters into body type and relative degree of ligamentous laxity or tightness are not available, and the physician or trainer who is involved in the care of these athletes must often use his own judgment in recommending or discouraging a particular sports activity for a particular child.

Because of the susceptibility of children to extremity and spine injury during the growth period, altering certain rules or tactics to decrease the risk of injury is indicated. Good examples of such measures are the Little League's pitching limit of six innings per week and rule changes in Pop Warner Football eliminating cross-body blocking or spearing. Children's sports, especially sports hitherto pursued by adults, need close screening to insure that the growing bones and joints of the children involved are not subjected to unacceptable levels of trauma and stress.

Coaching at this level should be concerned with the teaching of fundamentals and the development of basic game skills, with particular emphasis on long-term conditioning. Tactics such as face blocking or sliding into bases, which have increased the rate of injury in young athletes, should be discouraged.

The role of protective equipment in preventing injury in the young athlete has frequently been overemphasized.[6, 7] No protective equipment has yet been designed that adequately protects the knee of the young athlete in football competition. It is dangerous to think that increased use of protective equipment will allow youngsters to participate in adult-style games. On the other hand, the use of protective equipment such as helmets, faceshields, and mouth guards in hockey was initially a requirement only for children but one that has paved the way for the use of these safety devices at collegiate and professional levels.

Proper conditioning of the young athlete is certainly a factor in the prevention of unnecessary injury. Recent studies have shown that the child is capable of levels of cardiovascular training similar to those of the adult without the risk of injury.[34] In addition, weight training, if properly performed, can improve muscle strength and enhance the child's resistance to musculoskeletal trauma.[35]

The use of heavy weights or low repetition techniques must be avoided in training the child. Growth plate injuries have been reported in children involved in free weight lifting and, in particular, in children performing military presses.[36] In addition, we have observed musculotendinous ruptures in children lifting excessive weights, including a 9-year-old with an almost complete rupture of his quadriceps muscle resulting from an attempt to perform a full military press with free weight. If children weight lift under proper supervision using the low-weight, high-repetition technique, it can be done safely without significant risk of injury and can enhance injury prevention.[37]

Finally, techniques of athletic preparation that violate basic health principles, such as rapid weight reduction in wrestlers, may have a particularly deleterious effect on the child and should never be allowed.[38, 39] Coaching personnel must take specific steps to prevent these techniques.

Perhaps the most effective technique for injury prevention in the young athlete is the encouragement of a relaxed attitude toward sports. Children must be able to enjoy sports participation without being excessively pressured to win at all costs by adults who lack proper consideration for the development stage of these children's bones, joints, and emotions.

SUMMARY

The growth of organized competitive athletics for children increases the risk of injury to young athletes by two mechanisms: first, the recurrent microtrauma of excessive repetitive training; and second, exposure of growing bones and joints to excessive impact trauma in heavy contact sports.

There are four types of sports injuries generally seen in children: injuries to growth cartilage at (1) the growth plate, (2) bone ends, and (3) sites of tendon insertions; and (4) stress fractures due to excessive or rapid training techniques. Common anatomical sites of injury include the upper extremity, lower extremity, and spine of the child.

Techniques of injury prevention include matching the participant with the appropriate sport, formulating rules to limit risky activities, teaching fundamental skills, insuring sufficient physical conditioning, providing proper equipment, and adopting an unpressured approach toward sports. The main component of treatment is frequently just rest of the injured part.

STUDY QUESTIONS

1. Discuss factors involved in the increase of organized sports programs for children.

2. Discuss the pros and cons of organized sports versus free play activities for children.

3. What anatomical structure is responsible for growth of the long bones? Describe its composition.

4. Compare and contrast the physis (growth plate), epiphysis, and apophysis.

5. What are three possible results of growth plate injury?

6. Distinguish a stress fracture from a macrotrauma fracture.

7. Compare spondylolysis and Scheuermann's juvenile kyphosis.

8. Describe the mechanisms of injury in Little League elbow and discuss methods of prevention.

9. Describe the mechanism and prevention of musculotendinous avulsion. Does this occur in adults?

10. Discuss techniques of injury prevention in the young athlete.

REFERENCES

1. Haddon, W., Jr.: Principles in research on the effects of sports on health. J.A.M.A. *197*:885–888, 1966.
2. Godshall, R. W.: Junior League football: risks versus benefits. J. Sports Med. *3*(4):139–166, 1975.
3. Michener, J. H.: *Sports In America.* New York, Fawcett Crest, 1976.
4. Roser, L. A., and Clawson, D. K.: Football injuries in the very young athlete. Clin. Orthop. Rel. Res. *69*:212–223, 1970.
5. Peterson, T. C.: The cross-body block, the major cause of knee injuries. J.A.M.A. *211*:449–452, 1970.
6. Mueller, F. O., and Blyth, C. S.: North Carolina High School football injury study: equipment and prevention. J. Sports Med. *2*(1):1–10, 1974.
7. Garrick, J. G., and Requa, R. K.: Injuries in high school sports. J. Pediatr. *61*:465–469, 1978.
8. Micheli, L. J.: Trauma in childhood. *In* Ravitch, M. (ed.): *Pediatric Surgery.* Chicago, Year Book Medical Publishers, Inc., 1978.
9. Salter, R. I., and Harris, W. R.: Injuries involving the epiphyseal plate. J. Bone Joint Surg. *45*(A):587–622, 1963.
10. Collins, H. R.: Epiphyseal injuries in athletes. Cle. Clin. Quarterly *42*(4):285–295, Winter, 1975.
11. Larson, R. L.: Epiphyseal injuries in the adolescent athlete. Orthop. Clin. North Am. *4*:839–851, 1973.
12. McManama, G. B., and Micheli, L. J.: The incidence of sport related epiphyseal injuries in adolescents. Med. Sci. Sports *9*(1):57, 1977.
13. Green, W. T., and Banks, H. H.: Osteochondritis dissecans in children. J. Bone Joint Surg. *35*(A):26–47, 1953.
14. Brewer, B. J.: Injury to the musculo-tendinous unit in sports. Clin. Orthop. Rel. Res. *23*:32–38, 1962.
15. Clancy, W. E., and Foltz, A. S.: Iliac apophysitis and stress fractures in adolescent runners. Am. J. Sports Med. *4*(5):214–218, 1976.
16. Levi, J. H., and Coleman, C. R.: Fracture of the tibial tubercule. Am. J. Sports Med. *4*(6):254–263, 1976.
17. Devas, M. B.: Stress fractures in athletes. J. Royal Coll. Gen. Pract. *19*:34–38, 1970.
18. McBryde, A. M., Jr.: Stress fractures in athletes. J. Sports Med. *3*(5):212–217, 1975.
19. Walters, N. E., and Wolf, M. D.: Stress fractures in young athletes. Am. J. Sports Med. *5*(4):165–70, 1977.
20. Slocum, D. B.: The shin splint syndrome, medical aspects and differential diagnosis. Am. J. Surg. *114*:875–881, 1967.
21. Cahill, B. R., Tullos, H. S., and Fain, R. H.: Little League shoulder. J. Sports Med. *2*(3):150–53, 1974.
22. Wiltse, L. L., Widell, E. H., and Jackson, D. W.: Fatigue fracture: the basic lesion is inthmic spondylolisthesis. J. Bone Joint Surg. *57*(A):17–22, 1975.
23. Adams, J. E.: Injury to the throwing arm: a study of traumatic changes in the elbow joints of boy baseball players. Calif. Med. *102*:127–132, 1965.
24. Brown, R., Blazina, M. E., Kerlan, R. K., et al.: Osteochondritis of the capitellum. Am. J. Sports Med. *2*(1):27–47, 1974.
25. Lipscomb, A. B.: Baseball Pitching in Growing Athletes. J. Sports Med. *3*(1):25–34, 1975.
26. Tullos, H. S., and King, J. W.: Lesions of the pitching arm in adolescents. J.A.M.A. *220*:264–271, 1972.
27. Jackson, D. W., Wiltse, L. L., and Cirincione, R. J.: Spondylolisthesis in the female athlete. Clin. Orthop. Rel. Res. *117*:68–73, 1976.
28. Ferguson, R. J., McMaster, J. H., and Stanitski, C. L.: Low back pain in college football linemen. J. Sports Med. *2*(2):63–69, 1974.
29. Cahill, B. R.: Chronic orthopaedic problems in the young athlete. J. Sports Med. *1*(3):36–39, 1973.
30. Scheuermann, H.: Kyphosis dorsalis juvenilis. Orthop. Chir. *41*:305, 1921.
31. Mital, M. A., and Mitza, R. A.: Osgood-Schlatters disease: the painful puzzler. Phys. Sports Med. *5*(6):60–78, 1977.
32. Grossman, R. B., and Nicholas, J. A.: Common disorders of the knee. Orthop. Clin. North Am. *8*(3):619–640, 1977.
33. Lichtor, F.: The loose jointed young athlete. Recognition and treatment. J. Sports Med. *1*:22–23, 1972.
34. Shosky, G. B., and Hagerman, F. C.: Effects of conditioning on cardio-respiratory function in adolescent boys. J. Sports Med. *3*:97–107, 1975.
35. Cahill, B. R.: Pre-season conditioning in football. Presented to the American Orthopeadic Society for Sports Medicine, San Diego, Calif., 1977.
36. Ryan, J. R.: Fracture of the distal radial epiphysis in adolescent weight lifters. Am. J. Sports Med. *4*:26–28, 1976.
37. Jesse, J. P.: Olympic lifting movements endanger adolescents. Phys. Sports Med. *5*(9):61–67, 1977.
38. Ribisl, P. M.: Rapid weight reduction in wrestling. J. Sports Med. *3*(2):55–57, 1975.

39. Taylor, A. W.: Physiological effects of wrestling in adolescents and teenagers. J. Sports Med. *3*(2):76–84, 1975.
40. Nicholson, J. T.: *Epiphyseal Fractures About the Knee*. A.A.O.S. Instructional Course Lecture, Vol. 18. St. Louis., C. V. Mosby Company, 1961, p. 74.

FURTHER READINGS

Albinson, S. G., and Andrew, G. M.: *Child in Sports and Physical Activity*. Baltimore, University Park Press, 1975.
O'Donoghue, D. H.: *Treatment of Injuries in Athletes*. Philadelphia, W. B. Saunders Company, 1976.
Rang, M.: *Children's Fractures*. Philadelphia, J. B. Lippincott Company, 1974.
Tachdjian, M. O.: *Pediatric Orthopedics,* Vol II, Section 8, pp. 1532–1752. Philadelphia, W. B. Saunders Company, 1972.

20

FACTORS IMPORTANT TO WOMEN PARTICIPANTS IN VIGOROUS ATHLETICS

CLAYTON L. THOMAS, M.D., M.P.H.

SOCIAL FACTORS

Until quite recently, the social roles and domestic duties imposed on women limited their participation in sports. However, the blurring of male-female roles and the relaxation of sex stereotypes in the last few decades have given women a new freedom to follow their interests and talents. As a result, there has been a tremendous upsurge of interest in women's sports on both the amateur and professional levels.

Women's participation in sports has been aided by passage of federal legislation, Title IX of the Education Amendment of 1972, which mandated the provision of equal athletic facilities for girls in schools receiving federal funds. One result of this legislation is that girls have been permitted to play on boys' teams in most noncontact (and, in some instances, contact) sports. A landmark 16-month investigation by the New York State Education Department, reported in 1970, determined that no administrative or interpersonal difficulties were experienced when boys and girls competed on the same teams in golf, tennis, gymnastics, riflery, skiing, swimming, fencing, track, and cross-country foot racing.[1] There is a potentially negative aspect to this. Moyer notes: "We cannot continue to have a girls' bowling team dominated by boys as was the situation in Illinois in 1975, nor can we allow a boy on a girls' volleyball team to intimidate the girls on the opposite team as occurred in the Indiana State Girls Volleyball Championship in 1976."[2] However, problems engendered by these social and legal developments are insignificant in comparison to the benefits they have brought to females interested in athletics.

BIOLOGICAL FACTORS

The Suitability of Sports for Young Girls

We do not have data that would allow a precise and significant statement to be made concerning which sports are suitable for various age groups. Even though it has been customary to prohibit prepubertal girls from competing, there is ample evidence that some girls have competed during and before puberty and have not been harmed by this experience. For example, the average age of the girls who were members of the 1964 United States Olympic swimming team was 15½, and they had been competing for more than 5 years.[3] Obviously, many of the girls on the team had begun to train and compete prior to menarche.

Puberty and Sports

The biological differences between males and females have often been cited as a reason why females should limit or avoid participation in sports. These differences are real, but whether they lead to increased injury or limit performance is a matter of debate.

The physical capacity of young children is virtually the same for boys and girls prior to the onset of puberty.[4] Puberty occurs approximately two years earlier in the female than in the male, and it is felt that this is a contributing factor to the average increased stature of the adult male as compared with that of the adult female. The earlier puberty occurs, the earlier the epiphyses of the long bones close, preventing further linear growth. These changes at puberty are endocrine-mediated.

Rather extreme variation in body size and mass for individuals of both sexes may exist at the time the female experiences puberty. Thus, the maturation level of females in the 12- to 15-year age groups may be considerably greater than for males, and this should be taken into consideration when determining the suitability of the coeducational sports activities, particularly those involving contact. It would be possible for virtually mature adolescent girls to be involved in contact sports with relatively frail males of the same age.

The cause of the earlier onset of puberty in the female is not known, but Van Wyk and Grumbach[5] noted:

The female skeleton is normally, at all ages, somewhat advanced beyond that of the male, and pubescence likewise occurs earlier in girls than boys. These physiologic differences in timing are frequently exaggerated, since true sexual precocity occurs more commonly in females, whereas a physiologic delay in the onset of adolescence is predominantly a disorder of the male. Although ordinary methods of hormone assay fail to reveal significant sexual differences until the onset of pubescence, ovaries undergo greater enlargement and exhibit far more histologic activity during childhood than do testes; these histologic differences suggest that the prepubescent ovary also has more secretory activity than the infantile testis. Thus, the secretion of small amounts of estrogen throughout the prepubescent years could readily explain both the more rapid skeletal maturation and the earlier onset of pubescence in the female.

Physical, Biochemical, Endocrine, and Hematological Differences Between Men and Women

As Williams[6] has indicated, it is difficult to define "normal." An individual may have what appears to be an entirely normal laboratory value for certain chemical tests, but for another individual that value could be associated with illness. It is, therefore, quite important when discussing such values to define the variables such as age, sex, time of day the test was done, and metabolic and exercise state at the time of testing.

Prior to puberty, boys and girls are virtually equivalent in height, weight, and strength.[7, 8, 9] Postpubertal boys are taller, heavier, and stronger than girls on the average. Laubach[10] summarized an investigation of the strength of female subjects and compared his data with those developed by Kroemer[11] and Laubach and McConville[12] and stated:

> The data show that the "overall" total body strength of women as compared to men is about 63.5%; however, this value may range from 35 to 86%. Static strength in the upper extremities of women was found to be 59.5% that of men, ranging from 44 to 79%. Strength of the lower extremities of women was found to be 71.9% that of men with a range of 57 to 86%. Women's trunk strength was found to be 63.8% that of men with a range of 37 to 70%. The dynamic strength characteristics, which included lifting, lowering, pushing, and pulling tasks, of women was found to average 68.6% that of men, ranging from 59 to 84%.

Hematological and biochemical values for adult men and women are available in various publications.[13-16] Levels of cholesterol, total bilirubin, albumin, total protein, uric acid, and alkaline phosphatase are approximately the same in men and women. Women have lower levels of creatinine phosphokinase, inorganic phosphate, fasting blood glucose, acid phosphatase, 5-hydroxy indole acetic acid (in the urine), plasma testosterone, erythrocytes, hematocrit, hemoglobin concentration, serum iron, urine 17-ketosteroid excretion, urine 17-hydroxy steroid excretion, and basal metabolic rate. The levels of growth and luteinizing hormones are greater in men than in women.

The enzyme 2,3-diphosphoglycerate present in red blood cells is important in facilitating the exchange of oxygen from the red cell to tissues. The possibility that the level of this enzyme fluctuates with respect to the various phases of the menstrual cycle has been investigated. One study[17] indicated no change; another[17] reported that the enzyme was significantly higher in the last week of the menstrual cycle.

Anthropometric, Strength, and Growth Differences

Infant girls are, on the average, slightly shorter and lighter than boys. The heights and weights of children aged 6 to 11 years were obtained from a probability sample of 7417 children selected to represent approximately 24 million noninstitutionalized children in the United States. Height was obtained in stocking feet, and weight was measured in standardized clothing weighing less than two thirds of a pound. The study found that "American boys at age 6 are slightly taller and heavier than the girls; but by age 11 the girls are larger. This holds true for both white and Negro children analyzed separately and together."[19] Shortly after the onset of puberty, adolescent boys attain, on the average, greater height and weight than the girls.

The increase in individual muscle cell size in girls reaches a peak at about age 10½, but in boys the maximum rate of growth of muscle cells begins at 10½ and may continue to age 25. Until the onset of puberty, however, strength is quite similar in boys and girls of the same biological age.[20]

Rauh and Schumsky[21] reported that in children between 5 and 17, the average per cent of body fat is greater in females except during the period from approximately 7 to 10. In boys, per cent of body fat reaches a peak at age 11, but in girls it decreases from ages 5 through 7 and then increases continually through age 17.

Because of this greater percentage of body fat, girls are, at certain ages, relatively more buoyant than boys. This advantage has to be considered in light of buoyancy being gained at the expense of relatively less lean body mass and, therefore, less muscle mass. Even though contemporary champion girl swimmers have beaten the world and Olympic records held by men several decades ago, they have not equalled the current record times of males. The buoyancy advantage of girls is not sufficient to overcome their absolute deficit in muscle mass. In nonaquatic sports, the increased percentage of body fat in girls serves to place them at a disadvantage when competing against boys.

In summary, girls are, except for a short period, shorter and lighter and possess a greater percentage of body fat than boys.

THE FEMALE ATHLETE'S SPECIFIC PROBLEMS

Iron Metabolism

Prior to puberty, the daily dietary iron need is the same for boys and girls, but at menarche, with the subsequent loss of blood, the female's need for iron becomes considerably greater than that of boys. In the adult, the average daily requirement of iron for the female is almost twice that of the male. Pregnancy increases iron need by a factor of three or four times that of the male.[13] It is important for those concerned with the health and training of young girls to be aware of their special dietary needs.

The question often arises as to whether or not young girls should be allowed to donate blood during puberty. C. E. C. Harris[22] feels that during their adolescent years, neither boys nor girls should be allowed to be blood donors. Perhaps the female athlete should forego this humanitarian effort as long as she is involved in high-intensity training.

The use of the intrauterine contraceptive device (IUD) carries with it the potential for losing more than the normal amount of menstrual blood each period.[23, 24] Thus, it is essential that individuals who choose this method of contraception should be certain that their daily iron intake is sufficient to meet this potentially increased need.

Injuries and Protective Equipment

When boys and girls play the same sport, they generally experience the same types of injuries. However, Haddon and colleagues[25] and Ellison[26] found that women run a much greater risk of injury while skiing than men. They noted that the factors involved included less strength, less skill, and decreased bone density.

A type of sports injury peculiar to the female is that which can occur in water skiing. It is possible that while falling or while beginning to ski from a spread-leg, take-off position, water may be forced into the reproductive tract.[27, 28] The water may, by flowing from the vagina through the uterus and fallopian tubes, enter the peritoneal cavity, causing an inflammatory response. Occasionally in this type of injury, the water will rupture the vaginal wall and enter the peritoneal cavity by that route.

The vulval area, like other soft tissues, may be the site of bruises and contusions. To prevent these as well as the water-skiing injury, suitable protective clothing should be worn.

The Female Breast.   It is undoubtedly true that the volume of breast tissue is a factor in sports activity. Large or pendulous breasts could handicap girls whose sport activity involves running for a lengthy period, swimming, or the need for control of rotational forces as in gymnastics. Breast volume would be of less importance in sports such as sailing, equestrian events, golf, and track and field events not involving prolonged running.

With a properly engineered and designed brassiere, it is possible to contain the breast tissues so that the breasts will move synchronously with the chest wall rather than counter to its vertical motion during running. However, when this method of control is used, the breast may need to be bound so tightly as to interfere with pulmonary ventilation. Bayne[29] has described a protective brassiere. Such devices should be available in a multiplicity of sizes, but this has not been the case.

Breast volume is sensitive to hormonal influences and thus varies as the hormonal levels change during the menstrual cycle. Milligan and associates[30] have investigated changes in breast volume in normal menstrual cycles as well as those in subjects taking oral contraceptives. During normal menstrual cycles, the average change was an increase of as much as 100 ml, mostly during the latter half of the cycle. For those individuals taking oral contraceptives, the mean change was an increase of 66 ml, again in the latter half of the cycle.

It is logical to assume that the breasts of either sex will be subjected to trauma, especially in contact sports. The question of whether there is a relationship between trauma and the development of malignancy is a reasonable one. Monkman and co-workers[31] found no evidence that single uncomplicated trauma causes cancer.

Influence of the Menstrual Cycle on Behavior and Athletic Performance

At puberty, the female begins a cyclic hormone pattern, a rhythm not experienced by the male, which results in the establishment of the menstrual cycle. In the United States, for women between the ages of 18 and 34 surveyed between the years 1960 and 1970, the mean age of menarche was just several months short of 13 years. Menarche may occur as early as age 9 and as late as 17.[32] Approximately 50 per cent of women experience menopause by age 50.

There is hardly a single body function or system that is not influenced by the menstrual cycle. The psyche, skin, thermoregulatory system, gastrointestinal tract — all may be altered during various stages of the menstrual cycle. These changes have been comprehensively reviewed by Southam and Gonzaga.[33] Rogers[34] has reviewed the relationship between menstruation and systemic disease.

In England, Katharina Dalton investigated the influence of the menstrual cycle on criminal behavior in women,[35] scholastic performance of school girls,[36] accidents,[37] and hospital admissions for acute psychiatric illness.[38] Dalton felt that the negative aspects of this behavior were often associated with the the premenstural portion of the menstrual cycle. Sommer[39] critically examined Dalton's work and felt that her investigative techniques were deficient with respect to statistical methodology. Concerning one of Dalton's studies[40] having to do with scholastic performance, Sommer stated: "This assumption of causality is unwarranted; mediating factors have not been ruled out and lack of proper controls and statistical treatment were a serious question with respect to the validity and reliability of the findings."

The difficulties in investigating the influence of the menstrual cycle on various aspects of behavior were summarized as follows by Parlee:[41]

1. Psychological studies of the premenstrual syndrome have not as yet established the existence of a class of behaviors and moods, measurable in more than one way, which can be shown in a longitudinal study to fluctuate throughout the course of the menstrual cycle, or even a class of such behaviors which is regularly correlated with any particular phase of the cycle for groups of women. This is not to say that such a set of behaviors does not exist — many women spontaneously attest that they do — but that as a scientific hypothesis the existence of a premenstrual syndrome has little other than face validity.

2. Psychological studies of the premenstrual syndrome are difficult to interpret without control groups to establish a base line for describing changes in behavior in one sex and to determine the presence or absence of cyclic changes in the behaviors of nonmenstruating individuals. The use of control groups — automatic in most psychological studies — might yield

new data on rhythmic behaviors of hitherto unsuspected generality and, if so, would broaden the interpretation of those previously studied only in adult females.

3. Given the paucity of data showing actual changes in nonverbal behavior throughout the menstrual cycle, careful consideration should be given to the nature of the data in a particular study: Do they show what the subject says about menstruation or what she does — nonverbally — throughout the cycle? In view of the prevalence of culturally transmitted beliefs and attitudes about menstruation, this distinction is important in considering the relative influence of social and physiological factors both in interpreting the data and in formulating new hypotheses.

4. Given the variety of methods and the variable quality of data on the premenstrual syndrome, investigators proposing a physiological mechanism to explain hormone-behavior relationships should make clear both what behaviors they propose to account for and also the nature of the empirical and conceptual assumptions upon which their psychophysiological hypotheses rest.*

World-class athletes do not appear to allow the menstrual cycle to influence their performance. At the 1964 and 1968 Summer Olympiads, female members of the United States Olympic team won gold medals and set new world records during various phases of the menstrual cycle. However, these facts, though quite interesting, have little applicability to the great majority of athletes who do not reach the Olympic level of competition. Clearly, if training and competing during certain phases of the menstrual cycle represented a recurring deterrent to an athlete, she most probably would never reach the world-class level of performance. It is also possible that certain phases of the menstrual cycle exert a strong negative influence on many world-class athletes, but they have the mental and physical ability either to minimize those forces or to continue to compete and perform in the face of them. Bausenwein[42] stated that, in events of short duration, women have attained their best personal performance and even established Olympic and world records while menstruating. Yet, without presenting data, she contended that exercise during menstruation causes pelvic congestion and that strenuous exercise by younger girls may cause irreparable harm to ovarian function.

It is no doubt true that the determinants of championship performance involve a great number of physical and mental qualities and that even though certain phases of the menstrual cycle may be an important component of that complex, it is certainly not the only or all-important one.[42-44]

Physical Exercise and Reproductive Function

Just as important as the question of the influence of the menstrual cycle on performance is the question of the effect of athletic performance on reproductive function. This issue has received comprehensive treatment by Åstrand and colleagues.[7] Their study, as well as those of Hong and Rahn[45] and Anderson[46] — all involving swimming — are particularly apropos because of the virtual taboo against swimming during the menstrual cycle. In none of those investigations was swimming found to be the cause of obstetrical or gynecological difficulties in later life.

Excellent pictorial and narrative descriptions of Oriental women whose livelihood is provided by their skin-diving activities have been given by Maraini.[47] Concerning women in this occupation, Hong and Rahn[45] reported:

The Korean women dive even in winter, when the water temperature is 50 degrees Fahrenheit (but only for short periods under such conditions). For those who choose this occupation, diving is a lifelong profession; they begin to work in shallow water at the age of 11 or 12 and sometimes continue to 65. Childbearing does not interrupt their work; a pregnant diving woman may work up to the day of delivery and nurse her baby afterward between diving shifts. The divers are called ama. At present there are some 30,000 of them living and working along the seacoasts of Korea and Japan. About 11,000 ama dwell on the small, rocky island of Cheju off the southern tip of the Korean peninsula, which is believed to be the area where the diving practice originated. Archaeological remains indicate that the practice began before the fourth century. In times past the main objective of the divers may have been pearls, but today it is solely food. Up to the 17th century the ama of Korea included men as well as women; now they are all women. And in Japan, where many of the ama are male, women nevertheless predominate in the occupation. . . . The female is better suited to this work than the male.*

In a personal communication, S. K. Hong wrote concerning the diving ama: "Some years ago we made a survey on their menstruation, according to which they engage in usual daily diving work even during menstruation. As far as we learned, they use no particular menstrual protection. Our survey also indicated that their menstrual cycle is quite regular."

Javert[48] was interested in the question of whether or not physical activity was a factor in producing spontaneous abortion. He cited Potter as follows:

As well stated by Potter, the packaging of the child in utero is such that the tough skin, muscles, and fascia of the abdominal wall, the thick uterine muscle lined by membrane, and the amniotic fluid absorb physical trauma encountered in the daily routine of the mother to protect the growing fetus from ordinary harm.

Javert[48] concluded that "normal physical and mental activity do not predispose to spontaneous abortion. However, violent physical and mental trauma engendered by unexpected accidents are rare but significant factors in abortion."

The uterus, like the human brain, is well protected by being surrounded by aqueous material. The ability of this system to absorb and distribute forces is phenomenal. McCloy[49] discussed Paramore's work wherein the uterine protection was compared to that of an egg in a jar full of water. As long as the egg is not resting against the wall of the container and the container remains intact, it is not possible to break the egg by either hitting or dropping the jar.

The amount and type of exercise to be engaged in during pregnancy is an individual decision to be reached by a woman in consultation with her physician. They should be able to outline a program that will maintain her state of physical fitness if she is an athlete or even increase it if she has been completely sedentary prior to pregnancy.

In a study of 11 normal women, cardiac output and pulse rate were found to be elevated during most of the last two trimesters of pregnancy. Stroke volume progressively decreased during the same period. Cardiac output was investigated in six patients during light exercise (100 kilopond-meters per minute) and in five during moderate exercise (200 kilopond-meters per minute). In moderate exercise, there was a progressive decline in circulatory response as pregnancy advanced. This was not attributed by the authors to a change in cardiac function but rather to peripheral pooling of blood and obstruction to venous return by the large gravid uterus. Following exercise, cardiovascular function returned to resting levels as quickly during pregnancy as after delivery. To the extent that the results of this study could be applied to well-conditioned subjects, it is not surprising to find that championship-level athletes have competed until a few days prior to onset of labor and that one Olympic competitor won a bronze medal in swimming in the 1952 Games during her pregnancy.[51] Erdelyi[52] surveyed 729 Hungarian female athletes and found the incidence of cesarean section was only 50 per cent that of a control group.

Noack[44] investigated 10 women who continued their sports activity after delivery. He reported:

---

*From Hong, S. K., and Rahn, H.: The diving women of Korea and Japan. Scientific American, May, 1967, p. 34. Copyright © 1967 by Scientific American, Inc. All rights reserved.

Two retained their physical abilities, and eight clearly increased them. All the women reported that after the birth of a child they had become tougher, more enduring and stronger. It is striking to learn from this survey that everything went smoothly from the obstetrical point of view. The generally short duration of the delivery indicates that the frequently asserted rigidity of the soft parts . . . is insignificant. Certainly, the seven ruptures of the perineum are above the normal number. It cannot be excluded that the good activity of the abdominal muscles in the sports-trained woman was a disadvantage for the perineum. In spite of the desire to resume sports, breast feeding was apparently carried out for a normal length of time. It is especially significant and noticeable that six of these women won championships after delivery. We would not be able to find thirteen German Champions, three DDR-Champions, three Berlin Champions, and two Silver Medalists during the Olympic Games in 1948 in our German sports if these women had not resumed sports after delivery. We believe that this fact deserves attention in interested sports circles. Naturally, our material is small and selected, but the top performances are objective facts which should give food for thought.

It is recalled that the oldest female competitor at the 1948 Olympics was the 30-year-old runner, housewife, and mother of two children, Fanny Blankers-Koen. In her 7 days there, she ran 11 races, did not lose a heat, and won 4 gold medals.[53]

At the 1976 Olympics in Montreal, Irena Szewinska won the 400-meter race in the time of 49.29 seconds, thus setting a new world and Olympic record. She had previously competed in the 1964, 1968, and 1972 Olympics and in that time won six Olympic medals, including three gold medals. After the Mexico City Olympics in 1968, she retired to have a child (a son, born in 1970). In 1972 at the Munich Olympics, she finished third in the 200-meter race and then, as mentioned, came back to set a new world record in the 400-meter event in Montreal.[54]

The first two finishers in the Amateur Athletic Union women's marathon in 1974 were Judy Ikenberry and Marilyn Paul. Mrs. Ikenberry is the mother of three children, and Mrs. Paul has a young son.

The Female Runner[55] reported:

A distance runner from Colorado, Marcia Le Mire, tells of her experience while pregnant and while nursing: "I would like more female runners to know that neither of these conditions precludes running. I ran for nine months of my first pregnancy, with complete approval from my doctor, and seven months with my second pregnancy. Distances ranged from three to seven miles. I also began running again shortly after delivery (one and two weeks).

Many women feel exercise cuts down milk supply and therefore do not run and nurse at the same time. They do one or the other. This need not happen. I ran a marathon (3:53) when my first child was 10 months old and still nursing." Apparently the bigger problem for a mother of a young child is simply finding the time to get out of the house to run.*

Athletic Activity During Menstruation

Menstrual taboos[56] continue to influence the behavior of men and women during the bleeding phase of the menstrual cycle. These taboos have been invoked to prevent menstrual-age females from using sports facilities during the menstrual phase of their cycle. The general feeling has been either that the exercise would harm the individual or, with respect to swimming, that contamination of the pool would provide the potential for disease in those who shared the pool with menstruants. As will be shown, there is nothing to support these prohibitions. This is not to say that dysmenorrhea (pain with menstruation) does not exist and that some individual will not be inclined to participate in vigorous athletic activity during all phases of the menstrual cycle. Nevertheless, for those who wish to continue sports involvement during menstruation, no hindrances should be placed in their way.

---

*Copyright 1973 by Women's Running, published by World Publications, Box 366, Mountain View, Calif.

With respect to the question of swimming during menstruation, it is reasonable to inquire whether or not water flows freely in and out of the vagina of the submerged individual. Siegel[57] and Haselhorst[58] investigated this and found that the vagina is able to exclude water even when tested almost immediately following childbirth. However, even if there were a possibility of contamination of a pool by the free flow of water in and out of the vagina, this would not provide a source of pathogenic organisms. From the quantitative, as well as the qualitative, standpoint the skin and nasal and oral cavities represent a greater souce of potential contamination from pathogenic organisms than does the vagina. It is interesting to realize that a gram of tissue scraped from the skin contains as many as 530,000,000,000 bacteria.[59] This value is quite close to the number of bacteria and fungi found in a gram of fertile soil.

The possibility that swimming during the menstrual cycle adds an abnormal bacterial load to the water was investigated by Robinton and Mood.[60] They asked young women to swim at various stages of their menstrual cycle. In some cases the subjects used tampons for menstrual protection; in other tests they used no form of menstrual protection. The study was summarized, in part, as follows:

Five healthy young women swam in untreated water of known bacterial quality under a variety of hygienic conditions. Evidence based on bacteriological examination of water samples leads to the following conclusions:
1. There is a marked variation in the number and types of bacteria shed by a bather while swimming and the variations do not seem to be correlated to the differences in personal hygiene or the menstrual period. . . .

Women who participate in athletics, as well as those who provide instruction to young female athletes, should be aware of certain practical and basic information concerning menstruation and menstrual protection. The question of the type of product to use is, in general, a matter of personal choice and convenience. In aquatic sports, however, the external form of menstrual protection is useless. Menstrual tampons provide the only practical means of menstrual hygiene for those who swim.

Pain and Discomfort During the Menstrual Cycle (Dysmenorrhea)

There are few objective findings in dysmenorrhea. The symptoms include some or all of the following: lower abdominal cramps, backache, a feeling of fullness in the abdomen, headache, and, rarely, nausea and vomiting. The subjective nature of most of these is one of the reasons why the disorder has remained so poorly defined and understood. Harris[61] noted that the interviewer may have a strong influence on the responses of those being questioned concerning dysmenorrhea.

Attempts to investigate this subject have been, and are still, handicapped by the lack of methods for quantitating either premenstrual tension or dysmenorrhea. The bias introduced by self reporting was investigated by Ruble.[62] The problems of premenstrual tension and dysmenorrhea experienced by students and nurses are discussed in Sutherland and Stewart's report.[63] Of the 150 women (nullipara) they questioned, only 17 per cent were completely free from pain in relation to menstruation. Clitheroe[64] reviewed the literature and found that dysmenorrhea was reported as occurring in from 3 to 90 per cent of women. Bukowski[65] found that individuals who were warned in advance that they would be questioned about symptoms provided a greater number of positive responses than those not forewarned.

The possibility that severe dysmenorrhea will interfere with an athlete's exercise and training program is real. There is, however, evidence that persons who experience dysmenorrhea can receive relief from therapeutic exercise programs.[66, 67] Even though a specific therapeutic agent for dysmenorrhea is unavailable, some forms may be treated indirectly by preventing ovulation through use of hormonal antifertility agents. Primary dysmenorrhea is not present if ovulation does not precede the bleeding phase.

Even though hysteria has been reported to be contagious,[68] there are no data to support this author's feeling that the pyschological aspects of dysmenorrhea in young girls may also be contagious.

Menstrual Synchrony

The menstrual-age female has approximately a one in seven chance of being in the menstrual phase of her cycle on any given date provided she is not pregnant. It would be statistically reasonable to assume that this would apply to each member of a girls' athletic team. Evidence that this may not be entirely true has been presented by McClintock.[69] She reports that women living together in a college dormitory as roommates or close friends tend to develop synchronization of their menstrual periods. If this influence held true for athletes who were members of the same team, the menstrual phase of the entire team might be clustered in a portion of the month rather than being distributed by chance throughout the entire month.

Amenorrhea (Absence of Menstruation)

The only dependable characteristic of the menstrual cycle is its variability. This is true whether one is comparing menstrual cycle data in the same or different individuals. (This feature of the menstrual cycle was investigated by Vollman.[70]) For this reason, it is difficult to be certain whether a short series of missed periods is within the normal range of variability or is due to some pathological process. The menstrual cycle is sensitive to a variety of stresses. Wartime conditions and more common stressful events, such as entering college, have been shown to cause amenorrhea in healthy individuals.[71-73]

Data concerning the frequency of amenorrhea in individuals involved in strenuous athletic training programs are unavailable, but many coaches and athletes feel that this is a common occurrence. From the medical standpoint, there is little reason to be alarmed when an athlete becomes amenorrheic during a strenuous athletic training program; this most probably represents her reaction to that particular form of stress. The resumption of a regular menstrual pattern once training is reduced in intensity or terminated would be the expected outcome.

One most important note of caution: the most frequent cause of amenorrhea in the sexually active individual is pregnancy. This could come as startling news to a young athlete whose coaches and trainers had been quick to assure her that the amenorrhea was most probably due to her strenuous training program.

Influence of Sexual Activity on Women's Performance

There have been no controlled studies of the influence of sexual activity on subsequent performance in athletic events. Johnson[74] reported that sexual activity had no effect on muscular performance of men. Perhaps more important than the physical aspects would be the individual's emotional response to sexual activity. Weiler and Cavenar[75] have indicated that "feelings of relief, happiness, disappointment, sadness, guilt, contempt, anger, and powerfulness may be experienced in vary-ing degrees by both sexes after intercourse." Obviously, certain of these responses might have a negative influence on subsequent athletic performance, while others could enhance the athlete's feeling of well-being. With respect to energy expenditure during coitus, the work of Boas and Goldschmidt[76] indicates that the act represents a submaximum work load.

Masturbation, though the subject of much speculation,[77] has not been shown to be either harmful or beneficial to subsequent athletic performance.

Sexual Identification of Athletes

In the normal female, the cells contain 22 pairs of chromosomes called autosomes and two X (sex) chromosomes. The male has the same number of autosomes but has an X and a Y chromosome rather than two X chromosomes. In the female, one of the two X chromosomes appears as a dark-staining mass of chromatin at the inside edge of the nuclear membrane. This material, initially described by Barr, is present in 22 to 50 per cent of the cells. By use of this technique of cell examination, it is possible to distinguish genetic females from genetic males. The sexual phenotype (the anatomical and secondary sexual characteristics) of an individual may be discordant with respect to the genetic sex. Thus, it is possible for a genetic male to appear to be a female. If this individual were to compete as a female, unfair advantage over the true females could occur because male hormones produce greater strength and muscle mass. For this reason, the general feeling is that the apparent female who is in reality a genetic male or a male masquerading as a female (transvestite) should not be permitted to compete against women.

There are several types of genetic abnormalities that make it possible for a true male to appear to be an anatomical female or a true female to appear to be an anatomical male. However, not many of these disorders allow normal growth and development to an extent that would permit the person to compete in athletics.

A genetic female may develop an adrenal tumor that produces excess male hor-mones and subsequent changes in secondary sex characteristics such as hair growth, voice, and breast tissue. Even though this person might be mistaken for a male by the casual observer, she is actually a female. Occasionally, a true genetic male will develop an abnormality of the testis that will cause excess secretion of female hor-mones. This person might very well appear to be female but would still be a genetic male.

Drugs

Anabolic Steroids. There are no precise data concerning the extent of abuse of anabolic steroids by either males or females. Enjolras[78] stated, without indicating the source of information, that Russian athletes, both men and women, first used anabolic steroids in 1954. Talking to coaches and trainers leaves the impression that they have no doubt that female athletes do use these hormones in an attempt to enhance their performance.

The use of anabolic steroids by females, particularly those who are either prepu-bertal or have not attained full growth, is especially dangerous. The undesired side effects include masculinization[79-81] disruption of normal growth patterns,[79] voice changes[80-82] acne,[79-82] abnormal hair growth,[79, 80, 82] and enlargement of the clitoris.[79] The long-term effects on reproductive function are unknown, but anabolic steroids may be harmful in this area. Their ability to interfere with the menstrual cycle has been well documented.[79] For these reasons, all concerned with advising, training, coaching, and providing medical care for female athletes should exercise all persuasions available to prevent the use of anabolic steroids by female athletes.

Hormonal and Antifertility Agents.   Since the 1960's, various combinations of estrogenic substances and synthetic progestational agents have been available for the prevention of conception. Whether or not these hormones have the potential for enhancing or interfering with the quality of a female's performance by altering her strength, coordination, timing, endurance, or metabolism is not known. Kane [83] reported that clinical studies indicate that 10 to 40 per cent of oral contraceptive users experience mild to moderate depression.

Morris and Udry[84] compared the pedometer-measured activity of 8 women taking birth control pills with that of 26 who did not. The former walked an average of 4.2 miles (6711 meters) and the latter 4.9 miles (7821 meters) each day. These differences were statistically significant. The authors pointed out, however, that until a prospective study of women before and after taking the pills is done, their data will have to be regarded as only presumptive evidence that the use of various hormone agents as contraceptives causes women to be less physically active.

The various metabolic effects of contraceptive steroids have been thoroughly discussed in the volume edited by Salhanick and colleagues.[85] It would be somewhat surprising to find that these hormones did not alter performance. It is important to bear in mind that there are a variety of combinations of hormonal antifertility agents available and they are not identical in composition. If these drugs are prescribed for athletes, preparations containing the least amount of estrogen should be used so that fewer side effects result.[86-88]

PROSPECTS FOR WOMEN'S
PARTICIPATION IN ATHLETICS

The potential for women's participation in athletics is unlimited. The realization of this potential will, however, depend upon a great number of factors, not the least of which is the ability of women to influence their own progress and to overcome the traditional concepts of "a woman's place."

In the field of physical education, women have been studied to a much lesser extent than men.[89] It is essential that men learn more about women. Tiger[90] wrote:

It is curiously anomalous that while young males may be taught about the tax system, about the value of exercise, or about the poetry of Browning, they are unlikely to receive systematic knowledge about the specialized patterns of behavior of members of the sex with whom the great majority will spend a good deal of their adult lives. More realistic and analytic treatment of the different typical careers and life-chances of males and females might alleviate what appears to be frequent disharmony between what many females expect about their working and married lives and the extent to which communities help to meet these expectations. In particular, some objective discussion of the anti-female tradition and the nature of male exclusion of females from various male groups could simplify or clarify the problems women may feel who seek careers in predominantly male organizations.

The image of the female athlete and the risks she takes by winning when in competition with a man have been discussed by D. V. Harris,[61] who feels that many women take the easy route — that is, they avoid all participation in athletics. The deprecation of female athletes by themselves and their peers of both sexes is a powerful force that will have to be attenuated, if not abolished, before women are allowed, and indeed allow themselves, the opportunity to realize their full potential in sports endeavors.

For the assurance of a healthy gene pool, it is absolutely essential that members of neither sex continue to subscribe to a system that would provide inadequate opportunity for women to realize their full potential as vigorous, physically active beings. To do otherwise is to limit the potential of mankind.

SUMMARY

There are biological differences between the male and female, but there is no evidence to indicate that special rules and regulations need to be formulated with respect to sports participation by normal healthy girls. The young prepubertal girl is, when exercising vigorously, no more at risk from injury than is the prepubertal boy.

The "average" postpubertal female will have less strength and a greater per cent of body fat, will be of shorter stature, and will require more iron in her diet than the "average" male.

Special equipment is available for protecting the external genitalia of the male athlete—special protective brassieres are available for the female athlete.

A great number of bodily functions fluctuate in harmony with the menstrual cycle, but there is no evidence that such variation is an overriding consideration in determining the suitability of various sports, including swimming, for the female athlete. There is good evidence that championship performances have been attained by women while competing during all phases of the menstrual cycle. There is no evidence that having participated in vigorous athletic activity over a great length of time is harmful to those athletes who later bear children. Some athletes have attained their best performances subsequent to having borne children.

Pregnancy is usually a deterrent to the competitive athlete, particularly during the last six months. There is, however, no reason to restrict activity during pregnancy, unless so advised by the athlete's physician, who, of course, should be familiar with the physical demands of the sports in question.

The most frequent cause of amenorrhea is pregnancy, which should always be considered when evaluating this symptom in athletes.

Physical activity is basic to the health of humans. Thus, it is essential that men and women cooperate to be certain that women are provided with equal opportunities, incentives, and rewards for participating in athletic activity at all levels.

STUDY QUESTIONS

1. List the reasons why you feel women should or should not be allowed to participate in contact sports.

2. A high school has only one gym and both the boys' and girls' basketball teams need to use it for practice and training. How would you approach scheduling the two teams for using the gym?

3. At the college level, the strongest woman will not be as strong as the strongest man. Realizing this, how is it possible to justify allowing members of both sexes to play on the same team?

4. The authorities have learned that a scheduled competitor's team includes a male masquerading as a female. What action would you suggest?

5. A young boy is interested in becoming a member of the girls' synchronized swimming team. Discuss the reason why he should or should not be allowed to compete as the only male member of that team.

6. What is the influence of the menstrual cycle on athletic performance?

7. A young girl feels that in order to improve her performance she should take anabolic steroids. Discuss reasons why this would be inadvisable.

8. A young postpubertal female athlete complains that she has not menstruated in the last 4 months. List several possible causes of this problem.

FURTHER READINGS

Gerber, E., Felshin, J., Berlin, P., and Wyrick, W.: *The American Woman in Sport*. Reading, Mass., Addison-Wesley Publishing Company, 1974.
Ihalainen, O.: Psychosomatic aspects of amenorrhoea. Acta Psychiatr. Scand. (Suppl.)262, 1975.
Mathews,D., and Fox, E.: *The Physiological Basis of Physical Education and Athletics*, 2nd ed. Philadelphia, W. B. Saunders Company, 1976.
Michener, J.: *Sports in America*. Greenwich, Conn., Fawcett Publications, 1976.
Ullyot, J.: *Women's Running*. Mountain View, Calif., World Publications, 1976.
Vollman, R.: *The Menstrual Cycle*. Philadelphia, W. B. Saunders Company, 1977.
Wilmore, J.: *Athletic Training and Physical Fitness*. Boston, Allyn and Bacon, Inc., 1976.

REFERENCES

1. Grover, G. H.: Girls on boys' athletic teams. 12th Proc. Natl. Conf. Med. Aspects Sports, 1970.
2. Moyer, L. J.: Women's athletics — what is our future? JOPER *48*:52–54, 1977.
3. Counsilman, J. E.: Reflections on the 1964 Olympics. 6th Proc. Nat. Conf. Med. Aspects Sports, 1965, pp. 19–23.
4. Astrand, P.-O.: *Experimental Studies of Physical Working Capacity in Relation to Sex and Age*. Copenhagen, Ejnar Munksgard, 1952.
5. Van Wyck, J. J., and Grumbach, M. M.: Disorders of sex differentiation. *In* Williams, R. H. (ed.): *Textbook of Endocrinology*. Philadelphia, W. B. Saunders Company, 1968, pp. 559–560.
6. Williams, R. J.: *Biochemical Individuality*. New York, John Wiley and Sons, 1956.
7. Astrand, P.-O., Engstrom, L., Eriksson, B. O., Karlberg, P., Nylander, I., Saltin, B., and Thoren, C.: Girl swimmers. Acta Paediatr. Scand. (Suppl.)147, 1963.
8. Arena, J. M. (ed.): *Davison's Compleat Pediatrician*. Philadelphia, Lea & Febiger, 1969.
9. Werner, M., Tolls, R. E., Hultin, J. V., and Mellecker, J.: Influence of sex and age on the normal range of eleven serum constituents. Z. Klin. Chem. Klin. Biochem. *8*:105–115, 1970.
10. Laubach, L. L.: *Muscular Strength of Women and Men: A Comparative Study*. AMRL-TR-75-32, Wright-Patterson Air Force Base, OH, Aerospace Med. Res. Lab., Aerospace Med. Div., Air Force Systems Command, 1976 (AD A025793).
11. Kroemer, K. H. E.: *Push Forces Exerted in Sixty-Five Common Working Positions*. AMRL-TR-68-143, Wright-Patterson Air Force Base, OH, Aerospace Med. Res. Lab., Aerospace Med. Div., Air Force Systems Command, 1969 (AD 695040).
12. Laubach, L. L., and McConville, J. T.: The relationship of strength to body size and typology. Med. Sci. Sports *1*:189–194, 1969.
13. Wintrobe, M. M.: *Clinical Hematology*. Philadelphia, Lea & Febiger, 1974.
14. Castleman, B., and McNeely, B. U.: Normal laboratory values. N. Engl. J. Med. *283*:1276–1285, 1970.
15. Metropolitan Life Insurance Company: More about biochemical profiles. Statistical Bull. *52*:3–7, 1971.
16. Snyder, W. S., Cook, M. J., Nasset, E. S., Karhausen, L. R., Howells, G. P., and Tipton, I. H.: *Report of the Task Group on Reference Man*. International Commission on Radiological Protection No. 23. New York, Pergamon Press, 1975.
17. Macdonald, R. G., and Macdonald, H. N.: Erythrocyte 2,3–diphosphoglycerate and associated haematological parameters during the menstrual cycle and pregnancy. Brit. J. Obstet. Gynaecol. *84*:427–433, 1977.

18. Denis, P., Cazor, J. L., Feret, J., Weisang, E., and Lefrancois, R.: 2,3-Diphosphoglycerate red cell concentration changes during the menstrual cycle in women. Biomed. *25*:144–147, 1976.
19. Hamill, P. V. V., Johnson, F. E., and Grams, W.: *Height and Weight of Children.* Rockville, Md., Health Services and Mental Health Administration, DHEW Publication No. 1000, Series 11, No. 104, 1970.
20. Cheek, D. B.: Muscle cell growth in children. *In* Cheek, D. B. (ed.): *Human Growth.* Philadelphia, Lea & Febiger, 1968, pp. 337–351.
21. Rauh, J. L., and Schumsky, D. A.: Lean and non-lean body mass estimates in urban school children. *In* Cheek, D. B. (ed.): *Human Growth.* Philadelphia, Lea & Febiger, 1968, pp. 242–252.
22. Harris, C. E. C.: Blood donations by young women. Can. Med. Assoc. J. *104*:767, 1971.
23. Guttorm, E.: Menstrual bleeding with intrauterine devices. Acta Obstet. Gynecol. Scand. *50*:9–16, 1971.
24. Hefnawi, F., Younis, N., Zaki, K., Rassik, S. A., and Mekkawi, T.: Menstrual blood loss during oral contraceptive therapy and in I.U.D. users. Egypt. Population Family Planning Rev. *3*:1–4, 1970.
25. Haddon, W., Jr., Ellison, A. E., and Carroll, R. E.: Skiing injuries: epidemiologic study. *In* Haddon, W., Jr., Schuman, E. A., and Klein, D.: *Accident Research.* New York, Harper & Row, 1964, pp. 599–612.
26. Ellison, A. E.: Research techniques in ski medicine. 12th Proc. Natl. Conf. Med. Aspects Sports, 1970.
27. Pfanner, D.: Salpingitis and water-skiing. Med. J. Aust. *1*:320, 1964.
28. Ellsworth, H. S., de Vries, K. L., McQuarrie, H. G., and Harris, J. W.: Intravaginal pressures during physical activity and their possible relationship to pelvic disease. J. Sports Med. *9*:107–109, 1969.
29. Bayne, J. D.: Pro+Tec protective bra. J. Sports Med. Phys. Fitness *8*:34–35, 1968.
30. Milligan, D., Drife, J. O., and Short, R. V.: Changes in breast volume during normal menstrual cycle and after oral contraceptives. Brit. Med. J. *4*:494–495, 1975.
31. Monkman, G. R., Orwoll, G., and Ivins, J. C.: Trauma and oncogenesis. Mayo Clin. Proc. *49*:157–163, 1974.
32. MacMahon, B.: *Age at Menarche.* Rockville, Md., Health Resources Administration, National Center for Health Statistics, DHEW Publication No. (HRA) 74—1615, November 1973.
33. Southam, A. L., and Gonzaga, F. P.: Systemic changes during the menstrual cycle. Am. J. Obstet. Gynecol. *91*:142–165, 1965.
34. Rogers, J.: Menstruation and systemic disease. N. Engl. J. Med. *259*:676–681, 721–727, 770–775, 1958.
35. Dalton, K.: Menstruation and crime. Brit. Med. J. *2*:1752–1753, 1961.
36. Dalton, K.: Effect of menstruation on schoolgirls' weekly work. Brit. Med. J. *1*:326–328, 1960.
37. Dalton, K.: Menstruation and accidents. Brit. Med. J. *2*:1425–1426, 1960.
38. Dalton, K.: Menstruation and acute psychiatric illnesses. Brit. Med. J. *1*:148–149, 1959.
39. Sommer, B.: The effect of menstruation on cognitive and perceptual-motor behavior: a review. Psychosom. Med. *35*:514–534, 1973.
40. Dalton, K.: Menstruation and examinations. Lancet *2*:1386–1388, 1968.
41. Parlee, M. B.: The premenstrual syndrome. Psychol. Bull. *80*:454–465, 1973.
42. Bausenwein, I.: Frau und leistungssport. Sportaerztl. Praxis *3*:12–19, 1960.
43. Zaharieva, E.: Survey of sportswomen at the Tokyo Olympics. J. Sports Med. *5*:215–219, 1965.
44. Noack, H.: Die Sportliche Leistungsfahigkeit der Frau im Menstrualzyklus. Artz und Sport *79*:1523–1525, 1954.
45. Hong, S. K., and Rahn, H.: The diving women of Korea and Japan. Sci. Amer. *216*:34–43, 1967.
46. Anderson, T.: Swimming and exercise during menstruation. JOPER *36*:66–68, 1965.
47. Maraini, F.: *The Island of the Fisherwomen.* New York, Harcourt, 1962.
48. Javert, C. T.: Role of the patient's activities in the occurrence of spontaneous abortion. Fertil. Steril. *11*:550–558, 1960.
49. McCloy, C. H.: A study of landing shock in jumping for women. Arbeitsphysiologie *5*:100–111, 1931.
50. Ueland, K., Novy, M. J., Peterson, E. N., and Metcalfe, J.: Maternal cardiovascular dynamics. Am. J. Obstet. Gynecol. *104*:856–863, 1969.
51. Amateur Athletic Union of the United States: *Study of the Effect of Athletic Competition on Girls and Women.* San Francisco, Pacific Association of the Amateur Athletic Union of the United States, 1969.
52. Erdelyi, G. J.: Women in athletics. 2nd Proc. Nat. Conf. Med. Aspects Sports, 1961, pp. 59–63.
53. Greenspan, B.: Fanny Blankers-Koen. womenSports *4*:12–15, 1977.
54. Jordan, T.: Szewinska crushes Brehmer. Track and Field News *29*:79, 1976.
55. Warren, P.: *The Female Runner.* Mountain View, Calif., World Publications, 1976, pp. 23–24.
56. Crawfurd, R.: Notes on the superstitions of menstruation. Lancet *2*:1331–1336, 1915.
57. Siegel, P.: Does bath water enter the vagina? Obstet. Gynecol. *15*:660–661, 1960.
58. Haselhorst, G.: Das Vollbad vor und unter der Geburt. Arztl. Wochenschr., *4*:746–748, 1949.
59. Marples, M. J.: Life on the human skin. Sci. Amer. *220*:108–115, 1969.
60. Robinton, E. D., and Mood, E. W.: A quantitative and qualitative appraisal of microbial pollution of water by swimmers: A preliminary report. J. Hyg. *64*:489–499, 1966.

61. Harris, D. V.: The sportswoman in our society. *In* Harris, D. V. (ed.): DGWS Research Reports: Women in Sports. Washington, D.C., American Association of Health, Physical Education, and Recreation, 1971, pp. 1–4.

62. Ruble, D. N.: Premenstrual symptoms: a reinterpretation. Science *197*:291–292, 1977.

63. Sutherland, H., and Stewart, I.: A critical analysis of the premenstrual syndrome. Lancet *1*:1180–1183, 1965.

64. Clitheroe, H. J.: The etiology of primary dysmenorrhea. Obstet. Gynecol. Surv. *19*:649–659, 1964.

65. Bukowski, Z.: The premenstrual syndrome in student nurses. Pol. Tyg. Lek. *23*:1238–1241; abstracted in Hum. Reprod. *2*:1, 1969.

66. Clow, A. E. S.: Treatment of dysmenorrhea by exercise. Brit. Med. J. *1*:4–5, 1962.

67. Billig, H. E., Jr.: Dysmenorrhea: the result of a postural defect. Arch. Surg. *46*:611–613, 1943.

68. Ebrahim, G. J.: Mass hysteria in school children. Clin. Pediat. *7*:437–438, 1968.

69. McClintock, M. K.: Menstrual synchrony and suppression. Nature *229*:244–245, 1971.

70. Vollman, R. F.: *The Menstrual Cycle*. Philadelphia, W. B. Saunders Company, 1977.

71. Whitacre, F. E., and Barrera, B.: War amenorrhea. JAMA *124*:399–403, 1944.

72. Drew, F. L.: The epidemiology of secondary amenorrhea. J. Chronic Dis. *14*:396–407, 1961.

73. Matsumoto, S., Igarashi, M., and Nagaoka, Y.: Environmental anovulatory cycles. Int. J. Fertil. *13*:15–23, 1968.

74. Johnson, W. R.: Muscular performance following coitus. J. Sex Res. *4*:247–248, 1968.

75. Weiler, S., and Cavenar, J. O.: Postcoital feelings in men and women. Med. Aspects Human Sexual. *11*:69–81, 1977.

76. Boas, E. P., and Goldschmidt, E. F.: *The Heart Rate*. Springfield, Ill., Charles C Thomas, 1932.

77. Editorial: S. A. Tissot (1728–1797) layman's guide to health. JAMA *209*:1083, 1969.

78. Enjolras, O.: Utilite de l'emploi des steroides anabolisants chez les athletes. Nouv. Presse Med. *1*:2599, 1972.

79. Sanchez-Medal, L., Gomez-Leal, A., Duarte, L., and Guadalupe-Rico, M.: Anabolic steroids in the treatment of acquired aplastic anemia. Blood *34*:283–300, 1969.

80. Shahidi, N. T., and Diamond, L. K.: Testosterone-induced remission in aplastic anemia of both acquired and congenital types. N. Engl. J. Med. *264*:953–967, 1961.

81. Allen, D. M., Fine, M. H., Necheles, T. F., and Dameshek, W.: Oxymetholone therapy in aplastic anemia. Blood *32*:83–89, 1968.

82. Silink, S. J., and Firkin, B. G.: An analysis of hypoplastic anaemia with special reference to the use of oxymetholone ("Adroyd") in its therapy. Aust. Ann. Med. *17*:224–235, 1968.

83. Kane, F. J.: Evaluation of emotional reactions to oral contraceptive use. Am. J. Obstet. Gynecol. *126*:968–972, 1976.

84. Morris, N., and Udry, J. R.: Depression of physical activity by contraceptive pills. Am. J. Obstet. Gynecol. *104*:1012–1014, 1969.

85. Salhanick, H. A., Kipnis, D. M., and Vande Wiele, R. L.: *Metabolic Effects of Gonadal Hormones and Contraceptive Steroids*. New York, Plenum Publishing Corp. 1969.

86. Editorial: Oestrogens and thromboembolism. Brit. Med. J. *2*:189–190, 1970.

87. Editorial: Combined oral contraceptives: A statement by the Committee on Safety of Drugs. Brit. Med. J. *2*:231–232, 1970.

88. Inman, W. H. W., Vessey, M. P., Westerholm, B., and Engelund, A.: Thromboembolic disease and the steroidal content of oral contraceptives. Brit. Med. J. *2*:203–209, 1970.

89. Wyrick, W.: How sex differences affect research in physical education. *In* Harris, D. V. (ed.): DGWS Research Report: Women in Sports. Washington, D. C., American Association for Health, Physical Education, and Recreation, 1971, pp. 21–30.

90. Tiger, L.: *Men in Groups*. New York, Vintage Books, 1970.

21

HEAT ILLNESS AND ATHLETICS*

ROBERT J. MURPHY, M.D.

Clinical problems in athletes exposed to environmental heat can vary from temporary heat cramps to fatal heat stroke. It is probable that hundreds of heat stroke deaths, many of them unrecognized, have occurred in various sports over the past few decades. The only accurate records have been kept by the American College Football Coaches Association. From 1968 through 1972, there were 25 recorded deaths in American football. This dropped to four deaths over the next five years (Table 21-1). This dramatic decrease in deaths has been attained primarily through the use of *unlimited water on the field* and better understanding of physiological principles by physicians, trainers, and coaches.

TABLE 21-1. FOOTBALL FATALITIES FROM HEAT STROKE

1968–1972	1973–1977
1968 – 5	1973 – 2
1969 – 6	1974 – 1
1970 – 8	1975 – 0
1971 – 4	1976 – 0
1972 – 2	1977 – 1
25	4

PHYSIOLOGICAL CONSIDERATIONS

Muscular exercise produces internal heat. This heat diffuses from the muscle cell to capillary blood, which subsequently passes through the lungs. Some heat is lost through the lungs, but most is carried by blood into the general arterial circulation. The amount of blood reaching the skin is controlled largely by the temperature regulatory system (see Chapter 8). Heat is lost from the skin through conduction, convection, or radiation to the environment or through evaporation of sweat.

---

*Editor's note: The physiology of temperature regulation is discussed in detail in Chapter 8. Fluids and salt as part of the athlete's diet are discussed in Chapter 17.

Loss of sweat from the body is an important physiological consideration. Sweat is hypotonic. That is, it has a lower concentration of salts and other solutes than does blood. Profuse sweating causes excessive loss of body water. This leads to a decrease in blood volume and, if water is not replaced, a decrease in sweating rate and evaporative cooling. Decreased blood volume can lead to circulatory collapse, and decreased evaporative cooling can cause an excessive rise in body temperature.

Generally, a 3 per cent loss of body weight through sweating is safe, a 5 per cent loss is borderline, and anything over 7 per cent is dangerous. In football, a 200-pound athlete may lose as much as 10 pounds in a 90-minute practice. This represents a loss of 5 quarts of water, which results in a very dehydrated athlete. The amount of sodium and potassium lost is very low relative to the available body sodium and potassium, but the loss of this much fluid represents over 50 per cent of the available body water. The problems resulting from excessive weight loss, when an individual is exposed to environmental heat, are due to water deficit and not to salt deficit. Although it is important to replace salts from one day to the next, the important consideration before and during exercise is to provide plain water as the replacement fluid. Generally, the best way to replace salt is to salt foods to individual taste at mealtimes. Salt tablets, if taken without generous amounts of water, will actually compound the problem and should be used only after exercise, if at all.

CLINICAL DISORDERS

There are four recognizable heat disorders that may be encountered in the exercising athlete.

Heat Cramps

Heat cramps are painful spasms of skeletal muscle — most commonly of the gastrocnemius (calf). For years, the literature has suggested that this problem is due to salt loss. However, this author proposes that heat cramps are caused purely by a fluid volume problem and can be prevented by providing copious amounts of water throughout the exercise period. It is the author's experience that an athlete cannot "overhydrate" himself, so the problem of water intoxication, when fluid intake is controlled by the player himself, does not seem to exist.

Heat Fatigue

This syndrome affects many people after they have exercised in a hot environment. It is simply a feeling of weakness and tiredness, which usually improves promptly with rest and replenishment of the lost fluids.

Heat Exhaustion

This syndrome is characterized by extreme weakness, exhaustion, and sometimes unconsciousness. Headache, dizziness, and profuse sweating are usually present. These symptoms are due to a decrease in blood volume. The key features that differentiate heat exhaustion from heat stroke are (1) sweating skin and (2) normal body temperature. Affected individuals should be withdrawn from further activity for the remainder of that day. Fluids should be given by mouth when the athlete is able to swallow. If vomiting or unconsciousness ensues, hospitalization and intravenous administration of fluids are necessary. The athlete's fluid intake habits should be reviewed before further strenuous exercise is undertaken.

Heat Stroke

Heat stroke is a true medical emergency. It may occur suddenly without being preceded by any of the other clinical syndromes. The player collapses and becomes unconscious. Heat stroke is characterized by a hot, dry skin and a rising body temperature. When 50 to 100 per cent of the available body water is depleted, the brain stops further loss by shutting down the sweating mechanism. When sweating ceases, the body temperature can rise from 98.6° to 106° F within 20 minutes.

First aid treatment while awaiting transfer to a hospital consists of cooling the body with ice, immersing it in cold water, or using any other means available for immediate cooling. The object is to lower the body temperature as quickly as possible. Preventing death or serious damage is literally a matter of minutes. A temperature of over 106° F for more than a few minutes will result in irreversible changes in liver, kidney, or brain cells. In heat stroke, such temperatures are reached rapidly.

PREVENTION OF HEAT PROBLEMS

There are a number of preventive measures that physicians, coaches, and athletes should take in order to avoid heat problems.

Conditioning

A gradual exercise program should be started 7 to 21 days prior to actual participation in a sport. This conditioning should last only 30 to 45 minutes the first day, gradually increasing in length and intensity until a full program is established.

Effects of Environment and Clothing

Heat problems occur in athletes when both the environmental temperature and the humidity are high. Sweat then evaporates slowly, and cooling is reduced. Cooling by evaporation is proportional to the area of skin exposed. A football uniform covers most of the body, so sweating is less effective and greater in quantity — 70 per cent greater than in tennis players or track participants. If the weather is extremely hot and humid, football practice should be conducted with the players wearing shorts, or it should be postponed until later in the day.

Evaluate Environmental Conditions

The old saying, "It's not the heat that's bad, it's the humidity" is certainly applicable. Several football deaths have been reported when the temperature was under 75° F but the humidity was over 95 per cent. The greater the humidity, the more difficult it is for the body to cool itself.

It is absolutely essential for every coach or trainer to know both the temperature and the humidity. There is no room for guesswork. An inexpensive way to determine the environmental conditions on the field is by the use of a sling psychrometer, a unit that costs about 30 dollars. It measures dry-bulb temperature and wet-bulb temperature. By using these two measurements, the relative humidity can be read from a scale on the psychrometer.

The wet-bulb reading alone is a reasonably accurate measurement of the environmental conditions and can assist a coach or trainer in making decisions regarding training. Guidelines are as follows:

Wet-Bulb Temperature	*Field Precautions*
Under 66°	No precautions necessary except close observation of those squad members most susceptible to heat illness (those who lose over 3 per cent of their body weight as determined from weight chart).
67° to 77°	Insist that unlimited amounts of water be given on the field. Iced water is preferable. If desired, other dilute solutions very low in salt may be used (the electrolyte solutions).
Over 78°	Alter practice schedule to provide a lighter practice routine or have players practice in shorts. Withhold susceptible players from participation.

Any time the humidity is over 95 per cent, practice is altered as described for "Over 78°" or is postponed.

The use of a rubber sweat suit or, in fact, any kind of sweat suit in hot weather is vigorously condemned. There is a mistaken and highly dangerous impression that using a sweat suit will increase weight loss. It will, of course, increase water loss on a given day, but the athlete will replenish the fluids (and thus gain back the temporary weight loss) within a few hours. Any covering over the skin provides an environment of up to 100 per cent humidity for the skin, robbing the body of the only way it has to cool itself in hot weather. Whenever possible, clothing for athletes should be such that maximum skin surface is exposed. The net jerseys used in football, for example, permit maximum ventilation.

Identify Susceptible Individuals

Most of the serious heat problems develop in individuals who lose the most water. Those with large muscle mass (stocky individuals) seem to be more susceptible. The easiest way to identify susceptible individuals is to weigh them before and after each exercise session. Those who lose over 3 per cent of their body weight should be observed. Those who lose over 5 per cent must be warned of the danger in their weight loss problem.

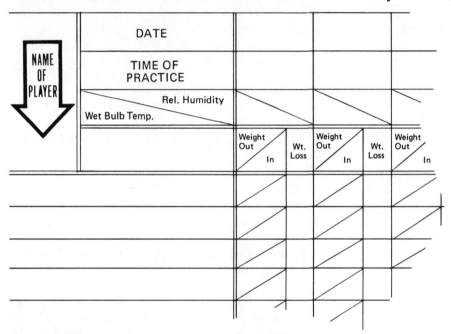

Figure 21–1. Example of a weight chart, with instructions, for prevention of heat illness.

Provide Water and Fluids on the Field

During the past 10 years, there has been a tremendous change in availability of water on the field. At Ohio State University, unlimited ice water is available to players throughout practice and games. On very hot days, the squad consumes 80 to 100 gallons of water during a practice session. Electrolyte solutions are available during breaks and after practice as an optional way to replenish lost electrolytes. Most athletes salt their own food to taste and replace the lost electrolytes by this means after each session.

Almost every eighth-grade student knows that if he is cast upon the ocean, he should not drink seawater. Seawater is hypertonic — it has a high concentration of salts. However, in many instances, coaches provide salt tablets and salted solutions to athletes while they exercise. This practice is to be condemned. A human can survive over 30 days without electrolytes as long as he has adequate water. He can rarely survive over 72 hours without water. Again, the main problem in exposure to environmental heat is water loss. Thus, attention must be directed to this loss.

BEFORE PRACTICE

1. Assign a trainer or manager to regularly maintain this chart.

2. Post chart on Locker Room wall near shower.

3. Place scales near the chart.

4. Weigh each player before practice in T-shirt and shorts.

5. Record weight in "out" section under day's practice. (If there are 2-a-day practices use 2 spaces.)

DURING PRACTICE

6. Measure wet bulb temperature and relative humidity by means of a sling psychrometer and record at beginning of practice and one hour later.

7. Record wet bulb temperature and relative humidity on chart.

8. Inform coach of condition which should be observed on the field. (See Wet-Bulb Guidelines).

AFTER PRACTICE

9. Weigh each player after practice and record in "in" space.

10. Record weight loss for each practice session for each player.

11. Inform coach of all players with any significant weight loss (over 3% of body weight).
    100 lbs.—3 lbs.   200 lbs.—6 lbs.
    133 lbs.—4 lbs.   233 lbs.—7 lbs.
    166 lbs.—5 lbs.   266 lbs.—8 lbs.

12. Offer water and replacement solutions after practice. Encourage use of salt at table during regular meal time.

Figure 21–1. *Continued.*

PROCEDURES TO BE FOLLOWED

Careful attention to factors related to heat stress is the responsibility of the physician, trainer, and coach. Often the coach or physical educator is the only person in daily contact with the athletes.

As stated previously, the simplest way to recognize athletes susceptible to heat problems is to weigh them before and after each practice. Figure 21–1 shows a portion of the weight chart used by the Ohio High School Athletic Association for the past 10 years. Use of the chart and the sling psychrometer in a football program is described. Such charts can be easily adapted to programs for both males and females in various sports, and it is strongly recommended that they be used widely. Similar charts are available from several companies that manufacture electrolyte solutions.

The well-hydrated athlete is a more efficient and effective athlete. It is of primary importance that everything be done to provide adequate hydration before, during, and after practice.

SUMMARY

During exercise in hot weather, much of the heat produced by the body is lost through evaporation of sweat. To promote such evaporation, as much skin as possible should be exposed to air. When environmental humidity is high, sweat cannot evaporate well and exercise may need to be postponed.

The main problem generated by sweating is that it removes water from within the body. The lost water is best replaced by allowing the athlete to drink as much water as he likes, whenever he wishes. The small amount of salt normally lost in sweat is adequately replaced by salting food to individual taste at mealtimes.

If body water is not adequately replaced, the athlete may develop heat cramps, heat fatigue, heat exhaustion, or heat stroke. Heat stroke is an emergency in which sweating stops and body temperature rises sharply within a few minutes. First aid consists of immediately cooling the victim with ice or cold water, before the high temperature causes brain damage or death.

STUDY QUESTIONS

1. What single factor is the most important in prevention of heat problems in athletes?

2. Heat cramps are best prevented by using copious amounts of water before and during exercise — true or false?

3. What disorders may occur when athletes are exposed to environmental heat?

4. What steps can a coach take to prevent these disorders?

5. How is heat exhaustion distinguished from heat stroke?

6. What is the primary first aid treatment for heat stroke?

FURTHER READINGS

Blyth, C. S., and Arnold, D. C.: Forty-fourth Annual Survey of Football Fatalities 1931–1977. Proceedings of the Annual Meeting, American Football Coaches Association, 1977.

Knochel, J. P.: Dog days and siriasis. How to kill a football player. J.A.M.A. 233:513–515, 1975.

Leithead, C. S., and Lind, A. R.: Heat Stress and Heat Disorders. Philadelphia, F. A. Davis Company, 1964.

Mathews, D. K., and Fox, E. L.: The Physiological Basis of Physical Education and Athletics. Philadelphia, W. B. Saunders Company, 1976.

Mathews, D. K., Fox, E. L., and Tanzi, D.: Physiological responses during exercise and recovery in a football uniform. J. Appl. Physiol. 26:611–615, 1969.

Murphy, R. J., and Ashe, W. F.: Prevention of heat illness in football players. J.A.M.A. 194:650–654, 1965.

Murphy, R. J., and Mathews, D. K.: Water is the key to heat problems. Med. Opinion, July 1976.

Round Table: balancing heat stress fluids and electrolytes. Phys. Sports Med. 3(8):43–52, August 1975.

Ryan, A. J.: Heat stress and the vulnerable athlete. Phys. Sports Med. 1:47–53, June 1973.

Shibolet, S., Lancaster, M. C., and Danon, Y.: Heat Stroke: A review. Aviat. Space Environ. Med. 47:280–301, 1976.

22

PERFORMANCE AT ALTITUDE

ROBERT F. GROVER, M.D., Ph.D.

PERFORMANCE DECREMENTS

Webster's *Third New International Dictionary* defines *sport* as " a diversion of the field (as fowling, hunting, fishing, racing, or athletic games)." In this broad sense, persons who engage in sports include not only the athlete, professional or amateur, but also those millions of individuals engaged in all forms of outdoor recreation, from back-packing and cycling to skiing and mountain climbing. Often the sportsman seeks his "diversion of the field" in the beauty and grandeur of mountainous areas. However, the sportsman soon learns that the aesthetic satisfaction of the mountain environment is combined with physical stress, including large fluctuations in temperature, intense solar radiation, low humidity, and the inescapable hypoxia (decreased oxygen) of high altitude. It is this hypoxia that is responsible for man's reduced capacity for physical and mental performance at high altitude.

Sea level is situated at the interface between two oceans, the obvious ocean of water and the less obvious ocean of air that envelopes the earth. Like water, this air also has mass and weight such that it exerts a pressure of over 1 ton per square foot (15 pounds per square inch) at sea level. This atmospheric pressure may also be expressed as the height of the column of mercury that it will support; such a measuring device is called a barometer. Thus, the atmospheric (or barometric) pressure is 760 mm mercury (mm Hg) at the bottom of the ocean of air, that is, at sea level. While ascending through the atmosphere, there is progressively less air above to exert pressure, so the atmospheric pressure is progressively less. At an altitude of 11,000 feet (3300 meters), the pressure (500 mm Hg) is only two thirds that at sea level. Since the atmosphere is essentially 21 per cent oxygen, the partial pressure of oxygen (Po_2) will be 21 per cent of the total atmospheric pressure. Thus, the Po_2 at sea level is about 160 mm Hg but decreases to 100 mm Hg at 3300 m altitude. Within the body, oxygen moves from regions of high Po_2 to regions of lower Po_2, and the ultimate "driving pressure" is the atmospheric Po_2. Consequently, as the atmospheric Po_2 decreases with increasing altitude, there is progressively less "driving pressure" to oxygenate the body. This is the physiological implication of atmospheric hypoxia.

Decrease in Aerobic Work Capacity

The performance of prolonged muscular exercise, as in long-distance running, requires a continuous supply of oxygen to the working muscles. A person's capacity for 327 such aerobic work is measured in terms of the maximum amount of oxygen his body can consume per minute, when the work is of only 5 to 10 minutes duration. This is the so-called "maximum oxygen uptake" ($\dot{V}O_{2max}$). Numerous investigators have reported that when $\dot{V}O_{2max}$ is measured in the same individual at both low and high altitude, there is a decrease at high altitude. Buskirk[1] collected a large number of such published reports, from which he established the general relationship between altitude and aerobic capacity (Fig. 22–1). From this relationship, it can be seen that $\dot{V}O_{2max}$ is not measurably altered by altitudes between sea level and about 1500 m.* However, at 1500 m a threshold is crossed, for above this there is a linear decrease in $\dot{V}O_{2max}$ at the rate of 10 per cent per 1000 m. Thus, when a man goes from sea level to 1500 m, his $\dot{V}O_{2max}$ remains unaltered; but if he ascends an additional 1500 m, then at 3000 m his $\dot{V}O_{2max}$ will be 15 per cent less than at sea level. This decrease in aerobic capacity will persist as long as he remains at 3000 m, with no improvement if his state of physical fitness and training does not change. The process is completely reversible upon return to sea level.

Although aerobic work capacity is measured during maximal effort of relatively brief duration, the decrease in aerobic capacity at high altitude is also reflected in more prolonged exercise of less severe intensity. Åstrand and Rodahl[2] have indicated that, whereas a man can work at 100 per cent of his aerobic capacity for five minutes, he can work at only 25 to 50 per cent of his capacity if the work is prolonged for eight hours. To illustrate: if a man at sea level has a $\dot{V}O_{2max}$ of 3000 ml O_2/min (during brief maximal effort), then he can perform work requiring about 1100 ml O_2/min for several hours. If, now, he goes to 3000 m altitude, his $\dot{V}O_{2max}$ will be reduced 15 per cent to about 2500 ml O_2/min. This means that he can now tolerate a prolonged work rate of only 900 ml O_2/min. Under all conditions, about 300 ml O_2/min is required to meet the basic metabolic requirements at rest. Therefore, only that oxygen consumed over and above 300 ml/min is available for work. Consequently, the excess oxygen available for prolonged work is reduced from 800 to 600 ml/min at 3000 m altitude (Fig. 22–2).

What does all this mean to the sportsman performing at high altitude? If he is a long-distance runner and attempts to run at the same speed (work rate) as at sea level, he will become exhausted sooner and will be unable to complete the prescribed distance

---

*1 meter = 3.3 feet.

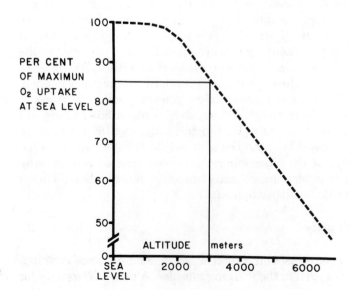

PER CENT
OF MAXIMUN
O_2 UPTAKE
AT SEA LEVEL

Figure 22–1. Aerobic work capacity at high altitude, expressed as a per cent of maximum oxygen uptake ($\dot{V}O_{2\ max}$) at sea level. Above 1500 m, $\dot{V}O_{2\ max}$ decreases at a rate of 10 per cent per 1000 m. Thus, at 3000 m, $\dot{V}O_{2\ max}$ is reduced to 85 per cent of the sea level value.

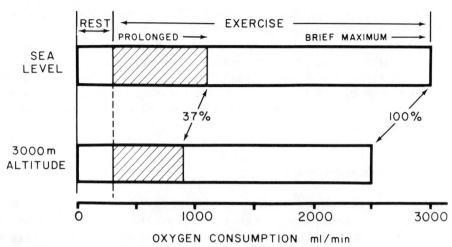

Figure 22–2. A man performing work that can be tolerated throughout an eight-hour day usually cannot exceed an average work intensity requiring him to consume oxygen at a rate greater than 37 per cent of $\dot{V}o_{2\,max}$. However, he must consume at least 300 ml O_2/ min at all times just to meet his resting metabolic requirements. Hence, the net oxygen available for external work (shaded area of bars) will be 37 per cent of $\dot{V}o_{2\,max}$ less 300 ml O_2/min. Consequently, a man's capacity for prolonged work is actually reduced 25 per cent at 3000 m altitude.

for the race. To compensate for his decreased aerobic capacity at high altitude, he must retrain and adopt a slower speed (lower work rate) that is tolerable for the distance to be covered. The obvious consequence will be poorer performance (longer time) than at sea level. If the sport is cross-country skiing, then one should plan on covering less distance in a given period of time. The intensity of effort is perceived in relation to aerobic capacity. Hence, if a task requires a fixed effort, that effort which seems only moderate at sea level may become severe relative to the lower work capacity at high altitude. For this reason, at high altitude, physical activity is generally more tiring, and the point of exhaustion is reached sooner. This is true even though muscle strength is not altered.

Impairment of Mental Function

While it is generally true that the consequence of atmospheric hypoxia is impaired tissue oxygenation at high altitude, some tissues are affected more than others. The brain is more sensitive to hypoxia than any other part of the body. As a result, complex mental tasks become more difficult. Arithmetic calculation, measuring, and the manipulation of numbers require more time, and errors are more frequent in spite of greater effort. Analyzing problems and making decisions become very difficult, and errors in judgment are common. When such errors occur during mountain climbing, the results can be fatal. In addition to diminished mental acuity, personality is altered; some individuals become very irritable and uncooperative, and discipline is more difficult to maintain. In group sports, such as soccer, team effort is less effective.

The retina of the eye is literally an extension of the brain. Consequently, vision is impaired by hypoxia, and it is more difficult to see in dim light at high altitude.[3] This constitutes an added hazard to the person who is trekking (back-packing) or cross-country skiing in the mountains and who is still on the trail at sundown.

Sleep at high altitude poses a special problem. One normal aspect of sleep is a decrease in ventilation. Whereas this is usually of no consequence at sea level, it makes hypoxia more severe at high altitude. This, combined with the common occurrence of periodic breathing, causes many people to wake up frequently. As a result, the person is deprived of deep, restful sleep.[4] This inability to sleep well at high altitude can lead to a state of chronic sleep deprivation that impairs mental function during the day. Sleep deprivation also augments the fatigue produced by physical exertion and becomes a major problem for many individuals spending prolonged periods at high altitude. As a consequence of these adverse effects of hypoxia on mental function, the accident rate is greater for all activities at high altitude, including sports.

Benefit from Reduced Air Density

The individual ascending to high altitude is exposed to a decrease in total atmospheric pressure. One consequence has been considered: the associated decrease in the partial pressure of oxygen (atmospheric hypoxia), with impaired tissue oxygenation and reduced aerobic work capacity. This has an adverse effect on prolonged muscular work, which is dependent upon a continuous supply of oxygen. As a consequence, the endurance athlete has a distinct handicap, and performance decrements result.

A second consequence of decreasing atmospheric pressure is a proportional decrease in air density. This means that wind resistance is less at high altitude, which provides a distinct advantage to the athlete who must perform at high speed, such as in skating or cycling. As further evidence for the advantage of reduced air density, all existing world records for horse racing over short distances have been established in Mexico City at an altitude of 2300 m where the air density would be one fourth less than that at sea level.[5]

PHYSIOLOGICAL ADAPTATION TO HIGH ALTITUDE

To perform sustained muscular work, the working muscles must receive a continuous supply of oxygen. Hence, the capacity of the human body to transport oxygen to the muscles will determine the aerobic work capacity. It follows that the decrease in aerobic work capacity ($\dot{V}o_{2max}$) observed at high altitude reflects a decreased capacity to transport oxygen. An analysis of the components of the body's oxygen transport system should reveal the "weak link" in the system; the answer is rather surprising.

Oxygen Transport System

Single-celled organisms living in water can obtain oxygen directly from their environment by simple diffusion. However, diffusion is efficient over only very short distances. Therefore, organisms with a large cell mass must be equipped with a specialized system for transporting oxygen from the environment to all tissues within the interior of the body. The system has four basic components: (1) a liquid vehicle to carry oxygen; (2) an organ where the liquid can take up oxygen from the environment; (3) a network of tubes for distribution of the oxygen-laden liquid to all tissues; and (4) a pump to circulate the liquid.

Blood. An aqueous solution would be a most inefficient vehicle for carrying oxygen in simple solution, since oxygen is relatively insoluble in water. When the red pigment hemoglobin is added to the solution, a much more efficient vehicle results because hemoglobin binds oxygen chemically but reversibly. In invertebrates, such as the earthworm, hemoglobin is simply dissolved in plasma. However, in higher an-

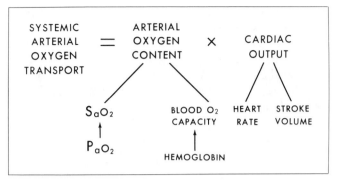

Figure 22–3. The determinants of systemic oxygen transport. (See text.)

imals, including humans, the hemoglobin is packaged in the red blood cells (RBC's), which in turn are suspended in plasma. One hundred milliliters of such human blood normally contain about 15 grams of hemoglobin, which can carry 20 ml of oxygen. Virtually all of this oxygen is chemically bound to the hemoglobin, while only 0.4 ml is in physical solution. Put another way, the oxygen-carrying capacity of whole blood is 50-fold greater than that of plasma alone, making blood a very effective vehicle for oxygen transport.

Lung. To oxygenate hemoglobin, the blood must be brought in close proximity to the atmosphere. Pumping blood through the capillaries of the skin serves this purpose in the earthworm and, to a significant extent, in the frog as well. However, mammals have developed a system of much greater capacity and efficiency: the lung. The functional unit of the lung is the alveolus or terminal air sac, about 250 micrometers (microns) in diameter. Capillaries in the alveolar walls carry the RBC's single file, allowing oxygen to diffuse from the alveolar air through the very thin alveolocapillary membrane into the blood. The adult human lung contains 300 million alveoli with a combined surface of between 40 and 80 square meters. This is an enormous area for oxygenation of the 300 ml of blood contained in the pulmonary capillaries at any one time.

Heart and Blood Vessels. Once oxygenated, the blood is pumped by the left heart through the arterial tree to all parts of the body. The quantity of oxygen presented to the body per minute (systemic oxygen transport) will then be determined

Figure 22–4. Exchange of O_2 and CO_2 between air and blood in the lung. At sea level, inspired air has an O_2 pressure (P_IO_2) of 150 mm Hg, which is much higher than the O_2 pressure of mixed venous blood ($P_{\bar{v}}O_2$) entering the lung. Hence, O_2 diffuses from air into blood until the pressure in alveolar air (P_AO_2) approximates that in arterial blood (P_aO_2). Concurrently, there is a reciprocal movement of CO_2 from blood to air, since the pressure of CO_2 in the mixed venous blood ($P_{\bar{v}}CO_2$) is about 45 mm Hg, whereas the pressure in inspired air (P_ICO_2) is virtually 0. Exchange proceeds until the pressures in alveolar air (P_ACO_2) and arterial blood (P_aO_2) are in equilibrium.

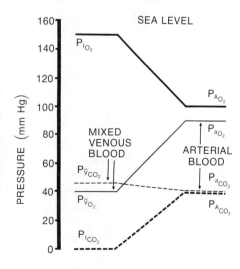

by the quantity of oxygen in each unit volume of blood (arterial oxygen content) and the number of units (liters) of blood pumped by the heart each minute (cardiac output) (Fig. 22–3). Depending on the oxygen demands of the body, somewhere between 20 and 80 per cent of the transported oxygen will be extracted from the arterial blood by the peripheral tissues. Thus depleted of oxygen, the blood drains by way of the veins to the right heart, which pumps it back into the lungs for reoxygenation. This same circulatory system serves to carry carbon dioxide, produced by oxidative metabolism, from the tissues to the lung for elimination.

As the venous blood with its low Po_2 and high Pco_2 enters the capillaries within the lung, it is exposed to the alveolar air, which is high in Po_2 and low in $Pco_2.$ These pressure gradients cause diffusion of O_2 from air to blood; alveolar Po_2 falls and blood Po_2 rises until equilibrium is reached. Simultaneously, there is diffusion of CO_2 in the opposite direction — from blood to air. The Pco_2 of alveolar air rises as the Pco_2 of blood falls, again until equilibrium is reached (Fig. 22–4). Therefore, it is the gas pressures in the alveoli (P_AO_2 and P_ACO_2), following equilibration with blood, that determine the partial pressures of these gases in the arterial blood (P_aO_2 and P_aCO_2). The Po_2 in the alveoli and arterial blood is always lower than the atmospheric Po_2 by an amount approximately equal to the Pco_2 in the alveoli and arterial blood.

Oxygen Transport at High Altitude

Pulmonary Ventilation. Ascent to high altitude, with the attendant decrease in atmospheric Po_2, produces a fall in alveolar, and hence arterial, $Po_2.$ As the "driving pressure" decreases, the P_aO_2 must also decrease. At the bifurcation of the carotid artery at the angle of the jaw, a tiny bit of specialized tissue called the carotid body monitors the $P_aO_2.$ When P_aO_2 falls, the carotid body sends more nerve impulses to the respiratory center in the brain, which in turn stimulates breathing; initially, each breath is deeper, followed by more rapid breathing. As a consequence, a greater volume of air enters (and leaves) the lung each minute. This greater volume of air compensates for the decrease in air density at high altitude. Although the physiological mechanisms do not adjust the quantity of oxygen moved, the end result is to maintain nearly constant the quantity (mass) of oxygen brought into the lung each minute. However, alveolar Po_2 cannot be restored to sea level values, and so there is a persistent reduction of arterial Po_2 at high altitude.

Normally, hyperventilation continues for as long as the individual remains at high altitude. Although the carotid body is probably responsible for the initial increase in ventilation, the mechanism that sustains hyperventilation for weeks and months or longer is not known. This hyperventilation is sensed as a feeling of "shortness of breath," and is most noticeable during exercise. However, at altitudes up to 4300 m, the respiratory apparatus is fully capable of moving the larger volumes of air required, even during maximal exertion. Because of this great reserve, ventilation, the first step in oxygen transport, is not the factor limiting oxygen uptake and is not responsible for the ultimate decrease in oxygen transport.

Blood Oxygenation. In water or plasma, the quantity of oxygen that enters physical solution is directly related to the oxygen pressure in a simple linear fashion. This is in contrast with the more complex chemical interaction between oxygen and hemoglobin in blood. The quantitative relationship between oxygen pressure and the resulting quantity of oxygen bound to hemoglobin is described by an S-shaped (sigmoidal) curve (Fig. 22–5). This curve defines both the uptake or "association" of oxygen with hemoglobin at higher pressures and the release or "dissociation" of oxygen from hemoglobin at lower pressures, since the chemical interaction is readily reversible. In

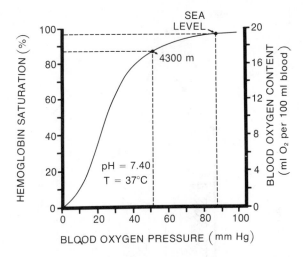

Figure 22–5. The hemoglobin-oxygen dissociation curve of human blood, indicating the extent to which hemoglobin is saturated with O_2 at various O_2 pressures in the blood. In spite of the large fall in arterial O_2 pressure with ascent to 4300 m altitude, hemoglobin remains well saturated at about 87 per cent. With a normal hemoglobin concentration of 15 grams per 100 ml of blood, the blood O_2 content would be lowered from 19.6 to 17.7 ml of O_2 per 100 ml of blood.

the literature this relationship is usually called the "hemoglobin-oxygen (Hb-O_2) dissociation curve." The quantity of bound oxygen is referred to as the *content* and is often expressed as milliliters of O_2 per 100 ml blood, or volumes per cent (vol %). The maximum amount of oxygen that the hemoglobin can bind is called the oxygen-carrying *capacity* of the blood. Hence, the content relative to the capacity defines the extent to which the hemoglobin is saturated, and is expressed simply as per cent *saturation*.

Examination of the Hb-O_2 dissociation curve (Fig. 22–5) reveals that when the oxygen pressure in the alveolar air ($P_A O_2$) produces a relatively high oxygen pressure in the arterial blood ($P_a O_2$), for example, 100 mm Hg as at sea level, the hemoglobin is almost fully saturated. The saturation of arterial blood ($S_a O_2$) will be about 96 per cent. With ascent to high altitude and a decrease in the "driving pressure" of oxygen, $P_a O_2$ must also fall, for example, to 50 mm Hg at 4300 m. However, because of the sigmoidal shape of the Hb-O_2 dissociation curve, the hemoglobin will still be quite well saturated (about 87 per cent) in spite of the large decrease in $P_a O_2$. With a normal hemoglobin concentration of 15 grams per 100 ml of blood, the oxygen-carrying capacity is 20 volumes per cent, since each gram of hemoglobin can bind 1.36 ml of oxygen. Consequently, at an $S_a O_2$ of 96 per cent, the oxygen content will be 19.2 volumes per cent. Even at 4300 m, where the $S_a O_2$ is 87 per cent, the oxygen content will still be 17.4 volumes per cent.

Obviously this is a very well-engineered system. Nevertheless, if oxygen transport were to remain unaltered, this 10 per cent reduction in blood oxygen content would require a compensatory 10 per cent increase in blood flow. In fact, this is the initial response to high altitude. Heart rate increases while the volume of blood pumped per beat (stroke volume) remains unaltered, producing an increase in cardiac output (Fig. 22–6). However, the maximal attainable heart rate, say 190, cannot be elevated, thus placing an upper limit on this compensatory mechanism. Hence, with the same maximum cardiac output but a reduced arterial oxygen content, maximum oxygen transport must be less, and this lowers $\dot{V}o_{2max}$. Thus, with *initial* ascent to high altitude, impaired blood oxygenation is the major cause for the decrease in aerobic work capacity.

The physiological processes of continued adaptation to high altitude modify this initial mechanism for preserving oxygen transport, perhaps because using a higher heart rate to pump more blood requires an inordinate expenditure of energy by the heart. The body instead "chooses" to correct the deficit in blood oxygen content by increasing the oxygen-carrying capacity, that is, by increasing the hemoglobin concen-

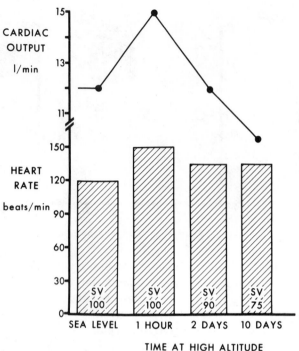

Figure 22–6. Time course of cardiac output response to high altitude. (Workload is unchanged.) The determinants of cardiac output are heart rate (HR) and stroke volume (SV). During the first hour of exposure to high altitude, HR increases, producing a rise in cardiac output with no change in SV. After two days, HR is less elevated, SV has begun to decrease, and cardiac output has returned to control values. With 10 days of adaptation, SV has decreased by 25 per cent, HR is only slightly elevated, and now cardiac output is significantly less than it was prior to ascent.

tration. Since the quantity of hemoglobin in each RBC is normally constant, the concentration of RBC's in the blood (hematocrit) must be increased. Stimulation of the bone marrow to produce more RBC's would eventually increase the total number of circulating RBC's. However, that process requires many weeks. The alternative is to reduce the plasma volume, so that the RBC's already in the circulation are then contained in a smaller total blood volume. In this manner, although the total number of RBC's remains unchanged, the concentration of RBC's in each 100 ml of blood is greater.

Normally, the body employs this latter alternative. During the first few days following ascent to high altitude, the hematocrit increases from 45 to 50 per cent, reflecting the decrease in plasma volume. This means a 10 per cent increase in hemoglobin concentration and oxygen-carrying capacity, that is, from 20 to 22 volumes per cent, which offsets the lower saturation of 87 per cent and restores the arterial oxygen content to 19.1 volumes per cent, which is the value present at low altitude. These changes are summarized as follows:

Condition	Oxygen-Carrying Capacity	$\times$	Hemo-globin Saturation	$=$	Arterial Oxygen Content
Sea level	20 vol %	$\times$	96%	$=$	19.2 vol %
High altitude					
Initial	20 vol %	$\times$	87%	$=$	17.4 vol %
Compensated	22 vol %	$\times$	87%	$=$	19.1 vol %

From the above chart we see that ascent to high altitude lowers arterial blood oxygen saturation. Initially, this reduces blood oxygen content. However, within a few days hematocrit increases to offset the lower saturation and fully restore arterial oxygen content to sea level values. Thus we must conclude that, following adaptation to altitudes up to 4300 m, blood oxygenation — the second step in oxygen transport — is also not the limiting factor in oxygen uptake.

Circulation. The third major component of oxygen transport is the circulation of oxygenated blood to the peripheral tissues, including the working muscles. This function is performed by the cardiovascular system. It is the heart that provides most of the pumping energy for the circulation. At rest, the heart contracts about 75 times each minute, and with each contraction an average of 80 ml of blood is delivered into the aorta, which is the "trunk" of the arterial tree. Hence, the quantity of blood pumped by the heart each minute at rest is about 6 liters (80 ml/beat × 75 beats/min = 6,000 ml/min). During heavy exercise, the heart rate may increase to 180 beats per minute, and the volume ejected per beat, the so-called stroke volume, may increase to 100 ml. Thus, the cardiac output will increase about threefold to 18 liters per minute (100 ml/beat × 180 beats/min = 18,000 ml/min). However, total body oxygen consumption may increase tenfold with exercise, and so in addition to increasing cardiac output (and hence oxygen transport) threefold, the extraction of oxygen from each unit of blood must also increase more than threefold (from 4.5 ml O_2/100 ml blood to 15.0 ml O_2/100 ml blood). This means that from the oxygen contained in arterial blood, 19.2 vol. %, only 4.5 vol % are extracted at rest, and the venous blood returning to the lungs is still about 73 per cent saturated. With exercise, extraction increases to 15.0 vol %, and only 4.2 vol % remains. Hence, venous saturation will be lowered to about 21 per cent with a Po_2 of only 20 mm Hg (Fig. 22–7). Under these conditions of strenuous exercise, virtually all of the original "driving pressure" of oxygen has been utilized, and no further oxygen extraction is possible.

Upon ascent to high altitude, the initial impact is a decrease in the "driving pressure" of oxygen, with a fall in $P_A O_2$ and $P_a O_2$ producing a decrease in saturation and oxygen content of arterial blood (Fig. 22–5). Since each unit of arterial blood now contains less oxygen, more units of blood must be pumped per minute if oxygen transport is to be maintained. This is achieved by an increase in heart rate, as mentioned previously. However, this initial response to hypoxia — the increase in heart rate — is only temporary, and with the passage of days at high altitude, heart rate slows to levels close to those present at sea level. Concurrently, hemoconcentration is occurring, which increases the hematocrit and restores arterial blood oxygen content. Although it might appear that these adjustments would augment the reduced oxygen transport, no such improvement occurs. The reason is that with hemoconcen-

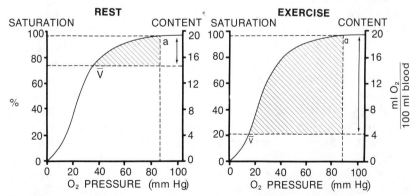

Figure 22–7. Extraction of oxygen from arterial blood at rest and during exercise. At sea level, arterial blood (a) 96 per cent saturated has an oxygen content of 19.2 vol per cent. From this, 4.5 vol per cent is extracted at rest and the mixed venous blood (v̄) returns to the lung 73 per cent saturated. During maximal exercise, oxygen extraction increases to about 15.0 vol per cent, lowering the mixed venous saturation to 21 per cent.

tration, there is a trade-off between greater blood oxygen content and less blood flow. Hemoconcentration is achieved by reducing total plasma volume while the total volume of RBC's remains unchanged. This means that total blood volume has been reduced. As a consequence, the cardiovascular system seems to perform as if it were "underfilled," and blood flow through the veins back to the right heart appears to be reduced. Obviously, the heart can pump no more blood than it receives, and so if venous return is less, then cardiac output must decrease. This does, in fact, occur. With adaptation to high altitude, cardiac stroke volume decreases, and with the return of heart rate to normal, cardiac output is reduced[6] (Fig. 22–6).

The phenomenon of a decrease in stroke volume at high altitude has been documented by a number of investigators. The physiological mechanisms involved are not fully understood. Since the rise in hematocrit and the fall in stroke volume occur simultaneously, the decrease in plasma volume, and hence a decrease in venous return, appears to be a plausible explanation. Furthermore, if hemoconcentration is prevented, there is neither a decrease in stroke volume nor a rise in hematocrit, but neither is there compensation for the arterial desaturation, so arterial oxygen content and oxygen transport remain decreased.[7] If this were the whole story, then one might expect a gradual increase in stroke volume with prolonged adaptation to high altitude. Long-term residents of Leadville, Colorado, at 3100 m altitude have a normal plasma volume and increased total RBC volume, and thus a total blood volume 10 per cent greater than that of sea level residents.[8] Nevertheless, they too have a stroke volume and cardiac output that is subnormal by sea level standards. Furthermore, they manifest a 15 per cent increase in stroke volume when they descend to sea level.[9] Therefore, the mechanisms responsible for the changes in stroke volume following changes in altitude require further investigation.

Obviously a smaller stroke volume per se would reduce maximum cardiac output even if maximum heart rate remained unaltered at high altitude. However, when some individuals adapt to altitudes in excess of 4000 m, there is also a significant decrease in maximum heart rate due to greater inhibitory activity of the vagus nerve.[10] This compounds the reduction in maximum cardiac output.

To summarize, aerobic work capacity ($\dot{V}_{O_{2max}}$) is directly related to oxygen transport, which has two major components, arterial oxygen content and cardiac output. Exposure to atmospheric hypoxia by ascending to high altitude decreases $\dot{V}_{O_{2max}}$ by lowering oxygen transport. Initially, it is the reduction in arterial oxygen content that is responsible, while maximum cardiac output remains unaltered. However, as hemoconcentration occurs, restoration of arterial oxygen content is traded for a decrease in cardiac output. Consequently, $\dot{V}_{O_{2max}}$ remains decreased because oxygen transport is still reduced. It is important to note that the factors responsible for the decrease in stroke volume and cardiac output are not fully understood. In some individuals the decrease in stroke volume is much less than in others, which is probably the basis for the observation that at a given altitude, $\dot{V}_{O_{2max}}$ is decreased more in some people than in others.[11]

Augmentation of Oxygen Transport. If it is true that $\dot{V}_{O_{2max}}$ is dependent upon maximum oxygen transport, and if reducing oxygen transport by some intervention such as ascent to high altitude lowers $\dot{V}_{O_{2max}}$, then increasing oxygen transport should raise $\dot{V}_{O_{2max}}$. Theoretically, oxygen transport could be augmented by increasing either cardiac output or arterial oxygen content. Cardiac output is determined by heart rate and stroke volume. However, the maximum effective heart rate of the young adult is about 200 beats/min, since this reduces to a minimum the time for effective cardiac filling between contractions. In fact, with physical training, maximum heart rate may even decrease somewhat.

Stroke volume is normally a function of the size of the heart, and heart size appears to be determined genetically. Hence, persons who are endowed with larger hearts that are otherwise normal will have larger stroke volumes and can achieve higher values of maximum cardiac output.[12] This gives them the potential for high values of $\dot{V}_{O_{2max}}$. In a very real sense, the potential endurance athlete is born (with a large heart) and not made. Conversely, the person born with a relatively small heart lacks the "machinery" for generating a large stroke volume, and hence must accept a relatively low $\dot{V}_{O_{2max}}$ as one of his physiological dimensions.

The stroke volume of the normal heart, that is, the volume of blood ejected during contraction, is related to the filling volume during the relaxation interval between contractions. Thus, if there is less filling during relaxation, then there will be a smaller stroke volume during contraction (Frank-Starling mechanism). Apparently this occurs at high altitude. However, as with all physiological mechanisms, this behavior of the heart has definite limits. Normally the heart operates near the upper limit of the Frank-Starling curve. Whereas less filling lowers stroke volume, more filling produces very little increase in stroke volume. Therefore, it must be concluded that it is not feasible to augment maximum oxygen transport by manipulation of cardiac output.

Arterial oxygen content is determined primarily by hemoglobin concentration and saturation. Lowering saturation will lower content, as with acute exposure to hypoxia. At sea level, however, saturation is nearly 100 per cent, so there is little room for improvement. Breathing 100 per cent oxygen may increase arterial oxygen content by no more than 10 per cent through added binding to hemoglobin and a greater amount in physical solution in plasma.

There remains the question of altering hemoglobin concentration to increase the oxygen-carrying capacity of the blood and thereby increase oxygen content at any given saturation. This occurs with adaptation to high altitude. However, once again we are faced with a trade-off, for increasing hematocrit not only raises oxygen content but also increases blood viscosity, which in turn impedes blood flow.[13] The interrelationships among hematocrit, viscosity, and flow are complex, but in general the adverse effects of viscosity are greater when the hematocrit is higher than 50 per cent. This suggests that in terms of augmenting oxygen transport, there is a net gain from increasing hematocrit up to about 50 per cent, whereas at higher hematocrits there is a net loss. This has been demonstrated as a temporary increase in $\dot{V}_{O_{2max}}$ by the autotransfusion of RBC's, so-called "blood doping."[14]

Just as increasing hemoglobin concentration should augment oxygen transport, so decreasing hemoglobin concentration should reduce it. Anemia is the obvious example of this situation. However, the inhalation of carbon monoxide from urban air pollution or cigarette smoking will have a similar effect. The hemoglobin molecule has a much greater affinity for carbon monoxide than for oxygen, so that when the binding sites on the molecule are occupied by carbon monoxide, they are unavailable to bind oxygen. Hence, that hemoglobin cannot participate in oxygen transport. It has been shown that a 20 per cent reduction in available hemoglobin (20 per cent carboxyhemoglobin) will produce a 23 per cent reduction in $\dot{V}_{O_{2max}}$.[15]

In an effort to increase $\dot{V}_{O_{2max}}$ by augmenting oxygen transport, attempts have also been made to facilitate oxygen extraction from the blood by reducing the affinity of hemoglobin for oxygen. With reference to Figure 22–5, this means shifting the dissociation curve to the right. At high values of P_{O_2}, this would reduce saturation very little. However, at a given low P_{O_2} of, say, 20 mm Hg, the corresponding saturation would be 20 per cent instead of the usual 30 per cent. Theoretically, then, extraction could be increased without further lowering P_{O_2}. Among the factors that shift the dissociation curve to the right is 2, 3-diphosphoglycerate (2,3 DPG), which is a normal constituent of the RBC. If one could induce an increase in the concentration of 2,3 DPG within the RBC, this might elevate $\dot{V}O_{2max}$ at either sea level or high altitude. The usual increase in 2,3 DPG in RBC's following ascent to high altitude[16] is indeed of value, for it does appear to facilitate oxygenation of the heart muscle.[17]

TRAINING AT ALTITUDE

Much controversy surrounds the question of training at altitude. In part this relates to the lack of agreement on how to measure the effects of training, apart from actual performance during competition. Usually the exercise physiologist measures $\dot{V}O_{2max}$ as the index of performance. From this viewpoint, training will increase $\dot{V}O_{2max}$, whereas altitude will decrease it. Therefore, if an untrained individual is taken to high altitude and trained there, a decrease in $\dot{V}O_{2max}$ following ascent will be measured with a subsequent increase in $\dot{V}O_{2max}$ resulting from training. Conversely, if a highly trained individual is taken to high altitude and he then stops training, an initial drop in $\dot{V}O_{2max}$ will be measured, followed by a further decline reflecting the loss of the training effect. Published reports include various combinations of these two situations.

In 1964 the high-school track team that won the Kentucky state championship that year was studied.[18] Initial measurements were made in Kentucky at an altitude of 300 m when the team was fully trained. They were then transported rapidly to 3100 m altitude in Leadville, Colorado, where they continued their training regimen for three weeks. Hence, degree of training was not variable. On the day following arrival at high altitude, $\dot{V}O_{2max}$ was 26 per cent less than at sea level, with no improvement over the three-week period of adaptation. Within one week following return to low altitude, $\dot{V}O_{2max}$ returned to 95 per cent of the preascent values. From this it can be concluded that following ascent to high altitude there is a prompt decrement in $\dot{V}O_{2max}$ that persists, unmodified, in spite of adaptation. Furthermore, the period of exposure to high altitude does not confer any measurable benefit in terms of $\dot{V}O_{2max}$ upon return to low altitude. The decrease in $\dot{V}O_{2max}$ at high altitude was reflected as poorer track performance; the time to run 1 mile was increased from 4:49 to 5:11 min. In contrast, sprints requiring less than 2:00 min and performed largely anaerobically showed slight improvement at high altitude, perhaps as a result of lower wind resistance.

One could ask if training for longer than three weeks at high altitude would eventually lessen the initial decrement. Buskirk studied athletes from Pennsylvania State University taken to an altitude of 4000 m in Peru.[1] Initially, $\dot{V}O_{2max}$ decreased nearly 30 per cent with only minimal improvement over seven weeks at high altitude. This more prolonged period of adaptation did not lead to superior performance upon return to sea level. We studied young athletes native to Leadville, Colorado, who had lived for 17 years at an altitude of 3100 m.[19] Their values of $\dot{V}O_{2max}$ were 24 per cent less than when measured three days following descent to sea level, a decrement virtually identical to that in the Kentucky athletes. Furthermore, the young men from Leadville were not superior to their Kentucky counterparts in terms of track performance at either high or low altitude. Therefore, it is difficult to make a case for training at high altitude.

A related question can be asked. If an athlete is going to compete at high altitude (as in the 1968 Olympic Games held in Mexico City at 2300 m), how long should he spend at high altitude prior to his event? Some argue that the athlete should compete the day he arrives, but that is debatable. After 24 hours, the decrement in $\dot{V}O_{2max}$ is established and subsequently does not change. Since the long-distance runner must cover a prescribed distance, he must lower his work rate (speed) in accordance with his reduced work capacity. If he retained his sea level work rate, he would reach exhaustion before completing the race. Therefore, following arrival at high altitude he must retrain to pace himself optimally for his altered work capacity. This would seem to be the dominant consideration in establishing the period of adaptation prior to competition.

Finally, it is important to recognize the individual variability in response to high altitude. At a given altitude the decrement in $\dot{V}o_{2max}$ is greater in some people than in others.[11] Hence, the handicap of altitude does not apply equally to all athletes. Unfortunately, this implies that the best competitor at sea level may not be the winner at high altitude. As would be expected, it is the losers and not the winners who complain about this "unfair handicap."

ADVERSE REACTIONS TO ALTITUDE

Acute Mountain Sickness

The vast majority of persons visiting mountainous areas will experience no serious adverse effects of high altitude. However, minor discomfort is not uncommon following rapid ascent to altitudes above 2600 m. Headache is the most frequent symptom, sometimes associated with feelings of lethargy and drowsiness but an inability to sleep soundly. Other symptoms are related to the digestive system and include loss of appetite, abdominal distension and "gas," an intolerance of fatty foods, and occasionally nausea and vomiting. This collection of symptoms is termed acute mountain sickness (AMS). The incidence of AMS, as well as the number and severity of the symptoms, increases at high altitudes. Nearly all persons ascending to 4300 m will be affected to some degree, but, paradoxically, at that altitude the initial reaction is often euphoria rather than discomfort, which comes later, particularly during the first night of attempted sleep. With continued sojourn at high altitude the symptoms of AMS subside, and marked relief and improvement usually occur within a day or two. Only rarely does an individual have persistent severe symptoms that necessitate his descent.

Gradual ascent (over several days) is the most effective way to avoid or minimize the symptoms of AMS. Other helpful measures include a diet high in carbohydrate and low in fat, the avoidance of strenuous exercise during the first day at high altitude, and aspirin or other mild analgesics for the relief of headaches. Diamox (acetazolamide) is also helpful because it stimulates and stabilizes breathing and thereby enables one to sleep better.[20] "Sleeping pills" should be avoided because they depress breathing and actually aggravate the symptoms of AMS. For most individuals, adaptation to high altitude will occur rapidly and without difficulty, and no medication is needed.

High-Altitude Pulmonary Edema

In contrast to AMS, which is common, a rare adverse reaction to the mountain environment is high-altitude pulmonary edema (HAPE). (Pulmonary edema is an accumulation of fluid in the lungs.) Among the millions of persons who visit the Rocky Mountains each year, only a handful of cases of HAPE are reported. The true incidence is unknown; mild cases of HAPE may go unrecognized. As with AMS, the incidence of HAPE appears to increase at higher altitude. In 1976, when 700 people attempted to climb Mt. McKinley (7000 m) in Alaska, 7 cases of HAPE occurred, or 1 out of 100.[21] However, the incidence is clearly much less at lower altitudes. Although HAPE is rare, awareness of it is important because it is life-threatening and can lead to death rapidly if not treated promptly. Fatal cases of HAPE have occurred at altitudes as low as 2700 m, and therefore HAPE is a potential threat in many mountainous areas within the continental United States as well as elsewhere.

Although HAPE occurs only in individuals who make rapid ascents above 2700 m (and only in humans), the actual cause of HAPE is unknown. There is something critical about the transition time from low to high altitude, for HAPE occurs only during the first one to four days following ascent, never later. It occurs in otherwise healthy individuals, and more frequently in children and young adults than in older persons. Oddly, the highest reported incidence is among children residing at high altitude who develop HAPE when they return home (reascent) after a brief visit to low altitude.[22] We know of no way to identify the rare individual who is susceptible to HAPE except by actual exposure to high altitude. The person who has been found to be susceptible is prone to develop some degree of HAPE each time he makes an ascent.

As previously stated, pulmonary edema is the abnormal accumulation of fluid in the lungs, which then interferes with the movement of air into the lungs. Consequently, the symptoms of HAPE include undue shortness of breath, excessive fatigue, and inability to keep up with one's companions. As the condition progresses, a persistent cough develops and the person often has sensations of fluid in his lung. Interference with breathing leads to insufficient oxygenation of blood, causing blueness of lips and fingernails, mental confusion, and loss of consciousness. Supplemental oxygen is essential for treatment, from an oxygen tank if available, but preferably by rapid descent to a lower altitude. Since exercise will aggravate HAPE, the person with HAPE should be carried, if possible, or at least assisted in walking slowly. HAPE can be avoided by gradual ascent with minimal exercise; Diamox may also be advisable. Most important is an appreciation of the fact that HAPE can be fatal. Hence, any person suspected of developing HAPE should be evacuated to lower altitude without delay.[23]

Cerebral Edema

The rarest but most lethal adverse reaction to high altitude is cerebral edema, that is, accumulation of fluid in the brain. The clinical picture is mental confusion progressing to coma and death. Most cases have occurred well above 4300 m, as in trekkers climbing to the base camp at 5500 m on Mt. Everest. The cause is unknown, but the treatment is clearly administration of oxygen and rapid descent.

Although AMS, HAPE, and cerebral edema have been described separately, they may in fact be related. For example, the common headache of AMS may be an early manifestation of mild cerebral edema. Fortunately, however, AMS almost always clears spontaneously without progressing to frank cerebral edema. Likewise, mental confusion and loss of consciousness occur in advanced cases of HAPE as well as in cerebral edema. Hence, the various adverse reactions to high altitude may well be differing manifestations of a common derangement of bodily function, all initiated by hypoxia.

Cold Injury

The environmental stress of mountain sport includes not only the atmospheric hypoxia of high altitude but frequently low ambient temperatures as well. In fact, it is climate rather than altitude per se that limits both plant and animal life in the mountains. Consequently, near the equator a favorable climate permits human populations to live permanently above 4300 m, and timberline is almost as high. As one moves away from the equator, either north or south, ambient temperatures fall progressively, the climate becomes more rigorous, and the maximum tolerable altitude for permanent survival of plants and animals, including man, is progressively lower. Timberline, the highest altitude at which trees can withstand the climate, is reduced to sea level as far northward as Alaska.

With the ever-increasing popularity of mountain sports, combined with the facility of travel to remote regions of the world, more and more people enter the mountain environment, often naively. Trekking in the Himalayas is no longer the exclusive domain of the experienced mountain climber. Literally millions of people flock to the Rocky Mountains each winter to ski the powder snow. How many are prepared for the climate above timberline, where high winds can combine with subzero temperatures to create a very hazardous chill factor? The sportsman should protect himself from the threat of frostbite under these conditions. Also, as explained earlier, high altitude accelerates fatigue, which, combined with intense cold, can lead to a dangerous fall in body temperature (hypothermia). When one considers the difficulty of moving an injured person over rough terrain in deep snow in the mountains, one must respect the potentially lethal combination of atmospheric hypoxia, hypothermia, and frostbite.[24]

The Person with Cardiopulmonary Disease

It is the nature of man to accept danger as part of the adventure of mountain sport. This is true not only of young, healthy individuals, but of older persons as well. It is not unusual to find men and women in their 50's and even 60's skiing above timberline at 3400 m or higher. In this age group cardiovascular disease often develops, and this might constitute an additional danger to mountain sport. However, the evidence does not indicate that this is true. Cardiovascular disease, particularly narrowing of the coronary arteries that carry blood to the heart muscle to supply it with oxygen, may limit the capacity of the heart to pump blood to the rest of the body. This in turn will reduce the person's capacity for exercise. High altitude will reduce his work capacity further. But in any situation, at low or high altitude, as long as the person recognizes his limitation and maintains the intensity of his exercise within those limits, he can function well. This is clear from studies of older skiers, even men who have had heart attacks in the past (healed myocardial infarction), who experience no ill effects from exercising (skiing) in the cold at high altitude. There is even evidence that residence at high altitude provides a degree of protection from cardiovascular disease.

In general, mountain sport is well tolerated as long as the body can deliver adequate amounts of oxygen to the working muscles. As discussed earlier, blood, which is the vehicle for transporting oxygen, contains normal quantities of oxygen even at altitudes as high as 4300 m. This is true provided that lung function is normal. Disease of the airways, such as emphysema and chronic bronchitis, interferes with the movement of air in and out of the lungs and can impair oxygenation of the blood even at sea level. Since larger volumes of air must be moved at high altitude to compensate for the reduced air density, it is obvious that the problems of airway disease will be compounded by high altitude. Persons with airway disease do poorly in the mountains and are advised to avoid such regions. This is borne out by statistics, which clearly show that altitude increases mortality from emphysema and chronic bronchitis.

Cigarette smoking, even before it produces airway disease, also impairs blood oxygenation. The carbon monoxide in cigarette smoke combines with the hemoglobin in blood to reduce the oxygen-carrying capacity of blood by 5 to 10 per cent. In addition, the irritant effect of cigarette smoke produces narrowing of the small airways, thereby interfering with the movement of air. The significance of these factors becomes apparent upon the realization that cigarette smoking at 3400 m impairs blood oxygenation to a degree equivalent to 4600 m. Clearly, smoking compounds the effects of high altitude. This impairment is proportionately greater in women as a consequence of their normally lower blood oxygen-carrying capacity (lower hemoglobin concentration).

SUMMARY

As altitude increases, the partial pressure of oxygen decreases and results in decreased performance of those activities (aerobic) that depend on a steady supply of oxygen. The saturation of hemoglobin by oxygen in arterial blood is decreased. An initial response of the body to altitude is to decrease plasma volume so that red blood cells become more concentrated and blood can carry more oxygen. Later, an increased number of red cells may be produced. However, too high a concentration of red blood cells can impair blood flow due to increased viscosity of blood.

Even after training at altitude for a number of weeks, performance generally remains impaired. Return to sea level can soon result in return to normal performance levels, but there seems to be no advantage to training at altitude for sea-level contests.

STUDY QUESTIONS

1. Give the approximate decrease in Vo_{2max} as altitude increases beyond 1500 meters.

2. What aspects of performance can benefit from high altitude?

3. What effect does ascent to 4300 m have on the arterial oxygen content of a normal individual?

4. Give one consequence of an increased hematocrit at altitude that might improve performance and one consequence that might impair performance.

5. Does the performance decrement observed shortly after reaching altitude generally improve with continued training at altitude for three weeks?

6. Describe several manifestations of impaired mental function at altitude.

7. Describe the symptoms of acute mountain sickness.

8. What age groups are most susceptible to high-altitude pulmonary edema?

9. What is the treatment for high-altitude cerebral edema?

10. Are older skiers placed at increased risk of cardiovascular disease when they ski at higher altitudes?

11. Are persons with emphysema and chronic bronchitis placed at increased risk at high altitude?

REFERENCES

1. Buskirk, E. R., Kollias, J., Picon-Reatigue, E., Akers, R., Prokop, E., and Baker, P.: Physiology and performance of track athletes at various altitudes in the United States and Peru. *In* Goddard, R. F. (ed.): *The Effects of Altitude on Physical Performance*. Albuquerque, Athletic Institute, 1967, pp. 65–71.
2. Åstrand, P. O., and Rodahl, K.: *Textbook of Work Physiology*. New York, McGraw-Hill Book Company, 1970, p. 292.
3. McFarland, R. A.: Review of experimental findings in sensory and mental functions. *In* Hegnauer, A. H. (ed.): *Biomedicine Problems of High Terrestrial Elevations*. Natick, Mass., U.S. Army Research Institute of Environmental Medicine, 1969, pp. 250–265.
4. Weil, J. V., Kryger, M. H., and Scoggin, C. H.: Sleep and breathing at high altitude. *In* Guilleminault, C. (ed.): *Sleep Apnea Syndrome*. New York, Alan R. Liss Inc., 1978.
5. Jokl, E., and Jokl, P.: The effect of altitude on athletic performance. *In* Jokl, E., and Jokl, P. (eds.): *Exercise and Altitude*. Basel, Switzerland, S. Karger, 1968, pp. 28–34.
6. Grover, R. F.: Influence of high altitude on cardiac output response to exercise. *In* Hegnauer, A. H. (ed.): *Biomedicine Problems of High Terrestrial Elevations*. Natick, Mass., U.S. Army Research Institute of Environmental Medicine, 1969, pp. 223–239.
7. Grover, R. F., Reeves, J. T., Maher, J. T., McCullough, R. E., Cruz, J. C., Denniston, J. C., and Cymerman, A.: Maintained stroke volume but impaired arterial oxygenation in man at high altitude with supplemental CO_2. Circ. Res. *38*(5):391–396, 1976.
8. Weil, J. V., Jamieson, G., Brown, D. W., and Grover, R. F.: The red cell mass-arterial oxygen relationship in normal man. J. Clin. Invest. *47*(7):1627–1639, 1968.
9. Hartley, L. H., Alexander, J. K., Modelski, M., and Grover, R. F.: Subnormal cardiac output at rest and during exercise in residents at 3,100 m altitude. J. Appl. Physiol. *23*(6):839–848, 1967.
10. Hartley, L. H., Vogel, J. A., and Cruz, J. C.: Reduction of maximal exercise heart rate at altitude and its reversal with atropine. J. Appl. Physiol. *36*(3):362–365, 1974.
11. Grover, R. F.: Adaptation to high altitude. *In* Folinsbee, L. J. (ed.): *Environmental Stress – Individual Adaptations*. New York, Academic Press, 1978.
12. Kjellberg, S. R., Rudhe, V., and Sjöstrand, T.: The relation of the cardiac volume to the weight and surface area of the body, the blood volume and the physical capacity for work. Acta Radiol. *31*:113–122, 1949.
13. Guyton, A. C., Jones, C. E., and Coleman, T. G.: *Circulatory Physiology: Cardiac Output and Its Regulation*. Philadelphia, W. B. Saunders Company, 1973, p. 408.
14. Ekblom, B., Wilson, G., and Åstrand, P. O.: Central circulation during exercise after venesection and reinfusion of red blood cells. J. Appl. Physiol. *40*(3):379–383, 1976.
15. Vogel, J. A., and Gleser, M. A.: Effect of carbon monoxide on oxygen transport during exercise. J. Appl. Physiol. *32*(2):234–239, 1972.
16. Rorth, M., Nygaard, S. F., and Parving, H. H.: Red cell metabolism and oxygen affinity of healthy individuals during exposure to high altitude. *In* Brewer, G. J. (ed.): *Hemoglobin and Red Cell Structure and Function*. New York, Plenum, 1972, pp. 361–372.
17. Grover, R. F., Lufschanowski, R., and Alexander, J. K.: Alterations in the coronary circulation of man following ascent to 3,100 m altitude. J. Appl. Physiol. *41*(6):832–838, 1976.
18. Grover, R. F., and Reeves, J. T.: Exercise performance of athletes at sea level and 3100 meters altitude. Schweiz. Zeitschr. für Sportmed. *14*(1):130–148, 1966.
19. Grover, R. F., Reeves, J. T., Grover, E. B., and Leathers, J. E.: Muscular exercise in young men native to 3,100 m altitude. J. Appl. Physiol. *22*(3):555–564, 1967.
20. Scoggin, C. H., McCullough, R. E., Jackson, D., and Weil, J. V.: Prevention of severe hypoxia during sleep at high altitude. Clin. Res. *26*(2):138A, 1978.
21. Baldwin, R.: The crisis on Denali. Off Belay *30*:2–10 (Dec.) 1976.
22. Scoggin, C. H., Hyers, T. M., Reeves, J. T., and Grover, R. F.: High-altitude pulmonary edema in children and young adults of Leadville, Colorado. N. Engl. J. Med. *297*(23):1269–1272, 1977.
23. Hultgren, H. N.: HAPE — high altitude pulmonary edema. Off Belay *26*:7–10 (April) 1976.
24. Paton, B. C.: Cold injury, hypothermia and frostbite. Summit *21*(10):6–13 (Dec.) 1975.

23

MEDICAL ASPECTS OF SCUBA AND BREATH-HOLD DIVING

RICHARD H. STRAUSS, M.D.

Swimming underwater while using a self-contained underwater breathing apparatus (*scuba*) is a noncompetitive sport enjoyed by a large number of people. More than 200,000 Americans are trained to scuba dive each year and do so in inland bodies of water as well as in the oceans. Scuba diving, like driving a car, is not particularly dangerous when done carefully, but it does require training. The hazards involved, other than drowning, are not obvious but must be kept in mind so they can be avoided. Many are related to increased pressure or changes in pressure. Breath-hold diving is simpler and less hazardous than scuba diving and is practiced by many persons who enjoy seeing the shallower depths (where most of the sea life is) without the complexity and expense of scuba gear.

BREATH-HOLD DIVING

Equipment

In breath-hold diving (skin diving), as in scuba diving, a face mask is worn for clear vision underwater. In air, most of the refraction (bending) of light takes place at the front of the eye where the cornea meets air. When the eye is submerged in water, this refraction is lost and vision is out of focus. Wearing a face mask (Fig. 23–1) traps a pocket of air in front of the eye so that focusing can occur. Refraction at the front of the mask underwater makes objects appear closer or larger than they actually are.

Persons who wear glasses can have special lenses attached to the inside of the mask. Contact lenses can be worn under a mask but are lost occasionally if water comes in contact with the eye, as it usually does.

Breathing is done at the surface, generally through a snorkel (tube) that runs from the mouth to the surface. This allows the diver to breathe without lifting his face from the water. Rubber swim fins are worn on the feet for added propulsion. An inflatable safety vest provides buoyancy at the surface in an emergency or when the diver wishes to rest.

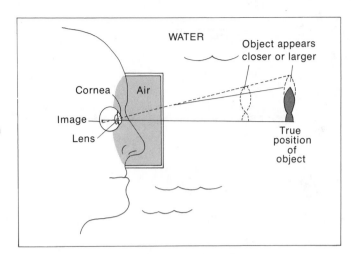

Figure 23–1. A face mask is worn for clear vision underwater.

Breath-hold Blackout

A diver can lose consciousness underwater if he hyperventilates (overbreathes) before diving.* Many swimmers and divers know that by breathing deeply a number of times before a dive they can delay the urge to breathe. This urge is caused primarily by an above normal rise in the level of carbon dioxide in the arterial blood. Hyperventilation delays such a rise because it gets rid of part of the carbon dioxide that is normally stored in the body. However, hyperventilation does *not* significantly increase the amount of oxygen stored in the body.

During a dive, oxygen continues to be used up. Low oxygen levels do not cause much urge to breathe, so the oxygen supply to the brain may fall low enough to produce unconsciousness before the carbon dioxide level has risen sufficiently to warn the diver to breathe. A number of swimmers and divers have drowned while trying to demonstrate how far they can swim underwater after hyperventilating. To avoid this problem, take only one or two deep breaths before a dive.

SCUBA DIVING

Equipment

The self-contained underwater breathing apparatus used by most sport divers consists of a tank containing compressed air and a regulator that delivers air through a mouthpiece when the diver inhales (Fig. 23–2). Air entering the mouthpiece is

*Hyperventilation is also discussed on pages 74 and 257.

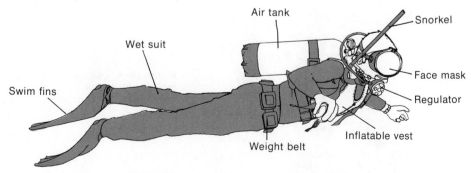

Figure 23–2. Equipment used in scuba diving.

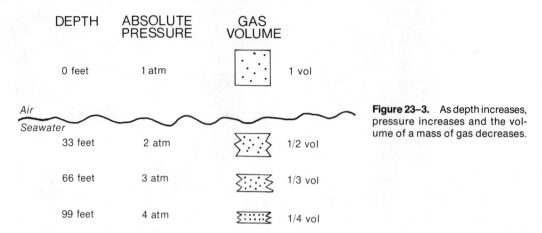

Figure 23–3. As depth increases, pressure increases and the volume of a mass of gas decreases.

automatically kept at about the same pressure as the surrounding water. Exhaled air is released into the water as bubbles.

In cold water, a foam rubber wet suit is worn for insulation. Lead weights compensate for the buoyancy of the air trapped within the foam rubber. The most frequent cause of death among scuba divers is drowning. Many of these drownings could have been prevented if the diver had simply remembered to unbuckle and drop his weight belt in a time of emergency. The inflatable safety vest rarely should be used for rapid ascent to the surface. Rather, it is inflated at the surface for flotation or air is added underwater to adjust buoyancy.

Ear Squeeze

The air pressure at sea level is termed *one atmosphere.* For every 33 feet of seawater through which a diver descends, pressure increases by 1 additional atmosphere (Fig. 23–3). The pressure of all soft tissues of the body, including the blood, is about the same as surrounding pressure. If, like many fish, a diver had no pockets of gas within him, pressure changes would cause few problems. However, as water pressure increases, the pressure within gas pockets of the body, such as the lungs and middle ears, must also increase or damage will result.

The scuba diver breathes compressed air at about the same pressure as the surrounding water. Normally, compressed air passes through the eustachian tube, which opens occasionally and "equalizes" the pressure within the otherwise isolated middle ear (Fig. 23–4). However, the eustachian tube is a bit like a piece of spaghetti

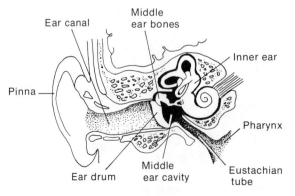

Figure 23–4. Air can pass through the eustachian tube so that pressure in the middle ear remains the same as surrounding pressure.

with a pinhole running through it. Swelling from a cold, allergy, or other problem may prevent easy opening. Then pressure within the middle ear will remain low even though water pressure increases. The result is *squeeze* (barotrauma) of the middle ear. The ear hurts immediately. Small blood vessels that line the middle ear may rupture and bleed because the blood within them is at a higher pressure. The eardrum may also break. If cold air enters the middle ear through the broken drum, dizziness (vertigo) can result and cause disorientation underwater. Bleeding within the eardrum or rupture of it can be seen by a physician examining the drum.

Ear squeeze is prevented by equalizing ear pressure during descent and by stopping descent if even mild ear discomfort occurs. Methods for opening the eustachian tube can be learned. Trying to exhale against the pinched nose may force air through the eustachian tube but occasionally leads to sudden hearing loss from damage to the inner ear. Avoidance of diving when suffering from a cold or allergies helps to prevent ear squeeze.

The treatment of moderate ear squeeze consists of avoiding diving for a few days until healing is complete. Decongestants (see page 256) may also be used. A small hole in the eardrum closes within a few days, but further diving should be delayed for several weeks. A large hole may require a surgical graft.

The sinuses of the head also may be "squeezed," causing facial pain. Eye goggles are not used in diving because they can result in eye squeeze. A face mask includes the nose and thus allows equalization of air pressure between the mask and nose.

Air Embolism

Cause. When pressure decreases, the volume of a given mass of gas increases (Fig. 23–3). If a scuba diver holds his breath while rising toward the surface, the trapped gas will tend to expand the lung beyond its normal size and cause tearing of tissue. (This does not happen during breath-hold diving, in which air is inhaled only at the surface.)

Embolism means that some material is carried by the blood stream to a location where it plugs a blood vessel. In air embolism, air bubbles are forced into torn blood vessels of the lung and carried to the heart, where they can be pumped in arterial blood to any part of the body. Bubbles travel to small arteries, where they get stuck, at least temporarily, and prevent blood flow beyond that point. This goes unnoticed in many parts of the body, but bubbles carried to the brain result in malfunction within seconds. The victim usually looks as if he had had a stroke. A typical case is that of the diver who was normal until he reached the surface, whereupon he suddenly sank back into the water, unconscious. If the diver regains consciousness, he may be confused, blind, or paralyzed on one side of the body. Unfortunately, air embolism kills a number of divers each year.

Problems other than air embolism may also result from tearing of lung tissue. If the tear involves the lung's surface, air will leak out and the lung will collapse (pneumothorax). Air may enter the central compartment of the chest (pneumomediastinum) or may dissect upward so that it can be felt under the skin of the neck (subcutaneous emphysema). Blood from a tear in the lung may mix with air and be coughed up, appearing at the mouth as pink froth. Lung tear can result from even shallow dives: several cases of air embolism have occurred during scuba training in swimming pools.

Prevention and Treatment. Air embolism is generally prevented by breathing normally during ascent or, in an emergency ascent, by exhaling continuously. Diving must be avoided when there is a lung disorder.

Air embolism is treated by moving the diver to a recompression chamber immediately (see further on). If the victim has not died within minutes after the accident, recompression with oxygen breathing may result in total recovery.

Decompression Sickness (The Bends)

Sport divers rarely die of decompression sickness, but damage can be severe, including paralysis.

Cause. The cause of decompression sickness is bubble formation within the body when pressure is decreased, somewhat like the formation of bubbles in a carbonated beverage when the top is removed. About four fifths of air is nitrogen. Nitrogen from a diver's lungs is carried, dissolved in blood, to the tissues, where it is stored in solution — not as bubbles.* The amount of nitrogen dissolved in tissues increases both as depth increases and, initially, as more time.is spent at depth. The nitrogen stored in tissues is not a problem until the diver decides to return to the surface. Then the decrease in pressure may result in bubble formation in blood or tissue. Tissue may be distorted and damaged. Bubbles in blood may obstruct flow both directly and by causing changes in blood such as formation of small clots.

Prevention. Decompression sickness can be prevented in three ways. (1) The sport diver who stays in water shallower than 30 feet will not be affected. (2) Divers who go deeper can still return directly to the surface if they limit their time at depth in accordance with established guidelines (no-decompression limits). (3) Beyond certain limits of depth and time, the accumulation of nitrogen is sufficient to require decompression. That is, return to the surface must be slow enough — over minutes or hours — to allow loss of nitrogen through the lungs without sufficient bubble formation to cause damage. Guidelines for safe decompression (decompression tables) have evolved over a number of years. An example of a dive that requires stopping at several depths is shown in Figure 23–5. Such dives require considerable training and experience. Sport divers generally should restrict their dives to those that require no decompression.

Diving at increased altitudes, such as in mountain lakes, requires special decompression schedules because the decreased atmospheric pressure leads to increased susceptibility to decompression sickness. Similarly, flying soon after diving can cause

---

*Other physiologically inert gases, such as helium and neon, can also cause decompression sickness.

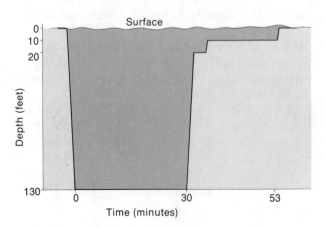

Figure 23–5. Example of decompression. After diving to 130 feet and remaining there for 30 minutes, the diver must stop at several depths during ascent in order to avoid decompression sickness (U.S. Navy Air Decompression Table).

decompression sickness. The recommended delay between diving and flying depends on the dive performed.

Signs and Symptoms.   A particularly dangerous type of decompression sickness among sport divers is that which strikes the spinal cord. The spinal cord transmits signals between the brain and the body. A typical case is that of a scuba diver who was exploring a sunken ship in 110 feet of water. After remaining on the wreck for what he thought was a reasonable time, he returned to the surface. Over the next several hours, he developed first a feeling of pins and needles in his legs, as though they had "gone to sleep" (Fig. 23–6). However, walking around to increase their circulation did not help. Next he noticed that walking was becoming difficult — weak and uncoordinated as if he were drunk, although he had not been drinking and his mind was clear. These problems were due to decompression sickness, which caused interference with nerve signals travelling through the spinal cord. For the same reason the diver could not urinate. The next stage in this progression is often paralysis, usually from the waist downward.

It is important for every diver to recognize the early manifestations of spinal cord decompression sickness — before paralysis — because immediate treatment in a decompression chamber may result in complete recovery, whereas delay in treatment may be associated with permanent nerve damage.

Another type of decompression sickness is manifested by pain in an arm or leg, particularly in the joints. This pain is usually steady, like a toothache. If untreated, the pain generally stops after a number of hours. However, it should be treated by recompression in order to decrease the chances of damage developing at a later time. In a delayed form of decompression sickness called osteonecrosis (bone death), damage goes unrecognized until a joint collapses months or years later. "The bends" is a term that developed among early compressed-air workers in caissons and tunnels who limped from the pain and damage of decompression sickness.

Since damage can involve almost any part of the body, the symptoms can mimic many medical disorders. When any unexplained symptom appears after a dive, decompression sickness should be considered until it is ruled out.

Treatment.   The treatment for decompression sickness is recompression in a chamber. Within the chamber, air pressure is raised, and the victim breathes oxygen intermittently by mask (Fig. 23–7). The elevated pressure causes bubbles to diminish in size. Oxygen breathing results in an increased gradient for the diffusion of nitrogen out of the body and also increases the availability of oxygen to tissues. Air breathing is peri-

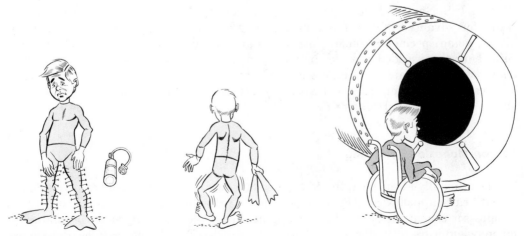

Figure 23–6.   Decompression sickness of the spinal cord can progress over a period of minutes or hours from a feeling of pins and needles in the legs to difficulty in walking and finally to paralysis.

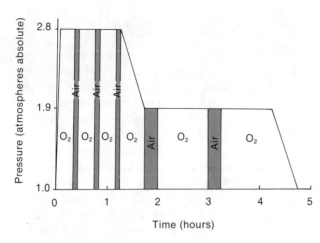

Figure 23–7. For treatment of decompression sickness, chamber pressure is raised and the victim breathes pure oxygen intermittently over several hours. (U.S. Navy Treatment Table 6 is shown.) (Redrawn from Strauss, R. H., and Prockop, L. D.: Decompression sickness among scuba divers. JAMA 223:640, 1973. Copyright 1973, American Medical Association.)

odically substituted for oxygen breathing in order to decrease the chances of oxygen toxicity. *Oxygen toxicity* is a problem that results from breathing oxygen at increased pressures. It can cause convulsions, which, in a chamber, are transient and not a major problem. Underwater, however, pure oxygen should not be breathed by sport divers because convulsions can result in drowning.

Decompression sickness (or air embolism) that affects the central nervous system or causes breathing problems or shock is a medical emergency. The victim should be transported to a recompression chamber by the fastest means available — by aircraft if necessary. In flight, cabin pressure should be kept as close to one atmosphere as possible. The victim should start to breathe oxygen immediately and continue doing so until reaching the recompression chamber.

Nitrogen Narcosis (Rapture of the Deep)

At high pressures, the nitrogen in air acts like an anesthetic gas such as ether. This effect gets worse as depth increases. "Martini's law" suggests that every 50-foot increment in depth acts like one Martini on an empty stomach. Divers at 100 feet or greater have some impairment of judgment, even though they frequently do not recognize this fact. Poor judgment underwater is clearly a hazard, and for deep diving, skill and caution should be made automatic through extensive training and experience.

The U.S. Navy and most sport-diving instructors limit scuba diving to 130 feet of water for advanced divers. For diving at depths greater than 190 feet, U.S. Navy divers, using special equipment, breathe a gas mixture that is mostly helium with sufficient oxygen added to keep the partial pressure of oxygen near normal. Helium does not act like an anesthetic gas, and thus it prevents narcosis. Helium does, however, cause decompression sickness as nitrogen does. In addition, it is too expensive to be used by sport divers.

Carbon Monoxide Poisoning

Occasionally in the past, the compressed air in a scuba tank has been contaminated with carbon monoxide. This can happen, for example, when the intake for the air compressor is near the exhaust of the engine. The diver breathing such contaminated air may suffer from headache, dizziness, and nausea. Finally, he may lose consciousness and drown. These problems occur mainly because carbon monoxide combines with hemoglobin and decreases the transport of oxygen in blood to the brain.

Carbon monoxide poisoning is prevented by insuring pure compressed air. Conscientious sellers of compressed air have their air quality checked periodically by state or commercial laboratories.

Carbon monoxide poisoning is treated by having the victim breathe oxygen immediately and on the way to the hospital. Oxygen breathing helps to increase oxygen transport to tissues and to drive carbon monoxide off the hemoglobin molecule. If a recompression chamber is available, breathing oxygen there at pressures above one atmosphere is the best treatment.

Other Problems

Panic, resulting in drowning, is probably the most frequent cause of death among divers. Panic generally is preventable through careful training, knowing one's own limitations, and familiarity with equipment and local conditions such as waves and currents.

Serious chilling, resulting in a drop in body temperature (hypothermia), is a severe stress encountered by divers in many areas. Hypothermia can impair physical and mental performance. It is prevented through the use of insulating suits and by limiting the length of the dive.

Although divers are rarely attacked by sea creatures, they may accidentally come in contact with stinging jellyfish, sea urchins, or fish with toxic spines. For a more complete discussion of these and other medical problems related to diving, the reader should consult advanced sources (see "Further Readings").

FITNESS FOR DIVING

The diver does not have to be a good athlete. The majority of sport divers spend most of their time swimming around slowly, sightseeing. However, the diver must be able to exercise strenuously for a moderate time in an emergency or, for example, in returning to the boat against a current. In practice, this means that the diver should be comfortable with a similar amount of exercise on land. In addition, the muscles used in kicking with swim fins are not entirely the same as those used for walking, so practice with fins in a pool or elsewhere is helpful. The diver should be strong enough to carry his own air tank and other gear.

Many scuba instructors require students to have clearance from a physician before initial scuba training. In particular, persons with the following conditions should not scuba dive because of a significant risk of death if the problem occurs underwater: epileptic seizures; syncope (passing out); and diabetes with the possibility of insulin shock. Persons with emphysema of the lung or active asthma should not scuba dive because air trapping in the lung may lead to air embolism. Certain other lung and ear problems may also lead to unacceptable risk. Persons who have had a heart attack (myocardial infarction) should consult carefully with their physician, keeping in mind the exertion required in an emergency and the fact that another heart attack is more likely to be fatal underwater than on land.

SUMMARY

Before a breath-hold dive, take only one or two deep breaths. Hyperventilation can result in blackout during the subsequent dive. During scuba diving, failure to equalize pressure in the middle ear can lead to ear pain and hemorrhage (squeeze).

The most important thing to remember in scuba diving is not to hold the breath while rising in the water, because such breath-holding may force air from the lungs into the blood stream and damage the brain (air embolism). Decompression sickness (the bends) can be avoided by following established depth and time guidelines. The manifestations of decompression sickness may include paralysis or pain. The treatment for both decompression sickness and air embolism is recompression with oxygen breathing in a chamber as soon as possible. Nitrogen narcosis can impair judgment at depth. Compressed air should be free of carbon monoxide and other contaminants. The diver should be in reasonably good physical condition but need not be an athlete.

STUDY QUESTIONS

1. Explain the mechanism and prevention of breath-hold blackout.

2. What is the most common cause of death among scuba divers? How can this be prevented?

3. Explain the mechanism and prevention of ear squeeze.

4. Give an example of an underwater act that could cause air embolism.

5. What are the signs of air embolism? How is it treated?

6. What causes decompression sickness? What are its signs, symptoms, and treatment?

7. How is decompression sickness prevented?

8. What is the usual, dangerous effect of nitrogen narcosis on divers? How can this be avoided?

9. Give several symptoms of carbon monoxide poisoning.

FURTHER READINGS

Bennett, P. B., and Elliott, D. H.: *The Physiology and Medicine of Diving and Compressed Air Work.* Baltimore, The Williams and Wilkins Company, 1975.
Empleton, B. E. (ed.): *The New Science of Skin and Scuba Diving.* New York, Association Press, 1975.
National Oceanic and Atmospheric Administration: *The NOAA Diving Manual.* Washington, D.C., U.S. Government Printing Office, 1975.
Strauss, R. H. (ed.): *Diving Medicine.* New York, Grune & Stratton, 1976.
U.S. Navy Diving Manual. Washington, D.C., U.S. Government Printing Office, 1973.

24

A COMPARISON OF SPORTS: PHYSIOLOGICAL AND MEDICAL ASPECTS

JACK H. WILMORE, Ph.D.
JOHN A. BERGFELD, M.D.

PHYSIOLOGICAL CHARACTERISTICS OF SELECTED SPORTS*

Recent trends in sports medicine and physiology include the widespread use of physiological and medical profiles to describe the qualities, characteristics, and associated medical problems of champion athletes in their various sports. Detailed physiological profiles have been established for track and field athletes, rowers, gymnasts, swimmers, speed skaters, wrestlers, weight lifters, jockeys, skiers, and basketball, baseball, football, ice hockey, tennis, and volleyball players. These profiles permit (1) a detailed analysis of the physical potential of the athlete for a particular sport; (2) an analysis of the physical conditioning needs of each athlete in his or her respective sport; and (3) an accurate individualized prescription for both in-season and off-season conditioning programs.

With a knowledge of the physical demands of any one sport or activity, the sports practitioner (elite or weekend athlete, coach, team trainer, or team physician) will be able to take a more scientific approach to the design and development of specific training and physical conditioning procedures. The work of Dr. David L. Costill and his associates at the Human Performance Laboratory, Ball State University, Muncie, Indiana, has focused on the long-distance runner. This work illustrates how research concentrated on a single activity can provide substantial practical and theoretical insight into that activity. Initially, the relationship between performance in distance running and various physiological variables was studied.[1] This was followed by investigations into the energetics of distance running,[2] the metabolic aspects of distance running,[3] maximal oxygen uptakes of elite marathon runners,[4] and the determinants of successful marathon running.[5] Later studies investigated the body composition

---

*By Jack H. Wilmore, Ph.D.

characteristics of marathon runners,[6] fluid ingestion during distance running,[7] muscle glycogen utilization during prolonged exercise,[8] glycogen depletion patterns in human muscle fibers during distance running,[9] and the psychological characteristics of the marathon runner.[10] Although the intent of this research was to advance theoretical knowledge about these various aspects of distance running, major benefits of a practical nature were also realized in areas such as prerace diet, fluid ingestion patterns, optimal composition of ingested fluid, and optimal training routines.

While many physiological aspects of performance have been quantified for selected athletes or small groups of athletes, there is more general data about the areas of body composition and physique; muscle fiber characteristics; strength, power, and muscular endurance; and cardiovascular endurance capacity. Each of these areas will be discussed briefly.

Body Composition and Physique

Total body weight can be divided into two components, lean body weight and fat weight. Lean body weight refers to the weight of all nonfat tissue such as bone, muscle, skin, and organs. The composition of body weight (lean versus fat weight) can be determined by several techniques. Probably the most accurate technique involves weighing the individual while he or she is totally submerged underwater. From this underwater weighing, body volume — and thus body density (mass/volume or weight/volume) — can be calculated accurately. Since the density of fat is known and the density of lean tissue is relatively constant among individuals, knowing total body density allows the calculation of lean body weight, fat weight, and relative fat (fat weight × 100/total body weight).[11]

Height, weight, and relative fat values for athletes in various sports are presented in Table 24–1. For reference purposes, the college-age male and female average 15 and 24 percent body fat, respectively.[12] From this table, certain facts are apparent: the female athlete is typically fatter than her male counterpart; the older athlete is fatter than the younger athlete; and athletes who are involved in endurance activities, or who must control their weight to meet a certain competitive weight classification, have very low relative body fats. It is generally felt that a low relative body fat is desirable for successful competition in almost any sport.

Body physique is traditionally expressed as the individual's somatotype. Somatotyping is a scientific procedure used to describe the morphology or shape of the body in a quantitative manner. Most somatotyping systems utilize the concept that the body has three major components or dimensions: muscularity, linearity (angularity), and fatness. These three components have been termed mesomorphy for muscularity, ectomorphy for linearity, and endomorphy for fatness. A rating system has been developed in which each person is given a rating in each of these three areas. The original system developed by Sheldon used a rating scale of from 1 to 7 to designate, on an increasing basis, the relative degree of each specific component. Later systems allow ratings above 7. As an example, a rating of 2–7–2 (endomorphy-mesomorphy-ectomorphy) would indicate an individual who had a preponderance of muscle, very little fat, and a stocky frame (lack of linearity).

Somatotypes of athletes in various sports are presented in Table 24–2. With the exception of the throwers in track and field, athletes are generally low in endomorphy. Mesomorphy values range from moderate in runners to high in athletes involved in activities that are dependent on strength. Ectomorphy values range from low in athletes who rely most on their strength to moderate in distance runners and jumpers.

TABLE 24–1. BODY COMPOSITION VALUES IN ATHLETES*

Athletic Group or Sport	Sex	Age (yr)	Height (cm)	Weight (kg)	Relative Fat (%)	Reference
Baseball	male	20.8	182.7	83.3	14.2	14
	male	–	–	–	11.8	15
	male	27.4	183.1	88.0	12.6	Unpublished data (Wilmore)
Basketball	male	26.8	193.6	91.2	9.7	Unpublished data (Wilmore)
	female	19.1	169.1	62.6	20.8	16
	female	19.4	167.0	63.9	26.9	17
Football	male	20.3	184.9	96.4	13.8	14
	male	–	–	–	13.9	15
Defensive backs	male	17–23	178.3	77.3	11.5	18
Offensive backs	male	17–23	179.7	79.8	12.4	18
Linebackers	male	17–23	180.1	87.2	13.4	18
Offensive linemen	male	17–23	186.0	99.2	19.1	18
Defensive linemen	male	17–23	186.6	97.8	18.5	18
Defensive backs	male	24.5	182.5	84.8	9.6	13
Offensive backs	male	24.7	183.8	90.7	9.4	13
Linebackers	male	24.2	188.6	102.2	14.0	13
Offensive line	male	24.7	193.0	112.6	15.6	13
Defensive line	male	25.7	192.4	117.1	18.2	13
Quarterbacks, kickers	male	24.1	185.0	90.1	14.4	13
Gymnastics	male	20.3	178.5	69.2	4.6	14
	female	19.4	163.0	57.9	23.8	17
	female	20.0	158.5	51.1	15.5	19
	female	14.0	–	–	17.0	20
	female	23.0	–	–	11.0	20
	female	23.0	–	–	9.6	21
Ice Hockey	male	26.3	180.3	86.7	15.1	Unpublished data (Wilmore)
Jockeys	male	30.9	158.2	50.3	14.1	Unpublished data (Wilmore)
Skiing	male	25.9	176.6	74.8	7.4	22
Swimming	male	21.8	182.3	79.1	8.5	22
	male	20.6	182.9	78.9	5.0	14
	female	19.4	168.0	63.8	26.3	17
Track and field	male	21.3	180.6	71.6	3.7	14
	male	–	–	–	8.8	15
Runners	male	22.5	177.4	64.5	6.3	22
Distance	male	26.1	175.7	64.2	7.5	6
	male	40–49	180.7	71.6	11.2	23
	male	50–59	174.7	67.2	10.9	23
	male	60–69	175.7	67.1	11.3	23
	male	70–75	175.6	66.8	13.6	23
	male	47.2	176.5	70.7	13.2	24
	female	19.9	161.3	52.9	19.2	25
	female	32.4	169.4	57.2	15.2	26
Sprint	female	20.1	164.9	56.7	19.3	25
Discus	male	28.3	186.1	104.7	16.4	27
	male	26.4	190.8	110.5	16.3	Unpublished data (Wilmore)
	female	21.1	168.1	71.0	25.0	25
Jumpers and hurdlers	female	20.3	165.9	59.0	20.7	25
Shot put	male	27.0	188.2	112.5	16.5	27
	male	22.0	191.6	126.2	19.6	11
	female	21.5	167.6	78.1	28.0	25
Tennis	male	–	–	–	15.2	15
Volleyball	female	19.4	166.0	59.8	25.3	17
Weight lifting	male	24.9	166.4	77.2	9.8	22
Power	male	26.3	176.1	92.0	15.6	27
Olympic	male	25.3	177.1	88.2	12.2	27
Body builders	male	29.0	172.4	83.1	8.4	27
Wrestling	male	26.0	177.8	81.8	9.8	27
	male	27.0	176.0	75.7	10.7	28
	male	22.0	–	–	5.0	20
	male	19.6	174.6	74.8	8.8	29
	male	15–18	172.3	66.3	6.9	30

*Adapted from Wilmore.[12]

TABLE 24–2. SOMATOTYPE VALUES FOR ATHLETES*

| Athletic Group or Sport | Sex | Age (yr) | Height (cm) | Weight (kg) | Somatotype | | | Reference |
					Endo	Meso	Ecto	
Swimming	male	19	179.3	72.1	2.1	5.0	2.9	31
	female	16	164.4	56.9	3.4	4.0	3.0	31
Track and Field								
Runners								
Marathon	male	26	168.7	56.6	1.4	4.3	3.5	31
	male	–	171.1	59.9	2.6	4.4	3.9	32
Long-distance	male	25	171.9	59.8	1.4	4.1	3.6	31
	male	–	174.4	60.8	2.7	4.2	4.3	32
Middle-distance	male	23	177.3	65.0	1.5	4.2	3.6	31
	female	20	166.9	54.3	2.0	3.3	3.7	31
Sprint	male	24	175.4	68.4	1.7	5.0	2.8	31
	female	21	165.0	56.8	2.7	3.9	2.9	31
Jumpers	male	24	182.8	73.2	1.7	4.4	3.4	31
Throwers	female	22	169.4	56.4	2.2	3.3	3.7	31
	male	27	186.1	102.3	3.5	7.1	1.0	31
	female	20	170.9	73.5	5.3	5.2	1.7	31
Weight lifting	male	27	168.0	76.6	2.4	7.1	1.0	31
Wrestling	male	26	169.3	70.6	2.2	6.3	1.6	31
	male	–	172.4	72.0	2.7	5.6	2.5	32

*Adapted from Wilmore.[12]

Muscle Fiber Characteristics

Muscle fiber types were discussed in Chapter 2. At the present time, only a few athletes have undergone muscle biopsies to determine their distribution of fast- and slow-twitch fibers. Since this is a relatively new technique, and has not been widely used owing to the inherent complexity of the subsequent analyses, few athletic populations have been studied. Table 24–3 provides data for those few athletic populations that have been studied. From this data it is clear that there is a direct linear relationship between the endurance nature of the activity and the percentage of slow-twitch fibers. Where data is available for both males and females in similar sports or events, there appears to be little difference between the sexes relative to fiber ratios, although males have larger fiber areas.

Strength, Power, and Muscular Endurance

Strength, power, and muscular endurance are critical factors for most athletes. However, data are limited to a few athletic populations and are primarily in the area of strength. Power and muscular endurance are more difficult to assess accurately, and the most complete data exists only for professional football players.[13] Table 24–4 lists selected strength values for various male athletic populations. Unfortunately, similar values do not exist for females. It is clear that strength is highly correlated to size. However, in those sports in which strength is not a major requisite for success (e.g., baseball), strength values are considerably lower for athletes of similar body size.

TABLE 24–3. MUSCLE FIBER CHARACTERISTICS OF ATHLETES

Athletic Group or Sport	Sex	Age (yr)	Height (cm)	Weight (kg)	Slow-Twitch Fibers (%)	Slow-Twitch Fiber Area (μ²)	Slow-Twitch Fiber Area (%)	Reference
Bicyclists	male	24	182	74.5	61.4*	–	–	33
	male	25	180	72.8	56.8	6333	59.7	Unpublished data (Costill)
	female	20	165	55.0	50.5	5487	47.6	Unpublished data (Costill)
Canoeists	male	26	181	74.0	61.4*	–	–	33
Orienteers	male	52	176	72.7	68.8*	–	–	33
Skiers, downhill	male	25	181	68.5	67.0*	–	–	34
	male	21	178	69.4	48.0*	–	–	34
Swimmers	male	21	181	78.3	57.7*	–	–	33
					74.3†			
Track and field								
Sprint runners	male	19	181	71.5	24.0‡	5878	23.5	35
	female	19	168	55.6	27.4‡	3752	26.8	35
Middle-distance runners	male	23	179	65.7	51.9‡	6099	46.5	35
	female	20	166	52.5	60.6‡	6069	60.4	35
Long-distance runners	male	25	180	67.8	61.8‡	6378	62.1	36
	male	24	180	70.8	69.4‡	6613	62.3	35
	male	26	179	63.9	79.0‡	8342	82.9	36
Runners	male	23	177	69.5	58.9*	–	–	33
	male	27	178	64.5	59.0*	–	–	34
Sprinters, jumpers	male	24	187	77.6	38.0*	–	–	34
Long-high jumpers	male	29	183	77.3	46.7‡	4718	38.8	35
	female	22	177	61.1	48.7‡	4163	44.0	35
Javelin throwers	male	25	176	83.6	50.4‡	5585	47.7	35
	female	21	169	65.3	41.6‡	4864	42.9	35
Shotput, discus throwers	male	27	198	129.0	37.7‡	7702	34.0	35
	female	24	171	77.0	51.2‡	5192	46.9	35
Weight lifters	male	25	171	81.3	46.1*	–	–	33
					52.6†			

*Biopsy from vastus lateralis.
†Biopsy from deltoid.
‡Biopsy from gastrocnemius.

TABLE 24–4.   SELECTED STRENGTH MEASUREMENTS IN MALE ATHLETES*

Athletic Group or Sport	Age (yr)	Height (cm)	Weight (kg)	One-Repetition Maximum Values†			
				BENCH PRESS (LB)	STANDING PRESS (LB)	CURL (LB)	LEG PRESS (LB)
Baseball	28	183.6	88.1	202	144	113	720
Basketball	26	196.6	91.2	207	161	–	576
Football							
Defensive backs	25	182.5	84.8	276	181	132	–
Offensive backs and wide receivers	25	183.8	90.7	285	203	156	–
Linebackers	24	188.6	102.2	343	215	174	–
Offensive linemen and tight ends	25	193.0	112.6	333	214	177	–
Defensive linemen	26	192.4	117.1	325	224	189	–
Quarterbacks, kickers	24	185.0	90.1	258	205	146	–
Ice Hockey	26	180.1	86.4	240	155	111	699
Jockeys	31	158.2	50.3	134	92	57	501

*Unpublished data from Wilmore.
†The maximum weight that can be lifted *only* one time.

Cardiovascular Endurance Capacity

As was discussed in earlier chapters, maximal oxygen uptake ($\dot{V}o_{2max}$) is the best overall index of cardiovascular endurance capacity. Table 24–5 presents maximal oxygen uptake values for male and female athletes in a variety of sports. It is apparent that in those sports that have a low aerobic or cardiovascular endurance requirement, the athletes have a relatively low $\dot{V}o_{2max}$. While their values range from the high 30's into the low 40's, the highly conditioned endurance athlete will have values in the high 60's to low 80's. Distance runners and cross-country skiers typically have the highest values.

In comparing male and female athletes, there is a considerable difference in $\dot{V}o_{2max}$ for most sports, the female usually being 15 to 30 per cent lower on the average. However, in distance running, the female who is training at the same level as the male has values that are much closer to those of her male counterpart. In fact, when $\dot{V}o_{2max}$ is expressed relative to lean body weight, there is less than a 5 per cent difference between the sexes.

TABLE 24–5.   CARDIOVASCULAR ENDURANCE CAPACITY OF
MALE AND FEMALE ATHLETES

Athletic Group or Sport	Sex	Age (yr)	Height (cm)	Weight (kg)	$\dot{V}o_{2max}$ ml/kg·min	Reference
Baseball	male	21	182.7	83.3	52.3*	14
	male	28	183.6	88.1	52.0*	Unpublished data (Wilmore)
Basketball	male	26	196.6	91.2	49.4*	Unpublished data (Wilmore)
	female	19	167.0	63.9	42.3†	17
	female	19	169.1	62.6	42.9†	16
Bicycling (competitive)	male	24	182.0	74.5	68.2†	33
	male	25	180.0	72.8	67.1†	Unpublished data (Costill)
	female	20	165.0	55.0	50.2†	Unpublished data (Costill)
Canoeing	male	26	181.0	74.0	56.8†	33

Athletic Group or Sport	Sex	Age (yr)	Height (cm)	Weight (kg)	$\dot{V}o_{2max}$ ml/kg min	Reference
Football	male	20	184.9	96.4	51.3*	14
Defensive backs	male	25	182.5	84.8	53.1*	13
Offensive backs, wide receivers	male	25	183.8	90.7	52.2*	13
Linebackers	male	24	188.6	102.2	52.1*	13
Offensive linemen, tight ends	male	25	193.0	112.6	49.9*	13
Defensive linemen	male	26	192.4	117.1	44.9*	13
Quarterbacks, kickers	male	24	185.0	90.1	49.0*	13
Gymnastics	male	20	178.5	69.2	55.5*	14
	female	19	163.0	57.9	36.3†	17
Ice Hockey	male	11	140.5	35.5	56.6†	37
	male	24	179.3	81.8	54.6†	38
	male	26	180.1	86.4	53.6*	Unpublished data (Wilmore)
Jockey	male	31	158.2	50.3	53.8*	Unpublished data (Wilmore)
Orienteering	male	52	176.0	72.7	50.7*	33
Skiing	male	26	176.6	74.8	62.3*	22
Speed skating	male	20	175.5	73.9	56.1*	39
	female	21	164.5	60.8	46.1*	39
Swimming	male	12	150.4	41.2	52.5†	40
	female	12	154.8	43.3	46.2†	40
	male	13	164.8	52.1	52.9†	40
	female	13	160.0	52.1	43.4†	40
	male	15	169.6	59.8	56.6†	40
	female	15	164.8	53.7	40.5†	40
	male	22	182.3	79.7	55.9†	40
	male	20	181.4	76.7	55.7* 54.6‡	41
	male	20	181.0	73.0	50.4†	42
	male	21	182.9	78.9	62.1*	14
	male	21	181.0	78.3	69.9†	33
	male	22	182.3	79.1	56.9*	22
Sprint	male	19	181.1	75.0	58.3*	43
Middle-distance	male	22	178.0	74.6	55.4*	43
Long-distance	male	21	179.0	74.9	65.4*	43
	female	19	168.0	63.8	37.6†	17
Track and field	male	21	180.6	71.6	66.1*	14
Runners	male	22	177.4	64.5	64.0*	22
	male	23	177.0	69.5	72.4*	33
Middle-distance	male	25	180.1	67.8	70.1*	36
Long-distance	male	26	178.9	63.9	77.4*	36
	male	27	178.7	64.9	73.2*	3
	male	32	177.3	64.3	70.3*	4
	male	35	174.0	63.1	66.6*	44
	male	40–49	180.7	71.6	57.5*	23
	male	50–59	174.7	67.2	54.4*	23
	male	60–69	175.7	67.1	51.4*	23
	male	70–75	175.6	66.8	40.0*	23
	female	32	169.4	57.2	59.1*	26
Discus	male	28	186.1	104.7	47.5*	27
	male	26	190.8	110.5	42.8*	Unpublished data (Wilmore)
Shot put	male	27	188.2	112.5	42.6†	27
Volleyball	female	19	166.0	59.8	43.5*	17
Weight lifting	male	25	171.0	81.3	40.1†	33
	male	25	166.4	77.2	42.6*	22
Power	male	26	176.1	92.0	49.5†	27
Olympic	male	25	177.1	88.2	50.7†	27
Body builders	male	29	172.4	83.1	41.5†	27
Wrestling	male	24	175.6	77.7	60.9*	45
	male	26	177.0	81.8	64.0†	27
	male	27	176.0	75.7	54.3*	28

*Treadmill test.
†Bicycle ergometer test.
‡Tethered swimming test.

PHYSIOLOGICAL EVALUATION OF PERFORMANCE
POTENTIAL*

Within the confines of the well-equipped exercise physiology laboratory, it is relatively easy to establish a detailed performance profile on the athlete or on the nonathlete who pursues exercise for health-related purposes. Fortunately, a profile can be established outside the laboratory, using tests that predict or estimate the various physiological parameters rather than measuring them directly. Various field tests that allow the estimation of body composition, strength, and cardiovascular endurance capacity will be described in this section. Results from these tests can then be compared with the respective values listed for various sports or activities in the preceding tables.

Body Composition

While the underwater weighing technique is considered by most authorities to be the most accurate for assessing body composition, anthropometric measurements can also be used. Skinfold thicknesses, body diameters or breadths, and body circumferences or girths have been used in the past with reasonable accuracy to estimate body composition.

For men, lean body weight (LBW) can be estimated from the equation

$$LBW = 10.3 + (0.8 \times weight) - (0.37 \times abdominal\ skinfold).[11]$$

For women, LBW can be estimated from the equation

$$LBW = 8.6 + (0.7 \times weight) - (0.16 \times scapula\ skinfold) - (0.1 \times triceps\ skinfold) - (0.05 \times thigh\ skinfold).[11]$$

---

*By Jack H. Wilmore, Ph.D.

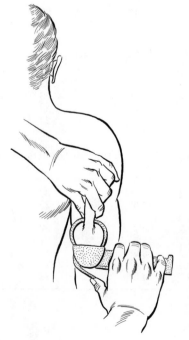

Figure 24–1. Technique for obtaining the triceps skinfold thickness using a skinfold caliper.

For both equations, the individual's weight is entered in kilograms (weight in pounds divided by 2.2), and the skinfold thicknesses are measured in millimeters with a skin-fold caliper, shown in Figure 24–1, at the sites illustrated in Figure 24–2.

Once LBW has been calculated, fat weight and relative fat can be calculated in the following manner:

$$\text{Fat weight} = \text{weight} - \text{LBW}$$

$$\text{Relative fat } (\%) = \frac{\text{fat weight} \times 100}{\text{weight}}$$

To convert kilograms to pounds, simply multiply the kilogram values by 2.2.

Strength

Strength can be assessed accurately by the one-repetition maximum test (1–RM). The basic muscle or muscle group to be tested is selected, and the individual is given a series of trials to determine the greatest weight he can lift just once. With inex-perienced weight lifters, this test is conducted largely through trial and error. Start with a weight that the individual can lift comfortably, then continue adding weight until he or she can lift the weight correctly just one time. If the weight can be lifted more than once, more weight should be added until a true 1-RM is reached. Proper positions for executing 1-RM strength tests are illustrated in Figure 24–3.

Cardiovascular Endurance Capacity

Aerobic or cardiovascular endurance capacity can be estimated on the basis of an endurance-run test. The 1.5 mile test is considered to be one of the best predictors of aerobic capacity and can be run on either a track or a 1.5 mile nonrepeating course. The latter assures each individual a full 1.5 mile course, and not a final distance that is a lap or two short. This test is run at the greatest possible speed and should be given only to those who are in good physical condition or who have been conditioned to run the distance. Pretraining is essential and will help eliminate possible problems of pacing. Those over 25 to 30 years of age should not be encouraged to take this test until

Figure 24–2. Skinfold (SF) measurement sites.

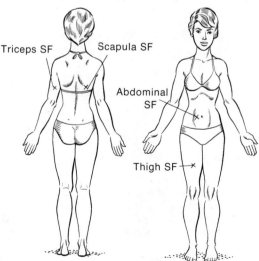

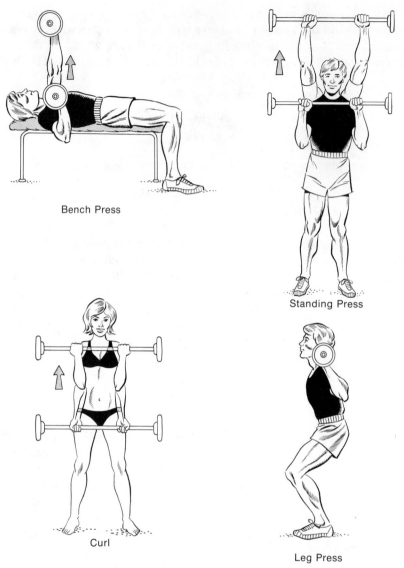

Bench Press

Standing Press

Curl

Leg Press

Figure 24–3. Proper positions for executing the 1-RM strength test.

they have obtained proper medical clearance, including a stress electrocardiogram. Estimated $\dot{V}_{O_{2max}}$ values from 1.5 mile run times are presented in Table 24–6.

MEDICAL PROBLEMS RELATED TO SPECIFIC SPORTS*

Almost all sports activities are potentially associated with medical problems. Generally, such problems can be divided in four categories:

1. Problems common to an age group, whether or not the individual engages in sports.
2. Problems of overuse: repetitive, forceful activities inherent in the nature of the sport, causing a breakdown of the musculoskeletal system.
3. Traumatic problems caused by abnormal extrinsic forces on the body.
4. Problems caused by the environment in which the sport is played.

*By John A. Bergfield, M.D.

The object of this section is not to discuss the diagnosis and treatment of various problems, but simply to create an awareness of them. Such awareness aids in the recognition and prevention of medical problems.

Age Group

The athlete cannot avoid the majority of illnesses common to his age group. Examples are: (1) in children — infectious diseases such as measles and mumps; (2) in adolescents—acne, psychological problems, scoliosis (curvature of the spine); (3) in young adults — mononucleosis, venereal disease; (4) in older adults — degenerative diseases. Such problems are not associated with any particular sport, but those in the remaining three categories can be related to specific sports.

Overuse

Overuse problems (tendinitis, bursitis, stress fractures) generally affect the musculoskeletal system. Other systems, such as the skin, may also be involved. These problems result from specific, repetitive activities required by a sport such as running. If the musculoskeletal system is not prepared for the demands placed upon it, it breaks down physically and an inflammatory reaction results. Examples of overuse problems include the sore arm experienced by amateur baseball players when spring training begins and tennis elbow in the unconditioned tennis player. Overuse syndromes can also occur in well-conditioned athletes—for example, stress fractures in long-distance runners.

Tendinitis is the most common overuse syndrome and has been described by Dr. Robert Kerlan of Los Angeles as "an inflammatory response to microscopic trauma."

TABLE 24–6. ESTIMATED $\dot{V}O_{2max}$ FROM 1.5 MILE RUN TIME

Time (min:sec)	Estimated $\dot{V}O_{2max}$ ml/kg·min
7:30 and under	75
7:31–8:00	72
8:01–8:30	67
8:31–9:00	62
9:01–9:30	58
9:31–10:00	55
10:01–10:30	52
10:31–11:00	49
11:01–11:30	46
11:31–12:00	44
12:01–12:30	41
12:31–13:00	39
13:01–13:30	37
13:31–14:00	36
14:01–14:30	34
14:31–15:00	33
15:01–15:30	31
15:31–16:00	30
16:01–16:30	28
16:31–17:00	27
17:01–17:30	26
17:31–18:00	25

Because of repetitive activity, the tendon eventually breaks down, producing inflammation that causes pain and tenderness. Bone structure may also break down, resulting in a stress fracture. A few sports commonly associated with overuse injury, and the sites of injury involved, include: swimming — shoulder rotator cuff; tennis — elbow; throwing sports — shoulder; crew — forearm musculature; running — lower leg (Achilles tendon) and foot (metatarsal bones); basketball — patellar tendon. Calluses develop on the hands of gymnasts as protection from friction against the bars and rings, but they can become troublesome if they tear or crack.

Overuse syndromes sometimes can be prevented (1) through use of proper equipment, such as special footwear for the runner; and (2) by preparing the musculoskeletal system for the specific demands to be placed on it. For example, conditioning is important for the elbow and arm musculature in a tennis player and for the lower leg musculature in a runner. Overuse syndromes tend to develop when demand exceeds the strength of the musculoskeletal system. This strength is increased by proper conditioning.

Trauma

Predictable injuries are caused by extrinsic trauma in certain sports. For example, ligaments of the knee are frequently injured in football. An awareness of such injuries is the first step toward prevention. Proper coaching, good equipment, and adherence to the rules of the game have all proven effective in preventing athletic injuries.

Environment

Finally, specific sport problems can be related to the environment in which a sport is played. Common examples are ear infections in swimmers, frostbite in skiers, and sea sickness in ocean racers. Artificial turf has created a new set of medical problems, including skin abrasions, foot injury, and bursitis.

Table 24–7 lists a number of sports and the medical problems commonly associated with each. Figure 24–4 illustrates a number of such problems.

INJURY PREVENTION*

Awareness of the medical problems encountered in the various sports helps to prevent injury. Other important factors are equipment, the physical examination, conditioning, environment, coaches, and officials.

Equipment must fit properly and be of high quality. In the past few years, partially because of legal liability, the quality control of athletic equipment has improved. A number of organizations† have completed independent evaluations of personal protective athletic equipment, playing surfaces, and the implements used in sports (bats, balls, rackets, etc.). Proper fitting of athletic equipment is an integral part of the certified athletic trainer's duties. The incidence of injuries from faulty, poor-fitting, or inadequate athletic equipment is decreasing.

---

*By John A. Bergfeld, M.D.

†Association for Standardization and Testing of Materials; National Organization for Control of Standardizatin of Athletic Equipment; American Orthopedic Society of Sports Medicine.

Text continued on page 369.

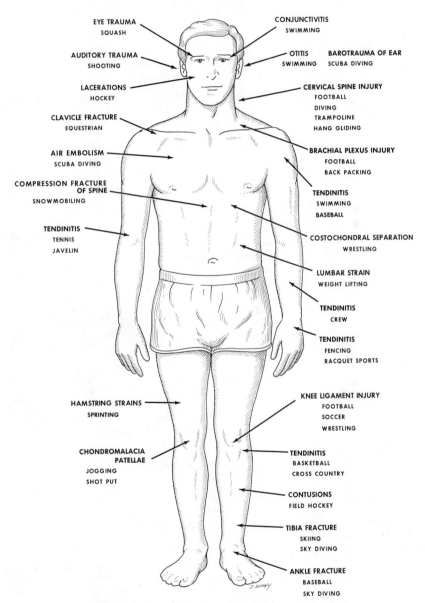

Figure 24–4. Injuries associated with specific sports.

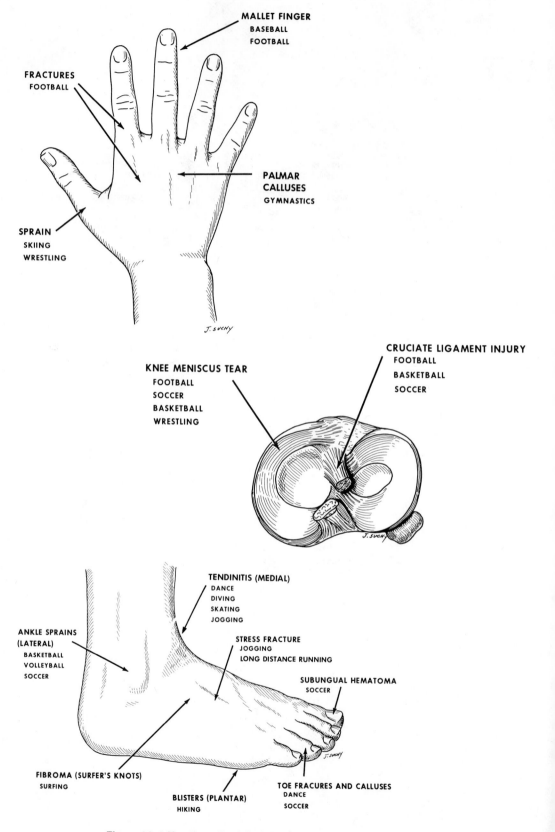

Figure 24–4 *(Continued).* Injuries associated with specific sports.

TABLE 24–7. MEDICAL PROBLEMS ASSOCIATED WITH SPECIFIC SPORTS*

Sport	Medical Problems
Auto racing	Heat exhaustion (E) Burns (E) Severe life-threatening trauma (T)
Back-packing	Brachial plexis (shoulder nerves) injury (T)
Baseball	Mallet (baseball) finger (T) Shoulder (rotator cuff) tendinitis (O) Little League elbow (O)
Basketball	Posterior tibial tendinitis at ankle (O) Ankle sprains (T)
Crew	Forearm tendinitis (O)
Cross country	Stress fracture (O) Knee tendinitis (O)
Dance	Flexor halluces (big toe) tendinitis at ankle (O) Toe fractures and calluses (O)
Diving (springboard)	Cervical (neck) spine sprain and fracture (T) Contusion from striking board (T) Flexor halluces (big toe) tendinitis (O)
Equestrian	Fracture of clavicle (collarbone) (T) Patellar (knee) tendinitis (O)
Fencing	Wrist tendinitis (O)
Field hockey	Contusions from stick and ball (T)
Football	Bursitis at elbow and knee (E) Cervical (neck) nerve pinch (T) Brachial plexus (shoulder nerve) injury (T) Ligament sprains at knee, shoulder, finger (T) Knee meniscus (cartilage) injury (T)
Gymnastics	Calluses on hands (O)
Hang gliding	Cervical fracture (T) Severe life-threatening trauma (T)
Hiking	Blisters of the feet (O)
Ice hockey	Lacerations (T)
Ice skating	Tendinitis of foot and ankle (O)
Javelin	Shoulder and elbow tendinitis (O)
Jockey	Weight control (E)
Jogging and distance running	Ankle and foot tendinitis (O) Stress fractures of tibia, fibula, metatarsals (O) Chondromalacia patellae (softening of undersurface of kneecap) (O)
Mountain climbing	Frostbite (E)
Pole vault	Fracture of humerus (O, T)

(Continued on next page)

TABLE 24–7. MEDICAL PROBLEMS ASSOCIATED WITH SPECIFIC SPORTS* (*Continued*)

Sport	Medical Problems
Sailing	Seasickness (E) Sunburn (E) Stress reactions (peptic ulcer) (I)
Scuba diving	Decompression sickness (E) Barotrauma (E) Air embolism (E)
Shooting (skeet)	Auditory trauma (E)
Shot put	Chondromalacia patellae (O, T)
Skate board	Contusions and abrasions of knees and elbows (T)
Skiing (snow) Alpine	 Tibial fractures (T) Thumb sprain (T)
Cross country	Frostbite (E)
Sky diving	Ankle fracture (T)
Snowmobiling	Compression fracture of thoracic spine (T)
Soccer	Hematoma under nail of big toe (T) Knee meniscus and ligament injury (T) Skin abrasion (E)
Sprint	Hamstring strains (O)
Squash	Eye injury (T)
Surfboard	Fibroma of knee and dorsum of foot (surfers' knots) (T)
Swimming	Eye irritation (conjunctivitis) (E) Ear infection (otitis externa) (E) Shoulder tendinitis (O) Drowning (E)
Tennis	Sprain of gastrocnemius (calf) muscle-tendon junction (O) Tendinitis of elbow (O)
Trampoline	Cervical (neck) spine fracture (T)
Volleyball	Elbow and knee contusions (T) Ankle sprains (T)
Water skiing	Knee ligament sprains (T)
Weight lifting	Lumbar (low back) sprains (O) Tendinitis (multiple locations) (O)
Wrestling	Hematoma of ear (cauliflower ear) (T) Skin infections (herpes, staphylococcal) (E) Costochondral (rib) separation (T) Weight control (E)

*The category into which each problem falls is indicated as follows: trauma (T); overuse (O); environment (E); and illness (I).

The *preseason physical examination* is now required in most organized sports. The main purpose of this examination is to restrict the participation of those individuals whose physical limitations present undue risk. Other purposes of this examination may include: providing a baseline of normal individual characteristics; protecting institutions against unwarranted liability; maintaining fair competition (size, maturity); and collecting statistical data concerning athletes. No matter how detailed the physical examination is, some abnormalities may go undetected and become evident at a later time.

Proper *conditioning* decreases the number of medical problems in sports. Many problems stem from the body's being unprepared to do what is asked of it. A classic example is the weekend athlete who plays two hours of touch football after having done nothing more than walk from his auto to his office during the week. Such persons are often beset with a variety of "day after" medical problems such as backache, tendinitis, shin splints, and sore muscles. Conditioning for sports should be specific for the sport, for example, interval training for soccer and strength training for wrestling.

Although the athletic *environment* can be controlled within massive indoor stadiums, there are still situations over which little control can be exercised. For example, outdoor sports may be played in high heat and humidity, an environmental condition that precludes heat dissipation and thus may cause various heat disorders (see Chapter 21); or exposure to subfreezing temperatures can cause frostbite. The athlete can sometimes be protected from the environment by postponing the contest, but high-cost factors or commercial commitments often make this nearly impossible. The athlete can also abuse an environment, for example, as in losing weight in a sauna or by exercising in a rubber suit. Other environmental problems of sports, such as storms in ocean sailing, will probably never be controlled. In fact, challenging environmental conditions sometimes create the sport, as in mountain climbing, surfing, or skiing. At present, efforts are being made to strike a balance between safety and the challenge of the environment.

Coaches can affect injury prevention. Blyth and Mueller[*] found that football coaches with certain characteristics of background and training were associated with a low injury rate. The important variables were age, college playing experience, coaching experience, and advanced degrees. These factors should be given consideration when selecting a coach. The same study showed that 3.8 per cent of all football injuries were caused by illegal acts such as clipping and spearing. Enforcement of rules can decrease the injury rate. School hockey has a much lower rate of injury than professional hockey, in part because of fewer illegal acts such as fights. If officials and coaches respect and support each other's roles, illegal acts and resultant injuries will diminish.

A knowledge of specific medical problems of sports, combined with a serious attempt to prevent predictable problems, will decrease the incidence of athletic injury.

SUMMARY

Physiological Aspects. Body fat can be estimated by underwater weighing or by measurement of skinfolds. Low relative body fat is desirable for most sports. In successful athletes, muscularity (mesomorphy) varies with the type of sport. Strength is highly correlated with body size except in sports in which strength is not particular-

---

[*]Football injuries. Phys. Sportsmed. *2*:21–26, 1974.

ly necessary for success. Endurance activities are associated with a higher percentage of slow-twitch fibers and high values for maximal oxygen uptake.

Medical Aspects. Medical problems associated with sports generally are a result of (1) usual diseases of the athlete's age group; (2) overuse of a body part; (3) trauma caused by an external force; or (4) the environment. Factors that can help prevent injury include proper equipment, thorough physical examination, adequate conditioning, control of the environment, and well-trained coaches and officials.

STUDY QUESTIONS

1. Identify the three components that constitute the basic somatotype. What does each of these represent?

2. What is the predominant somatotype component for almost all athletes?

3. For a sport of your choice, compare male and female athletes, physiologically.

4. Explain the basic relationship between cardiovascular endurance capacity and muscle fiber types.

5. How does one distinguish between fat weight and lean weight?

6. What is the usual relationship between strength and body size? Give several examples in which this generalization does not apply.

7. List several medical problems related to age that are common among athletes.

8. Give three examples of overuse injury and a sport associated with each.

9. Choose a sport not listed in Table 24–7 and give possible injuries associated with it.

10. Discuss several methods of minimizing injury in football.

REFERENCES

1. Costill, D. L.: The relationship between selected physiological variables and distance running performance. J. Sports Med. 7:61–66, 1967.
2. Costill, D. L., and Fox, E. L.: Energetics of marathon running. Med. Sci. Sports 1:81–86, 1969.
3. Costill, D. L.: Metabolic responses during distance running. J. Appl. Physiol. 28:251–255, 1970.
4. Costill, D. L., and Winrow, E.: Maximal oxygen consumption among marathon runners. Arch. Phys. Med. 51:317–320, 1970.
5. Costill, D. L., Branam, G., Eddy, D., et al.: Determinants of marathon running success. Int. Z. Angew. Physiol. 29:249–254, 1971.
6. Costill, D. L., Bowers, R., and Kammer, W. F.: Skinfold estimates of body fat among marathon runners. Med. Sci. Sports 2:93–95, 1970.
7. Costill, D. L., Kammer, W. F., and Fisher, A.: Fluid ingestion during distance running. Arch. Environ. Health 21:520–525, 1970.
8. Costill, D. L., Bowers, R., Branam, G., et al.: Muscle glycogen utilization during prolonged exercise on successive days. J. Appl. Physiol. 31:834–838, 1971.
9. Costill, D. L., Gollnick, P. D., Jansson, E. C., et al.: Glycogen depletion pattern in human muscle fibers during distance running. Acta Physiol. Scand. 89:373–383, 1973.
10. Morgan, W. P., and Costill, D. L.: Psychological characteristics of the marathon runner. J. Sports Med. Phys. Fitness 12:42–46, 1972.
11. Behnke, A. R., and Wilmore, J. H.: *Evaluation and Regulation of Body Build and Composition.* Englewood Cliffs, N.J., Prentice-Hall, 1974.

12. Wilmore, J. H., Brown, C. H., and Davis, J. A.: Body physique and composition of the female distance runer. Ann. N.Y. Acad. Sci. *301*:764–776, 1977.
13. Wilmore, J. H., Parr, R. B., Haskell, W. L., Costill, D. L., Milburn, L. J., and Kerlan, R. K.: Athletic profile of professional football players. Phys. Sportsmed. *4*:45–54, 1976.
14. Novak, L. P., Hyatt, R. E., and Alexander, J. F.: Body composition and physiologic function of athletes. J.A.M.A. *205*:764–770, 1968.
15. Forsyth, H. L., and Sinning, W. E.: The anthropometric estimation of body density and lean body weight of male athletes. Med. Sci. Sports *5*:174–180, 1973.
16. Sinning, W. E.: Body composition, cardiovascular function, and rule changes in women's basketball. Res. Quart. *44*:313–321, 1973.
17. Conger, P. R., and Macnab, R. B. J.: Strength, body composition and work capacity of participants and nonparticipants in women's intercollegiate sports. Res. Quart. *38*:184–192, 1967.
18. Wickkiser, J. D., and Kelly, J. M.: The body composition of a college football team. Med. Sci. Sports *7*:199–202, 1975.
19. Sinning, W. E., and Lindberg, G. D.: Physical characteristics of college age women gymnasts. Res. Quart. *43*:226–234, 1972.
20. Pařizková, J.: Body composition and exercise during growth and development. *In* Rarick, G. L., (ed.): *Physical Activity: Human Growth and Development.* New York, Academic Press, 1973, pp. 97–124.
21. Pařizková, J., and Poupa, D.: Some metabolic consequences of adaptation to muscular work. Brit. J. Nutr. *17*:341–345, 1963.
22. Šprynarová, S., and Pařizková, J.: Functional capacity and body composition in top weight-lifters, swimmers, runners, and skiers. Int. Z. Angew. Physiol. *29*:184–194, 1971.
23. Pollock, M. L., Miller, H. S., and Wilmore, J.: Physiological characteristics of champion American track athletes 40 to 75 years of age. J. Gerontol. *29*:645–649, 1974.
24. Lewis, S., Haskell, W. L., Klein, H., Halpern, J., and Wood, P. D.: Prediction of body composition in habitually active middle-aged men. J. Appl. Physiol. *39*:221–225, 1975.
25. Malina, R. M., Harper, A. B., Avent, H. H., and Campbell, D. E.: Physique of female track and field athletes. Med. Sci. Sports *3*:32–38, 1971.
26. Wilmore, J. H., and Brown, C. H.: Physiological profiles of women distance runners. Med. Sci. Sports *6*:178–181, 1974.
27. Fahey, T. D., Akka, L., Rolph, R.: Body composition and $\dot{V}o_{2max}$ of exceptional weight-trained athletes. J. Appl. Physiol. *39*:559–561, 1975.
28. Gale, J. B., and Flynn, K. W.: Maximal oxygen consumption and relative body fat of high-ability wrestlers. Med. Sci. Sports. *6*:232–234, 1974.
29. Sinning, W. E.: Body composition assessment of college wrestlers. Med. Sci. Sports *6*:139–145, 1974.
30. Katch, F. I., and Michael, E. D.: Body composition of high school wrestlers according to age and wrestling weight category. Med. Sci. Sports. *3*:190–194, 1971.
31. de Garay, A. L., Levine, L., and Carter, J. E. L.: *Genetic and Anthropological Studies of Olympic Athletes.* New York, Academic Press, 1974.
32. Tanner, J. M.: *1964: The Physique of the Olympic Athlete.* London, George Allen and Unwin Ltd., 1964.
33. Gollnick, P. D., Armstrong, R. B., Saubert C. W., IV, Piehl, K., and Saltin, B.: Enzyme activity and fiber composition in skeletal muscle of untrained and trained men. J. Appl. Physiol. *33*:312–319, 1972.
34. Thorstensson, A., Larsson, L., Tesch, P., and Karlsson, J.: Muscle strength and fiber composition in athletes and sedentary men. Med. Sci. Sports *9*:26–30, 1977.
35. Costill, D. L., Daniels, J., Evans, W., Fink, W., Krahenbuhl, G., and Saltin, B.: Skeletal muscle enzymes and fiber composition in male and female track athletes. J. Appl. Physiol. *40*:149–154, 1976.
36. Costill, D. L., Fink, W. J., and Pollock, M. L.: Muscle fiber composition and enzyme activities of elite distance runners. Med. Sci. Sports *8*:96–100, 1976.
37. Cunningham, D. A., Telford, P., and Swart, G. T.: The cardio-pulmonary capacities of young hockey players: age 10. Med. Sci. Sports *8*:23–25, 1976.
38. Seliger, V., Kostka, V., Grusová, D., Kovác, J., Machovcova, J., Pauer, M., Pibylová, A., and Urbánková, R.: Energy expenditure and physical fitness of ice hockey players. Int. Z. Angew. Physiol. *30*:283–291, 1972.
39. Maksud, M. G., Wiley, R. L., Hamilton, L. H., and Lockhart, B.: Maximal $\dot{V}o_2$, ventilation, and heart rate of Olympic speed skating candidates. J. Appl. Physiol. *29*:186–190, 1970.
40. Cunningham, D. A., and Eynon, R. B.: The working capacity of young competitive swimmers, 10–16 years of age. Med. Sci. Sports *5*:227–231, 1973.
41. Magel, J. R., and Faulkner, J. A.: Maximum oxygen uptakes of college swimmers. J. Appl. Physiol. *22*:929–938, 1967.
42. Charbonnier, J. P., Lacour, J. R., Riffat, J., and Flandrois, R.: Experimental study of the performance of competition swimmers. Eur. J. Appl. Physiol. *34*:157–167, 1975.
43. Shephard, R. J., Godin, G., and Campbell, R.: Characteristics of sprint, medium and long-distance swimmers. Eur. J. Appl. Physiol. *32*:99–116, 1974.
44. Costill, D. L., Thomason, H., and Roberts, E.: Fractional utilization of the aerobic capacity during distance running. Med. Sci. Sports *5*:248–252, 1973.
45. Nagle, F. J., Morgan, W. P., Hellickson, R. O., Serfass, R. C., and Alexander, J. F.: Spotting success traits in Olympic contenders. Phys. Sportsmed. *3*:31–34, 1975.

FURTHER READINGS

Physiological Aspects

Behnke, A. R., and Wilmore, J. H.: *Evaluation and Regulation of Body Build and Composition*. Englewood Cliffs, N. J., Prentice-Hall, 1974.

deVries, H. A.: *Physiology of Exercise for Physical Education and Athletics*, 2nd ed. Dubuque, Iowa, William C. Brown Company, 1974.

Edington, D. W., and Edgerton, V. R.: *The Biology of Physical Activity*. Boston, Houghton Mifflin Company, 1976.

Mathews, D. K., and Fox, E. L.: *The Physiological Basis of Physical Education and Athletics*, 2nd ed. Philadelphia, W. B. Saunders Company, 1976.

Wilmore, J. H.: *Athletic Training and Physical Fitness: Physiological Principles and Practices of the Conditioning Process*. Boston, Allyn and Bacon, 1977.

Medical Aspects

O'Donoghue, D.: *Treatment of Injuries to Athletes*. Philadelphia, W. B. Saunders Company, 1976.

25

PHYSICAL ACTIVITY
AND AGING

WAYNE D. VAN HUSS, Ph.D.

It may appear presumptuous to develop a chapter on physical activity and aging when (1) it is not known what aging is,[1, 2, 3] and (2) the evidence regarding the effectiveness of exercise in delay of the aging process[4] and in prevention of cardiovascular disorders is all indirect.[5, 6, 7] However, the public is bombarded by persuasive advertisements designed to sell exercise devices, programs, or food supplements for which exaggerated claims are often made. So much misinformation prevails that the average individual is unable to sort fact from fiction in making personal decisions. Thus, there is a professional responsibility to review the literature regarding exercise and aging, and to provide the reader with a base for decision making about personal life style. In the following material, changes that may be attributed to aging are reviewed. Then, specific questions of interest to college-age students are presented.

CHANGES ATTRIBUTED TO AGING

A major problem faced by all investigators studying aging is the task of attempting to sort out age-related changes from life-style changes.[8-15] The most common view regarding aging is that advances in medicine have lengthened the human life span. Neither biological evidence nor vital statistics support this supposition. What has happened is that medical advances have improved treatment in the early years of life; thus, life expectancy has increased. The human life span, however, has changed but little.[16] Owing to medical advances, more people may be approaching an age that may be a fixed life span.[1] If heart disease, stroke, and cancer were eliminated, it is estimated that about 20 years of additional life might be expected.[17] Before conclusions can be drawn, some of the recent data and theories of aging must be examined.

Theories of Aging

Recent work on cell aging has shown that what was once believed to be firm evidence supporting the potential immortality of vertebrate cells in culture appears to have been in error. It has been demonstrated recently that normal cells grown in culture under the most favorable conditions underwent about 50 population doublings 373 before dying. Their death was due to an inherent property of the cells themselves.[18, 19] Human embryo cells were found to be capable of about 50 population doublings, whereas the doublings of cells from normal human adults were fewer, depending upon the age of the donor.[18] Across species, the capacity for cell population doubling also appears to be related to the life span of the species.[1]

There are numerous theories of aging, none of which appear to be mutually exclusive.[1, 2, 20] Currently, it is believed that there are organ "clocks" that control aging in much the same manner that maturation and development are controlled. Recent data by Wright and Hayflick indicate that the "clock" is located in the nucleus.[21, 20] Nuclei from young and old cells were inserted into opposite, aged cytoplasts, yielding viable whole cells. The cells containing the younger nuclei were capable of more population doublings than the cells containing the older nuclei. These results suggest that the nucleus contains the "clock" that determines the proliferation capacity. Aging, by these concepts, is a "playing out" of the genetic program.[1]

It would appear likely that in most instances the life span of the individual is not reached and that the programmed "playing out" does not occur. Rather, the organism seems to succumb before this occurs, owing to multiple insults from radiation, temperature stress, emotional stress, disease, aberrant free radicals, lack of adequate exercise, and excessive food, smoking, alcohol, or drugs. With reduction of these insults, it is likely that man might extend his life span somewhat because information molecules would be able to "play out" without premature failure. At this time, the maximum age range is not known and the validity of this clock concept is not completely clear.

Changes Associated with Aging

Figure 25–1 shows the changes with age of selected anthropometric, biochemical, and functional parameters from data on women aged 20 to 69 years.[14] Figure 25–2

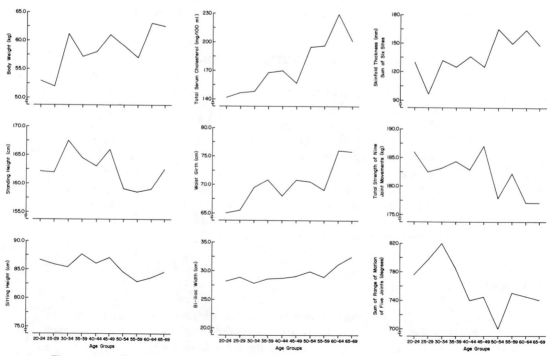

Figure 25–1. Changes in women aged 20 to 69 years. (Modified from Wessel, J. A., et al.[15])

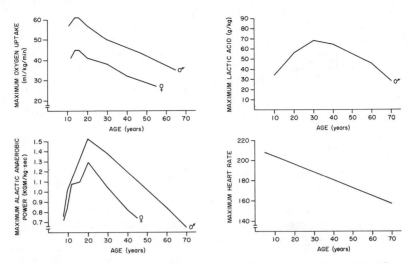

Figure 25–2. Changes in heart rate and metabolic measures with age (Modified from data of Cerretelli,[55] Bar-Or and Buskirk,[54] and Robinson.[56])

shows trends by age for several parameters of energy metabolism and for maximum heart rate. These patterns of response are typical of those observed by other investigators.[10, 11, 22] Strength decreases, joint range of motion decreases, and height decreases. In women, body dimensions change, with increases in body weight, waist girth, hip width, and body fatness. In terms of performance in untrained subjects, the maximum oxygen intake decreases; less lactic acid can be produced; the alactic anaerobic power (the oxygen debt capacity without lactate formation) decreases; and the maximum heart rate decreases over the years. Figure 25–3 shows, by age, the percentage of males with insufficient blood flow to the heart during exercise.

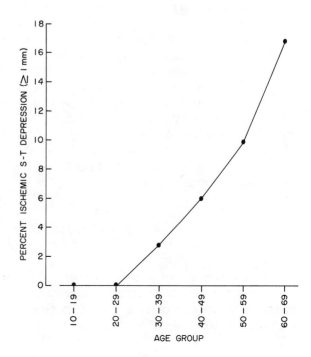

Figure 25–3. Percentage of males showing ischemic (insufficient blood flow) changes in the electrocardiogram under exercise conditions. (Modified from Montoye.[25])

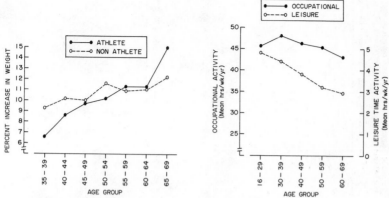

Figure 25–4. Changes in physical activity levels and body weight with age. (Modified from Montoye[25] and Montoye et al.[29])

Anatomically, in the aging cell the nucleus shrinks, the nucleolus enlarges, and vacuoles accumulate. Collagen, the principal substance in connective tissue, shows increased rigidity. Nerve conduction velocity decreases, the cardiac index (the amount of blood pumped per minute divided by the body surface area) decreases by 30 per cent, and the maximum breathing capacity decreases by about 50 per cent. There are decremental changes in the sensory processes, that is, vision, hearing, taste, and smell; and in psychometric performances, that is, reaction time, speed and accuracy, and complex performance. Also observed are decreases in mental capacity—learning, problem solving, and creativity — and added cautiousness in decision making.[23, 3] Participation in leisure activities decreases, as does the intensity of leisure activities.[24, 25] Decreases in both occupational and leisure physical activity are associated with increases in body weight (Fig. 25–4).

Contributing Factors

What portion of decremental change is due to aging and what portion is attributable to life-style changes as one grows older? This question is unresolved. The relationship of age to oxygen uptake at standard work loads has been examined. The more active subjects performed work more economically, regardless of age. In older women, work performance was more closely associated with physical activity level than with age.[15] The decrements shown in Figures 25–1, 25–2, and 25–3 reflect the real world. However, capacities have been maintained in trackmen who, as a result, have had running performances in their early forties that were equal to the best performances achieved in their twenties.[26] It appears that, prior to age 50, life style rather than age is the major factor in influencing change.

RELEVANT QUESTIONS REGARDING EXERCISE AND AGING

1. WILL PARTICIPATION IN COMPETITIVE ATHLETICS ADVERSELY AFFECT THE INDIVIDUAL IN TERMS OF LENGTH OF LIFE OR THE AMOUNT OR TYPES OF ILLNESSES?

On the basis of studies in which sufficient mortality and morbidity experience is available, the answer is no.[27-31] These studies, however, report data based upon athletic participation in the 1930's or before. Both the intensity and duration of the training required for successful athletic participation today are many times that required in the 1930's. Although the effects of the more intensive training and competition have not yet been absolutely determined, no negative trends are evident with continuing research.

The capacities achieved during athletic competition cannot be stored unused. Inactive former athletes cannot be distinguished from nonathletes in middle and old age. However, individuals who were active in sports respond more favorably than nonathletes to an exercise regimen after age 40.

Similar results have been obtained in longitudinal studies of animals.[33] An enhanced ability to respond to training is retained, but the capacities themselves cannot be stored.

2. WILL REGULAR PARTICIPATION IN EXERCISE INCREASE THE LENGTH OF LIFE?

There are no definitive human studies that indicate that regular exercise increases the length of life. Two animal studies, however, show enhanced longevity.[34, 35] In one, moderate endurance exercise was administered regularly to both male and female rats. The exercised animals lived significantly longer than sedentary control animals.[36] In the other study, mild endurance exercise administered in young and middle-aged animals resulted in enhanced longevity.[34] If regular exercise contributes to the prevention of the major cardiovascular disorders — as the data suggest but do not prove[5, 6, 7] — it is likely that the longevity of man should be increased somewhat.[17]

Before proceeding further, the type of exercise under discussion should be identified. Exercise is not a single entity. It can elicit a continuum of very different, specific anatomical and physiological adaptations. Table 25-1 identifies characteristics of five levels of fitness. It is not intended to be all-inclusive. Undoubtedly, there are many other levels that cannot be adequately identified as yet. The type of fitness for which most evidence is available in regard to aging is level 5, which requires primarily aerobic responses at a steady state for 20 to 30 minutes. The long-term effects of the other levels are not as well known. Much of the confusion that exists about "exercise" effects is due to the wide differences in adaptations acquired from vastly different activities. For our purposes, exercise is defined as the level 5 type.

3. WHY SHOULD ONE EXERCISE REGULARLY?

Should one exercise regularly? The answer is an unequivocal yes. Endurance training produces alterations (Table 25-2) — particularly in circulatory mechanisms — that are opposite to changes attributed to aging (Figs. 25-1 to 25-4). Such training results in an ameliorative effect on aging, with a better maintenance of physical capacity and greater joy of living. Indirect evidence suggests that there is a delay of the aging process[4] and a reduced incidence of cardiovascular disorders, but as yet the data are not conclusive.[5, 6] Clearly, however, from the standpoint of long-range health it is prudent to exercise regularly.

Advancing technology has markedly lessened the amount of physical work involved in both occupational and nonoccupational activity. It is questionable whether the daily physical activity of many people is adequate for their physical maintenance. Additional, regular physical activity appears to be necessary for the physical maintenance of most individuals.[36] It is becoming increasingly evident that the average

TABLE 25-1. THE CHARACTERISTICS OF FIVE SPECIFIC FITNESS LEVELS*

	Level 1	Level 2	Level 3	Level 4	Level 5
Approximate time of maximum performance (min: sec)	0–0:08	0:12–0:30	0:30–1:30	3:00–7:00	35:00–240:00
Event:					
Runners	60 yds	200 m	400 m	1500 m	Marathon
Swimmers	–	50 m	100 m	400 m	10,000 m
Energy metabolism:					
Oxygen intake	None	Low	Low-moderate	High	High
Oxygen debt	Low	Moderate	High	High	Low
Arterial lactate	Low	Moderate	High	High	Low
Relative contribution of major energy sources for muscular contraction:					
Endogenous ATP and PC†	High	Moderate	Moderate	Low	Very low
Muscle glycogen	Low	High	High	High	Low
Blood glucose	None	None–very low (?)	Low (?)	Moderate (?)	Moderate (?)
Free fatty acids	None	None	Very low	Low-moderate	High
Approximate percentages of muscle fiber types	10–25 ST†(?) 75–90 FT†	25 ST 75 FT	30 ST (?) 70 FT	57 ST 43 FT	80 ST 20 FT

*Examples drawn from data on high-performance athletes.
†ATP = adenosine triphosphate; PC = creatine phosphate; ST = "red" slow-twitch fibers; FT = "white" fast-twitch fibers; (?) = not resolved or not known.

individual should plan for and perform daily endurance exercise as routinely as the teeth are brushed.

4. WHAT TYPES OF EXERCISE SHOULD BE INCLUDED IN A PROGRAM FOR PHYSICAL MAINTENANCE?

Endurance. The most important component is a rhythmical endurance exercise of at least 20 minutes duration. The activity may be jogging, swimming, cycling, fast walking, rope skipping, or any other activity of a rhythmical type. The intensity or duration of the exercise required to produce beneficial effects is not known. A recent study by Paffenbarger of 16,936 men 35 to 74 years of age indicates that the incidence of coronary heart disease is related to the level of energy output.[41] If the energy output was low, the incidence of coronary heart disease was greater. The duration of physical activity necessary to achieve such beneficial effects is most likely somewhere between 20 minutes to one hour of steady-state work. The desired intensity must be tailored to the age and relative fitness of the individual. Steady-state pulse rates of 110 to 120 bpm (beats per minute) probably are adequate for middle-aged individuals, whereas younger individuals may wish to work at steady-state pulse rates of 140 to 160 bpm.

In the author's opinion, it is the rhythmical endurance exercise that produces the preventive benefits. If one wishes to continue with other types of exercise programs such as handball, tennis, squash, volleyball, and so on, they should be included only as additions to the rhythmical endurance program. These games are competitive and promote overexertion. First, a reasonable fitness level should be maintained using the basic endurance program. Then, if one wishes to participate in competitive activities,

TABLE 25–2. CHRONIC EFFECTS OF ENDURANCE TRAINING*

Organ or Function	Effect
Heart:	
Size	↑ (children, young adults)
	↓ (old adults)
Stroke volume	↑
Maximum cardiac output	↑
Resting heart rate	↓
Exercise heart rate (standard submaximal work)	↓
Maximum heart rate	(?)
Rate of pulse rate response to exercise	↑
Rate of pulse rate recovery following work	↑
Arterial–venous oxygen difference	↑
Energy metabolism:	
Oxygen uptake during standard work	↓
Oxygen debt following standard work	↓
Oxygen debt following maximal work	↑
Maximum oxygen uptake	↑
Substrate metabolized:	
Fat	↑
Carbohydrate	↓
Protein	(?)
Muscle:	
Blood flow	↑
Mitochondria number	↑
Aerobic enzymes	↑
Size (overall)	↓
Percentage content of "red" muscle fibers	(?)
Number of muscle fibers	(?)
Strength	0 or ↓
Myoglobin	↑
Bones:	
Strength and density	↑
Ligaments:	
Strength	↑
Blood:	
Volume	↑
Total hemoglobin	↑
Relative hemoglobin	(?)
Acid-base buffers	(?)

*References 37, 38, 39, 40.
↑ = increase; ↓ = decrease; 0 = no effect; (?) = not resolved.

less risk is involved. Ideally, the endurance program is performed for five days weekly, the minimum being three days weekly. The program should be progressive in its overload.

Flexibility. Joint flexibility is lost with age and nonuse. Selected exercises for the maintenance of joint flexibility are shown in Figure 25–5. One execution per week of each of the exercises should be sufficient to maintain range of motion. There is no hard and fast rule. If range of motion is being lost, as evidenced by difficulty in moving in a given range, then the exercise can be repeated several days each week with some added repetitions until the range of motion is regained. Do not force the motion. Rather, move until the stretch is felt and then slacken efforts. It is better to gain a little bit each day than to experience soreness from overdoing.

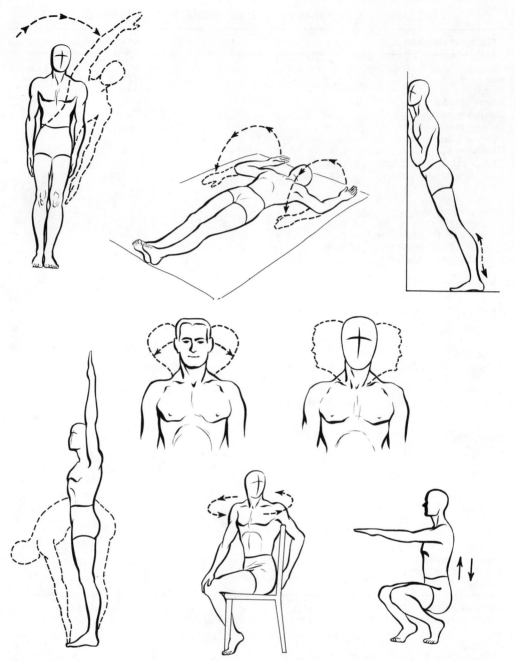

Figure 25–5. Recommended exercises for maintenance of flexibility. (Modified from Van Huss et al.[36])

Strength. No specific strength exercises are included because circulatory capacity and maintenance of flexibility are the primary goals. With the previously mentioned activities, sufficient strength should be maintained. Strength is not to be discounted, since strength of the abdominal and lower back muscles is particularly important. However, in the author's experience, additional strength exercises are not needed for general physical maintenance. Adequate endurance exercise with flexibility maintenance is usually sufficient. A general, all-around weight program for additional strength could be added if one wishes, but lifting the heavy weights is not recommended.

In recommending types of exercise, an attempt has been made to interpret the literature and determine the optimal program based on current knowledge. Less is known about the effects of sports participation or about exercise in general. Certain data indicate that individuals in occupations requiring more physical activity show a reduced incidence of coronary heart disease.[3, 36] (There are also some indications that negative effects may result from too much physical activity.) These data, however, are not sufficiently definitive to identify the types of activities that produce beneficial effects. The evidence is much clearer for rhythmical endurance activities.

The benefits of sports participation may be more psychological than physiological. Meeting one's psychological needs (e.g., satisfaction) can be important. This need not conflict with the recommendation of 30 minutes or more of rhythmical endurance activity at least three times per week with added flexibility maintenance. However, it is the author's firm belief that participation in any sports program as one grows older should be an extension of the rhythmical endurance program, not a substitute for it.

5. AT WHAT AGES MAY EXERCISE PROGRAMS BE INITIATED?

Ideally, the rhythmical endurance program is participated in regularly throughout life, and the individual never becomes completely sedentary. However, the program may be initiated at any age. There is some evidence that a threshold age[34] and prior experience[32] are factors in training individuals past 60 years of age. However, the preponderance of evidence indicates that individuals past 60 years of age respond favorably to the initiation of training.[8, 42–44] Particularly in the older age groups, training programs should increase gradually.

Legislation, social practices, and values have prolonged the period during which young people are treated as if they were immature and irresponsible. The child of today is excessively sheltered both physically and socially in spite of the fact that the people most likely to be creative and to act as leaders are those who have faced and overcome adversity and who have withstood considerable stress. As a result of these stresses, patterns of adaptation are developed that enable the individual to adjust rapidly to new situations.[45] There is no passive solution. A person develops adaptive mechanisms only by experiencing stress. It has been reported that, once adaptation to a stressor is achieved, the individual will respond more favorably to the same and other stressors.[46, 47] Enhanced ability to respond to the same type of stressor is fairly well documented, but the ability to respond more favorably to a different type of stressor is still open to question.[48] The body, however, is vulnerable to two heavy stresses applied simultaneously.[48] Although most of the evidence is indirect, and in some instances fragmentary, it appears that exercise-stressed individuals subsequently are more adaptable to stresses of different types. The optimal ages at which to apply the exercise stress are not known.

It is clear that cardiovascular degeneration starts early in Western societies. How early is still controversial. The results of autopsies performed on American servicemen killed during the Korean War were compared with those of a similar age group of Japanese killed in accidents. Atherosclerosis, the fatty degeneration of the circulatory system, was present in many Americans but not in the Japanese. Most astounding was the fact that the average age of the Americans was 22.1 years![49] At that time, the incidence of coronary heart disease in Japan was approximately one tenth that of the United States.[50] In the Japanese who moved to Hawaii or elsewhere in the United

382

States, the incidence of atherosclerosis and of coronary heart disease was similar to that observed in U.S. citizens. These results have been attributed to the American life style, with its high level of emotional stress, high-fat diet, and physical inactivity. Today, some investigators believe that the basis for this deterioration is established in early childhood.

It is not precisely known at what ages exercise programs should be initiated. The most prudent approach would seem to be to maintain a reasonable capacity for rhythmical endurance exercise over the life span.

6. HOW SHOULD THE EXERCISE PROGRAM BE INITIATED?

If the individual has been sedentary, any program should be preceded by a routine medical examination. For individuals over 30 years of age, ideally the medical examination should include an exercise stress test. In such a test, the electrocardiogram is monitored for coronary ischemia (insufficient blood flow as reflected by S-T segment depression $\geq$ 1 mm); and ectopic beats (beats originating other than through the usual conductive pathway).[51, 52, 53] Today, most cardiologists are knowledgeable about stress testing and exercise prescription. The stress test provides valuable information for exercise prescription, since heart rate and blood pressure responses to progressively greater exercise loads have been recorded. Thus, a personalized program may be outlined.

The establishment of the exercise intensity level is the key issue. One approach is to take the maximum heart rate for the individual's age, subtract the resting heart rate, multiply the difference by 0.5, and add this to the resting heart rate to arrive at a recommended exercise heart rate. For example, if the maximal heart rate for one's age were 165 bpm and the resting heart rate were 75 bpm, the recommended training heart rate would be 120 bpm.*

A pulse rate of 120 bpm, however, may be higher than necessary. Training responses in men over 60 years of age can be elicited at pulse rates of 95 to 99 bpm, and even well-conditioned men above 60 years of age need to raise their heart rates to only 103 to 106 bpm to provide a training stimulus.[43] The point is: be cautious. Training changes are produced at far lower exercise intensity levels than was originally thought, so start low and increase progressively.

The ultimate fitness goal is not known. The level of fitness needed to ameliorate cardiac and other health risk factors is an important but unanswered question. It is the author's view that the type of endurance exercise is not critical, although jogging and swimming are both excellent. Rather, the intensity level of the steady, rhythmical exercise is the vital factor. Initially, pulse rate should be monitored carefully.

The young man can proceed fairly fast in increasing load. The older man, over 60 years of age, should probably recheck with his physician about every six weeks early in the program. A very simple, yet effective, program of walking and jogging has been used by de Vries.[43, 44] It starts the first day with five sets of "run 50 steps — walk 50 steps." Each succeeding exercise day the number of sets is increased by one until 10 sets are reached, at which time the walk interval is reduced to 40 steps, and so on. The rate of running and walking can be adjusted to the pulse rate goal by monitoring pulse rate either during the walk phase or immediately after the run phase.

An important point to remember in any training program is that retrogression usually precedes improvement. In other words, one gets poorer before getting better.[36] Knowledge of this principle tends to prevent discouragement in, and premature quitting by, individuals naive about training.

---

*165 bpm − 75 bpm = 90 bpm; 90 bpm × 0.5 = 45 bpm; 75 bpm + 45 bpm = 120 bpm.

7. HOW MAY A PERSONALIZED PROGRAM PLAN BE DEVELOPED?

The first step is to select a rhythmical endurance activity and, assuming at least average health status, perform the exercise regimen for at least 30 minutes three times each week. Implement the program gradually and make it a habit.

Next, take some time to consider the multiple factors involved in planning a personal physical maintenance: future occupation, likely future place of residence, probable weight gain pattern, interests, and present physical, emotional, and social needs. Consider how much activity you are likely to have in your future occupation and how much emotional stress is involved. What types of activity could be continued in your likely place of residence? On the basis of your body type, what kind of weight gain pattern are you liable to have and what can you do about it?[36] What do you really like to do? Do you need any specific development programs now? Do your activities satisfy you? Do you have skills that will provide for social interaction, and are you sufficiently skilled in such activities for participation to be satisfying?

Consider the above factors and determine: (1) the activities through which the rhythmical endurance capacities can be maintained after leaving college (jogging, swimming, cycling, rowing, rope skipping, etc.); and (2) the sports skills necessary to satisfy social, emotional, or other needs. These should be learned or improved upon during the college years. The sports should be satisfying, should cover all four seasons of the year, and should be available in the future place of residence.

In the college years, one tends to feel that life is eternal and that one is invincible. Aging somehow happens to someone else. The author's advice is to take personal physical maintenance seriously and plan wisely for the future.

SUMMARY

The human life span has changed but little. Currently it is believed that aging is controlled by organ "clocks" programmed into the nucleus. According to these concepts, aging is a "playing out" of the genetic program. However, it appears likely that the programmed "playing out" rarely occurs and that the organism succumbs prematurely to the multiple insults of lack of adequate exercise and excessive food, alcohol, tobacco, and so on. It is difficult to separate aging from life style. In the general population, capacities decrease with aging. However, physical capacities may be maintained for an indeterminate period if the individual continues to be active. Thus, regular, rhythmical endurance exercise of at least 20 minutes daily has been recommended for personal physical maintenance. This has been shown to add "life" to years and likely years to life. Procedures for initiating endurance exercise regimens and specific exercises for the maintenance of joint flexibility are described. It has not been resolved whether exercise will delay the aging process, but a conservative assessment of current research shows that it clearly is prudent to exercise regularly in endurance-type exercise programs.

STUDY QUESTIONS

1. Has the human life span changed in recent years?

2. What is meant by organ "clock"? Of what significance is this to aging?

3. What is the relationship of age to most anthropometric, biochemical, and functional parameters?

4. What is the major problem in studying aging?

5. Will participation in competitive athletics affect longevity?

6. Will regular participation in exercise increase the length of life?

7. What types of exercises should be included in your physical maintenance program? Why?

8. In an individual older than 30 years, what steps are recommended prior to the initiation of any exercise program?

9. How may the intensity level of the exercise program be established?

10. Why are rhythmical endurance programs recommended for personal physical maintenance?

REFERENCES

1. Hayflick, L.: The cell biology of human aging. N. Engl. J. Med. *295*:1302, 1976.
2. Hayflick, L.: Theories of biological aging. *In* Scheinberg, P. (ed.): *Cerebrovascular Disease.* New York, Raven Press, 1976, p. 339.
3. Wallace, D. J.: The biology of aging: 1976, an overview. J. Am. Geriatr. Soc. *25*:104, 1977.
4. Jokl, E.: *Alter und Leistung.* Berlin, Springer-Verlag, 1954, p. 75.
5. Fox, S. M., and Haskell, W. L.: Physical activity and the prevention of coronary heart disease. Bull. N.Y. Acad. Med. *44*:950, 1968.
6. Fox, S. M., and Naughton, J. P.: Physical activity and the prevention of coronary heart disease. Prevent. Med. *1*:92, 1972.
7. Fox, S. M., and Skinner, J. S.: Physical activity and cardiovascular health. Am. J. Cardiol. *14*:731, 1964.
8. de Vries, H. A.: Physiological effects of an exercise training regimen upon men aged 52 to 88. J. Gerontol. *25*:325, 1970.
9. Jokl, E. (ed.): *Physical Activity and Aging.* Baltimore, University Park Press, 1970.
10. Norris, A. H., and Shock, N. W.: Exercise in the adult years. *In* Johnson, W. R., and Buskirk, E. R. (eds.): *Science and Medicine of Exercise and Sport,* 2nd ed. New York, Harper and Row, 1974, p. 346.
11. Skinner, J. S.: Age and performance. *In* Keul, J. (ed.): *Limiting Factors of Physical Performance.* Stuttgart, Georg Thieme, 1973, p. 271.
12. Wessel, J. A., Small, D. A., Van Huss, W. D., Heusner, W. W., and Cederquist, D. C.: Functional responses to submaximal exercise in women, 20–69 years. J. Gerontol. *21*:168, 1966.
13. Wessel, J. A., Small, D. A., Van Huss, W. D., Anderson, D. J., and Cederquist, D. C.: Age and physiological responses to exercise in women 20–69 years. J. Gerontol. *23*:269, 1968.
14. Wessel, J. A., Ufer, A., Van Huss, W. D., and Cederquist, D. C.: Age trends of various components of body composition and functional characteristics in women aged 20–69 years. Ann. N. Y. Acad. Sci. *110*:608, 1963.
15. Wessel, J. A., and Van Huss, W. D.: The influence of physical activity and age on exercise adaptation in women. J. Sp. Med. *9*:173, 1969.
16. Comfort, A.: *Aging: The Biology of Senescence.* New York, Holt, Rinehart, and Winston, 1964.
17. U. S. Bureau of Census (1973): Some demographic aspects of aging in the United States. *Current Population Reports,* Ser. P–23, No. 43. Washington, D. C., U. S. Government Printing Office, 1973.
18. Hayflick, L.: The limited *in vitro* lifetime of human diploid cell strains. Exp. Cell Res. *37*:614, 1965.
19. Hayflick, L., and Moorhead, P. S.: The serial cultivation of human diploid cell strains. Exp. Cell Res. *25*:585, 1961.
20. Wright, W. E., and Hayflick, L.: Nuclear control of cellular aging demonstrated by hybridization of anucleate and whole cultured normal human fibroblasts. Exp. Cell Res. *96*:113, 1975.
21. Wright, W. E., and Hayflick, L.: Contributions of cytoplasmic factors to *in vitro* cellular senescence. Fed. Proc. *34*:76, 1975.
22. Bafitis, H., and Sargent, F.: Human physiological adaptability through the life sequence. J. Gerontol. *32*:402, 1977.
23. Okun, M. A.: Adult age and cautiousness in decision. Hum. Dev. *19*:220, 1976.

24. Cunningham, D., Montoye, H. J., Metzner, H., and Keller, J.: Active leisure time activities as related to age among males in a total population. J Gerontol. *23*:551, 1968.

25. Montoye, H. J.: *Physical Activity and Health: An Epidemiologic Study of an Entire Community.* Englewood Cliffs, N. J.: Prentice-Hall, 1975.

26. Bidon, A.: Le viellissement des athletes et la longevite sportive. Med. Educ. Phys. et Sport *2*:187, 1949.

27. Dublin, L. I.: College honor men long lived. Stat. Bull. Metropolitan Life Ins. Co. *13*:5, 1932.

28. Greenway, J. C., and Hiscock, I. C.: Preliminary analysis of mortality among athletes and other graduates of Yale University. Yale Alumni Weekly *35*:1086, 1926.

29. Montoye, H. J., Van Huss, W. D., Olson, H. W., Pierson, W. R., and Hudec, A. J.: *The Longevity and Morbidity of College Athletes.* Indianapolis, Phi Epsilon Kappa, 1957.

30. Montoye, H. J., Van Huss, W. D., Olson, H. W., Hudec, A. J., and Mahoney, E.: Study of the longevity and morbidity of college athletes. J.A.M.A. *162*:1132, 1956.

31. Polednak, A. P., and Damon, A.: College athletics, longevity, and cause of death. Hum. Biol. *42*:28, 1970.

32. Hollman, W.: Changes in the capacity for maximal and continuous efforts in relation to age. *In* Jokl, E., and Simon, E. (eds.): *International Research in Sport and Physical Education.* Springfield, Ill., Charles C Thomas, 1964.

33. Van Huss, W. D., Heusner, W. W., Weber, J., Lamb, D., and Carrow, R.: The effects of prepubertal forced exercise upon postpubertal physical activity, food consumption and selected anatomical and physiological parameters. *In* Antonelli, F. (ed.): *Psicologia Dello Sport, Proceedings of the 1st International Congress of Sport Psychology,* Rome, 1966, p. 734.

34. Edington, D. W., Cosmos, A. C., and McCafferty, W. B.: Exercise and longevity: evidence for a threshold age. J. Gerontol. *27*:341, 1972.

35. Retzlaff, E., Fontaine, J., and Furata, W.: Effect of daily exercise on the life span of albino rats. Geriatrics *21*:171, 1966.

36. Van Huss, W. D., Niemeyer, R. K., Olson, H. W., and Friedrich, J. A.: *Physical Activity in Modern Living,* 2nd ed. Englewood Cliffs, N.J., Prentice-Hall, 1969.

37. Astrand, P. O., and Rodahl, K.: *Textbook of Work Physiology.* New York, McGraw-Hill Book Company, 1970, p. 378.

38. Scheuer, J., and Tipton, C. M.: Cardiovascular adaptations to physical training. Ann. Rev. Physiol. *39*:221, 1977.

39. Steinhaus, A. H.: Chronic effects of exercise. Physiol. Rev. *13*:103, 1933.

40. Steinhaus, A. H.: Exercise — a review. Ann. Rev. Physiol. *3*:695, 1941.

41. Paffenbarger, R. S., Wing, A. L., and Hyde, R. T.: Contemporary physical activity and incidence of heart attack in college men. Circulation *56*:(Suppl III):15, 1977.

42. Cureton, T. K.: *The Physiological Effects of Exercise Programs on Adults.* Springfield, Ill., Charles C Thomas, 1969.

43. de Vries, H. A.: Exercise intensity threshold for improvement of cardiovascular-respiratory function in older men. Geriatrics *26*:94, 1971.

44. de Vries, H. A.: Prescription of exercise for older men from telemetered exercise heart rate data. Geriatrics *26*:102, 1971.

45. Dubos, R. J.: Adaptability for survival and growth. Mich. Health, Oct. 1960, p. 27.

46. Selye, H.: *The Chemical Prevention of Cardiac Necrosis.* New York, Ronald Press, 1958.

47. Zimkin, N. V.: Stress during muscular exercise and the state of man — specifically increased resistance. Sechenov. Physiol. J. USSR *47*:741, 1961.

48. Simonov, P. V.: Psychophysiological stress of space flight. *In* Marburger, J. P., and Vasil'yev, P. V. (eds.): *Foundations of Space Biology and Medicine,* Vol. II, Book 2. Washington, D. C., U. S. Government Printing Office, 1975, p. 549.

49. Enos, W. F., Holmes, R. H., and Beyer, J.: Coronary disease among United States soldiers killed in Korea. J.A.M.A. *152*:1090, 1953.

50. Keys, A., Kimura, N., Kusukawa, A., Bronte-Stewart, B., Larsen, N. D., and Keys, M. H.: Lessons from serum cholesterol studies in Japan, Hawaii and Los Angeles. Ann. Intern. Med. *48*:83, 1958.

51. Ellestad, M. H.: *Stress Testing: Principles and Practices.* Philadelphia, W. B. Saunders Company, 1975.

52. American Heart Association: *Exercise Testing and Training of Apparently Healthy Individuals.* New York, 1972.

53. Jones, N. L., Campbell, E. J. M., Edwards, R. H. T., and Robertson, D. G.: *Clinical Exercise Testing.* Philadelphia, W. B. Saunders Company, 1975.

54. Bar-Or, O., and Buskirk, E. R.: The cardiovascular system and exercise. *In* Johnson, W. R., and Buskirk, E. R. (eds.): *Science and Medicine of Exercise and Sport.* New York, Harper and Row, 1974, p. 121.

55. Cerretelli, P.: Exercise and endurance. *In* Larson, L. (ed.): *Fitness, Health and Work Capacity.* New York, Macmillan, 1974, p. 112.

56. Robinson, S.: Experimental studies of physical fitness in relation to age. Arbeitsphysiologie *10*:251, 1938.

26

HEART DISEASE AND THE CLINICAL USES OF EXERCISE

L. HOWARD HARTLEY, M.D.

Exercise physiology has relevance not only to sports activities but also to clinical medicine. Studies of the physiological adjustments that take place during exercise have provided the basis for the exercise stress test, and exercise conditioning has potential value in the prevention of heart disease and the rehabilitation of victims of it. These uses of exercise will be reviewed in this chapter.

EXERCISE TESTING

Background

During exercise, the heart and blood vessels are capable of increasing the delivery of blood by more than fivefold the resting amount. In doing so, the heart contracts more rapidly and vigorously. Most of the blood flows to exercising muscles because their arterioles dilate, thus decreasing resistance. If the arterioles cannot widen, or if the vigor of contraction is weak, the blood supply may not provide sufficient oxygen or nutrients.

The cardiovascular system has a large reserve; hence, the supply of blood at rest may be adequate despite extensive disease. One important use of the exercise test is to discover disease early — when it can be detected only during the stress of exercise. Most importantly exercise may reveal ischemia (insufficient blood supply). Other goals of exercise testing are an assessment of the amount of work that can be safely performed, an opportunity to examine a patient when symptoms occur, and a determination of the progress of a disease.

Types of Tests

The exercise test should have the following characteristics: graded intensities, an accurate electrocardiogram, an identifiable end point, and a measurement of working capacity. The treadmill and bicycle ergometer are used widely.

Conduct of Tests

The exercise test is preceded by a resting evaluation. This evaluation insures that it is safe to proceed and provides a baseline with which the exercise data can be compared. The electrocardiogram is recorded before exercise and is monitored for potentially dangerous irregularities during the test using an oscilloscope. At intervals, the electrocardiogram is recorded for later interpretation. The blood pressure is measured frequently during exercise and recovery. Exercise starts at a low intensity with work periods of three to four minutes. The intensity after each period increases until the end point of the test is reached. After exercising the subject is observed until recovery is complete.

Although complications are rare, the possibility of heart stoppage (cardiac arrest), heart attack (myocardial infarction), or other problems must be anticipated. A physician should be in the immediate area during exercise testing to manage problems if they develop.

End Points

The usual reasons for stopping an exercise test are leg fatigue or the achievement of a certain heart rate. Other more troublesome reasons include chest pain, difficulty in breathing, a fall in blood pressure, or irregularities of the heartbeat.

Chest pain is an important symptom because it may indicate that the myocardium (heart muscle) lacks oxygen owing to insufficient blood supply. This pain is called angina pectoris. Oxygen deficiency is potentially dangerous because either a heart attack or a cardiac arrest may occur if exercise continues. Hence, if the clinician regards chest pain of the test subject as suggestive of angina pectoris, the exercise should cease.

Shortness of breath (dyspnea) may indicate that the heart is not functioning normally during exercise. An increase in the rate and depth of breathing normally occurs during exercise, but shortness of breath implies difficulty in breathing. In some cases, the bronchi (air ducts to lungs) contract and make movement of air difficult. In other cases, fluid accumulates in the lungs owing to the high pressure in pulmonary veins. The high venous pressure is due to an inability of the heart to pump the blood that is returned to it.

A fall in blood pressure during exercise also indicates abnormal heart function. The relationship between the arterial blood pressure and the quantity of blood that the heart pumps (cardiac output) can be expressed mathematically as:

$$\text{Arterial Pressure} = \text{Cardiac Output} \times \text{Systemic Vascular Resistance}$$

During exercise, local metabolic events lead to dilation of arterioles within exercising muscle. This dilation leads to a decrease in vascular resistance, which would be expected to cause a fall in pressure. However, since cardiac output increases during exercise, pressure is maintained. If the heart is not functioning normally, the pressure may fall. A fall in pressure is significant because it indicates that the heart is not functioning normally and also warns that a hazardous condition exists. That is, the low pressure may lead to lack of oxygen for either the brain or the heart. Hence, blood pressure should be measured frequently during the exercise test. (Irregularities of the heartbeat are discussed further on.)

Measurement of Work Capacity

Work capacity may be measured and expressed in several ways. As was reviewed in Chapter 5, the value of maximal oxygen uptake is the best indicator of the physiological state of the circulatory system. However, measurement of maximal oxygen uptake is not feasible for routine clinical evaluation because the procedure is costly, time-consuming, technically difficult, and poorly accepted by both patients and physicians. The most commonly used techniques for assessing work capacity in clinical settings are measurement of the maximal attainable work intensity, determination of the work load at which a certain heart rate is reached, and determination of the heart rate in response to a certain work intensity. The first two methods are used in most laboratories.

A maximal test in clinical laboratories is one that proceeds until the subject cannot continue or until a clinical reason for stopping the test is detected. In most apparently healthy subjects, the end point is leg fatigue. Since endurance depends in part upon the availability of oxygen, the intensity of exercise at which the legs become fatigued reflects the state of the circulation. The intensity at which individuals can work is also determined by the tolerance of leg discomfort. Hence, maximal achievable intensity is a measurement of both physiological and psychological factors.

Since heart rate increases almost linearly with work intensity, capacity can be expressed in other ways. In Figure 26–1, subjects A and B are compared in two ways: (1) by heart rate responses when both perform the same intensity of work (points a and b); and (2) by the work intensities at which a certain heart rate is reached (points a and c). The heart rates used for target values are usually near maximal and are at least equal to those recommended by the Scandinavian Heart Association (190 minus the age). The mean maximal heart rate decreases by about one beat per year and has a standard deviation of 15 beats per minute. Thus, the target heart rate must be corrected for age. Certain medications or the presence of heart disease may reduce the maximal heart rate. In such cases, exercise must be stopped because of leg fatigue.

All methods of measuring work capacity have a broad range of normal values. Age and sex have a marked effect on work capacity. Females have lower values than males, and work capacity decreases with advancing age. However, even when corrected for age and sex, the range of normal values is wide. Because of variability among patients, these measurements are used principally to assess the progress of a patient. In this way, progression of a disease or response to treatment can be quantified. Whether these tests can be reproduced is therefore important, and all methods of assessing work capacity seem to be about equally reproducible.

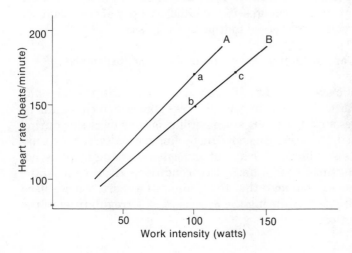

Figure 26–1. The work capacities of two individuals (A and B) can be compared in two ways: by the heart rates observed at a given work intensity (points a and b); or by the intensities of work at which both subjects reach a given heart rate (points a and c). The work capacities of one individual at two different times can be compared in the same way.

Evidence for Heart Disease

The exercise test must be evaluated for evidence of heart disease. Just as the arterioles dilate in exercising skeletal muscle, so do they widen for the heart muscle when its work load increases. The mechanism of dilation is not known, but maintenance of adequate oxygen supply is the end result. If the arteries that supply the heart muscle (coronary arteries) are diseased and cannot dilate normally in response to the increased need for oxygen, myocardial ischemia develops. This condition is referred to as either ischemic heart disease or coronary heart disease.

Angina Pectoris. Ischemia of the heart muscle can cause chest pain (angina pectoris) or abnormalities of the electrocardiogram, or both. The characteristics of angina pectoris are: its location in the anterior part of the chest near or under the sternum (breastbone), its appearance with exercise and relief after about five minutes of rest, and its occurrence with emotional stress. The nature of the chest pain may vary from one individual to another, but the characteristics just noted are constant. These symptoms alone do not confirm heart disease, but they provide evidence that may lead to a diagnosis when used in conjunction with other clinical findings.

Electrocardiogram. The electrocardiogram may show changes that are indicative of heart disease. In order to understand these changes, a few fundamentals of electrocardiography should be learned. It is beyond the scope of this chapter to teach the reader to interpret the electrocardiogram, but an understanding of the principle of electrocardiography is within the grasp of the interested student.

The electrocardiograph is a sensitive voltmeter that measures the electrical activity of the heart by means of electrodes on the surface of the body. The body acts as an electrical conductor, and differences in electrical potential are generated owing to the migration of ions into and out of the myocardial cells. The physiological processes can be divided into depolarization and repolarization (see also Chapter 2). Depolarization includes those processes that begin when the heart muscle is stimulated and ion shifts occur. Depolarization leads to contraction of the heart muscle, which for a short time, will not respond to further stimulation. Repolarization consists of those processes that prepare the heart for another contraction. Depolarization and repolarization generate potential differences through ion shifts — a pattern of voltage changes that can be recorded as the electrocardiogram. Combinations of electrodes on the body surface "see" the electrical activity from different vantage points.

Figure 26–2 shows a normal electrocardiogram. The deflections are assigned letters. The P wave is due to the depolarization of the atrial chambers of the heart, and the QRS wave complex is generated by the depolarization of the ventricles. The S-T

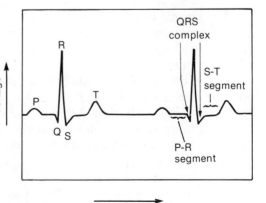

Figure 26–2. Example of a normal electrocardiogram.

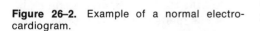

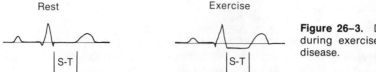

Figure 26–3. Depression of S-T segment during exercise suggests coronary heart disease.

segment is the electrical activity when the ventricles are depolarized, and the T wave is generated during their repolarization. The P-R segment is considered the baseline of the electrocardiogram.

Depression of the S-T segment below the P-R segment during exercise (Fig. 26–3) either indicates the presence of, or predicts the development of, coronary heart disease. Experimental work indicates that S-T depression occurs when the myocardium is ischemic. It is not known why the S-T segment is depressed. In fact, the P-R segment may be elevated instead. The following guidelines are used in exercise electrocardiography:

1. A normal test does not exclude the presence of coronary heart disease.
2. One millimeter of S-T depression indicates an increased probability for having or developing coronary heart disease.
3. Two millimeters of S-T segment depression is virtually diagnostic of coronary heart disease.

Arrhythmias. Irregularities of the heartbeat (arrhythmias) occur both at rest and during exercise. Most of these irregularities are harmless. The detection of the arrhythmias that are potentially harmful is important because the exercise test should be terminated and the individual instructed to keep activity levels below that which precipitates the abnormality. Unlike S-T segment depression, arrhythmias are of little value in diagnosing specific heart diseases.

Certain patterns of premature ventricular contractions lead to sustained irregularities that can cause either a fall of blood pressure or even cessation of the coordinated heartbeat (ventricular fibrillation). Premature ventricular contractions originate abnormally — in the wall of the ventricle. If the beats begin to occur in sequence, fatal irregularities may follow. Sequences of more than three premature beats are called ventricular tachycardia, and this arrhythmia may lead to a fall of blood pressure. Most premature ventricular contractions are harmless, as are most arrhythmias that originate above the ventricles.

EXERCISE DURING OTHER DIAGNOSTIC TESTS

Individuals are sometimes asked to exercise in order to enhance the diagnostic value of procedures other than formal exercise tests. Cardiac catheterization is one example. In cardiac catheterization, a long tube is threaded from a blood vessel of an extremity into the heart, where blood samples can be taken for later analysis and blood pressure can be measured. When the ventricular muscle contracts (systole) the pressure inside the left ventricle rises to about 120 mm Hg (40 mm Hg in the right ventricle). Almost all of the blood in the ventricles is expelled into the arteries. The ventricles then relax (diastole), and the pressure falls to 1 or 2 mm Hg. When the pressure in the ventricles falls below that of the atria, blood flows into the ventricles and pressure rises to about 8 to 10 mm Hg just before the next systole.

During exercise, the muscles of the legs contract and pressure increases in the deep veins of the legs. Because of one-way valves in the veins, blood flows toward the heart with each muscular contraction. When more blood returns to the ventricles, the walls are increasingly stretched, causing the heart to contract with more vigor (Starling's law of the heart). Also, as a result of the stimulation of the sympathetic nervous system during exercise, hormones called norepinephrine and epinephrine are released into blood and stimulate the heart muscle to contract more vigorously. Consequently, the heart continues to empty the ventricles completely, even with a greater supply of blood, and the pressure in the ventricles during diastole remains unchanged from rest. During systole, the pressure in the left ventricle normally rises from 120 mm Hg at rest to a maximum of 190 mm Hg during exercise.

If the function of the heart is abnormal, the heart cannot respond to the exercise with the same vigor. The heart does not empty completely with each contraction, and the diastolic pressure in the ventricles increases. Hence, the diastolic pressure may be normal at rest but abnormal during exercise.

The amount of blood that the heart pumps is called the cardiac output and is usually expressed as liters per minute. At rest, the cardiac output remains constant even with advanced disease states. Therefore, measurement of cardiac output is not as informative as measurement of cardiac pressures in most cases. With advanced disease states, the cardiac output may also become abnormal — with exercise values showing abnormality before resting values do.

EXERCISE CONDITIONING AS A CLINICAL TOOL

Exercise conditioning causes a number of changes that are beneficial to the cardiovascular system. This section deals with such changes and with the prescription of exercise for patients.

Effects of Exercise Conditioning

Stroke volume is the amount of blood that is ejected during each heartbeat, usually expressed in milliliters. After exercise conditioning, the stroke volume is increased. Also, the heart volume may become larger because the walls get thicker. Cardiac output during maximal exercise is greater. Most physiologists believe that these findings indicate a stronger and more vigorous heart. The large heart size sometimes observed in athletes ("athlete's heart") is a normal adaptation to exercise conditioning. It does not lead to heart disease later in life.

Exercise is popularly believed to promote health and well-being. This belief is based largely on anecdotal information, on scientific studies that produce reasons why exercise is expected to benefit health, and on studies indicating that active populations have better health than sedentary populations. The final proof that exercise benefits health can be provided only by demonstrating that the health of an inactive population improves with regular physical activity. Such a study is likely to cost millions of dollars and still be indefinite if conducted with present technology. Much research is being done in this field; however, final answers probably will not be known for a number of years.

Some effects of exercise conditioning are clearly beneficial. The increase of work capacity is important for the athlete, since the trained person can do more work and can sustain any exercise intensity for a longer period of time. This same benefit accrues to any person who regularly engages in heavy exertion either at work or during recreation. The importance of this benefit depends upon the circumstances of the person involved and, for some individuals, might be of little value.

Another potentially beneficial effect of exercise conditioning is on the psychological profile of the participant. Exercise conditioning is frequently associated with a feeling of well-being. This effect has been measured on psychological tests, which indicate lower mental depression indices and better body image. Authorities with extensive experience in exercise conditioning almost uniformly attest to the feeling of well-being that regular exercise engenders.

Coronary Risk Factors

Inactivity has been linked with the development of coronary heart disease. In addition to inactivity, a number of "coronary risk factors" have been associated with a tendency to develop coronary heart disease. The risk factors that are reversible include increased blood pressure, cigarette smoking, obesity, increased blood lipid concentrations, and sedentary life style. Other factors that are important but not reversible are: age, sex, family history, and certain psychosocial factors. Personality types contribute to the psychosocial factors, but the reversibility of these patterns has not been demonstrated.

Physical activity has a demonstrable effect on risk factors other than sedentary life style. Resting arterial blood pressure is often lower after conditioning, especially in persons with elevated blood pressure. Blood lipid concentrations are also reduced, including both cholesterol and triglyceride levels. Regular physical activity also improves compliance with weight reduction programs and aids in the cessation of smoking. Unfortunately, the effects on other risk factors are small, and results are difficult to predict in any individual.

Exercise by Patients with Coronary Heart Disease

Exercise conditioning is also used in the management of patients with coronary heart disease, which is caused by an imbalance between the oxygen supply and demand of the heart muscle. The cause of the imbalance is a narrowing of the coronary arteries that supply the myocardium. Exercise conditioning has the potential benefit of either increasing oxygen supply or decreasing demand.

The blood supply to the heart muscle of experimental animals with partially closed coronary arteries was found to be higher in active animals than in sedentary animals. The greater blood supply was due to new channels of blood (collaterals) around the constriction. Collaterals form in man when the coronary arteries become narrowed; however, exercise has not been demonstrated to accelerate this process in humans.

Exercise conditioning has a clear effect on myocardial oxygen requirements. Heart rate, blood pressure, and circulating norepinephrine levels are major determinants of myocardial oxygen demand, and all are reduced both at rest and during exercise following exercise conditioning. As a result of this effect, the amount of oxygen deficiency (ischemia) for any work intensity is less after conditioning than it is during the sedentary state.

One way to understand the reduction in myocardial oxygen demand is to examine Figure 26-4. The product of systolic blood pressure and heart rate is on the vertical axis, indicating oxygen demand. Work intensity, performed on an ergometer, is on the horizontal axis. Two studies were performed, one before and one after exercise conditioning. The work was stopped on both occasions because of the development of chest pain and of electrocardiographic changes indicating myocardial ischemia. The re-

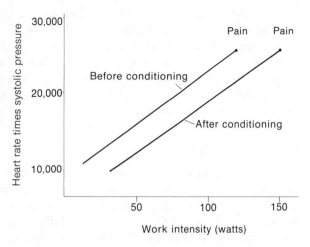

Figure 26–4. Effect of conditioning on myocardial oxygen demand. The product of heart rate and systolic blood pressure (vertical axis) is sometimes used as a convenient indicator of the oxygen requirement of the heart. For any work intensity (horizontal axis), the myocardial oxygen demand is reduced following exercise conditioning. Accordingly, more work can be done before the onset of pain.

sponse to exercise includes an increase in blood pressure and heart rate both before and after conditioning. However, the product of heart rate and blood pressure is less for any work load after conditioning. This indicates lesser myocardial oxygen demand for each work load. Even though ischemia occurs at the same level of heart rate and pressure, the individual is able to do more work after conditioning. This is beneficial for the myocardial oxygen demand-supply balance.

Studies have indicated that regular physical activity can increase the life span and decrease the probability of deterioration of individuals with coronary heart disease. However, the association of an improved prognosis with increased activity does not prove a cause-and-effect relationship. Since the least healthy group of individuals will probably remain inactive, there is thus a strong bias in favor of a better outlook for active patients.

Risks of Exercise Conditioning

Exercise conditioning does carry some risk. Injuries to bones and joints are related to the terrain, the type of exercise, the intensity of the work, and the preparation of the individual. Cardiovascular complications during high-intensity exercise are rare in apparently normal populations. Sudden deaths that occur usually do so in middle-aged males who are prone to develop coronary heart disease. The usual cause for sudden death is cessation of the heartbeat due to ventricular fibrillation. This complication occurs during exercise testing in about 1 of 5000 tests in laboratories that test individuals suspected of having heart disease.

Exercise Prescription

Certain precautions are currently used to minimize the probability of complications when prescribing exercise. A complete physical examination should be conducted to be certain that no medical condition exists for which exercise might be detrimental. After the age of 30 to 35 years, an exercise test will help determine individuals with latent heart disease who may be at increased risk for sudden death during exercise. If evidence of myocardial ischemia or potentially harmful irregularities of the heartbeat occur during exercise, then an activity that will avoid these problems should be prescribed. This is usually accomplished by maintaining the intensity of work below that which precipitates the undesirable finding.

Individuals who have coronary heart disease present a special problem for exercise prescription. In programs in which the patients exercise by jogging, potentially lethal irregularities of the heartbeat occur at the rate of about 1 in 5000 man-hours of exercise. In these programs, prompt medical attention has saved almost all of the persons who were stricken. However, the outcome would have been uniformly fatal if the patients had been exercising alone. These individuals therefore require special attention. Activity should be rigidly controlled, or programs that provide medical coverage should be used. After a person has tried the exercise for several months, it is permissible for him to exercise alone.

Guidelines for individuals who are apparently normal may be more general than those for patients with heart disease. The exercise should begin with a warmup at low intensity to loosen the joints and tendons in preparation for strenuous exercise. The main portion of the exercise should consist of walking or jogging for 20 minutes at an intensity that is about 70 per cent of maximal oxygen uptake. This intensity is recommended because it is effective for increasing work capacity and is well tolerated. Intensity may be judged by counting heart rate. Maximal heart rate is about 220 minus the age, and 70 per cent of maximal oxygen uptake corresponds to a pulse of 80 per cent of the maximal heart rate.

Pulse counting is considered by many individuals to be tedious and difficult. For such persons, general instructions will suffice. An individual exercising at 70 per cent of maximal oxygen uptake will find that he becomes exhausted in about 40 minutes. Exercising at this level for only 20 minutes avoids exhaustion but allows significant exertion.

Heavy exertion is probably not dangerous for completely normal persons. However, for the nonathlete, excessively strenuous workouts are undesirable for several reasons. An individual's enjoyment of the activity will be enhanced if exhaustion is avoided. Lower intensities of work are associated with fewer leg injuries and other orthopedic complications. Also, it is often difficult to ascertain whether the heart is normal, so exercise should be prudent. Exercising at the intensity recommended is sufficient to generate desirable physiological and psychological changes.

SUMMARY

Exercise is used in clinical medicine for diagnostic, preventive, and therapeutic purposes. Muscular exercise increases the demand for oxygen by myocardium (heart muscle), and the ability of the coronary arteries to supply oxygen-carrying blood may be exceeded. When this occurs, symptoms, signs, or electrocardiographic evidence of myocardial ischemia (insufficient blood supply) may appear. Exercise tests provide important information about the work capabilities of an individual, and these measurements are useful in determining progress, regression, or the response of disease to therapy.

Beneficial psychological and physiological changes occur as a result of exercise conditioning. In addition, exercise helps to decrease certain risk factors associated with coronary heart disease. However, only circumstantial evidence exists to show that health maintenance is improved by exercise conditioning.

Exercise conditioning is of benefit to the patient with coronary heart disease because it favorably affects the balance between oxygen supply and demand. Reductions in heart rate, blood pressure, and norepinephrine levels in the blood lessen the amount of oxygen that the heart muscle requires. As in individuals with apparently normal hearts, the preventive value of exercise conditioning is supported by circumstantial evidence only.

Exercise conditioning has a risk of complications that can be lessened by careful medical clearance, exercise testing, and correct guidelines for prescribing exercise. Overstressing should be avoided.

STUDY QUESTIONS

1. What vessels supply oxygen to heart muscle, and how do they accommodate to increased demands during exercise?

2. What is myocardial ischemia, and why may it develop during exercise when it is not present at rest?

3. What are the purposes of clinical evaluation prior to exercise testing?

4. In what ways can work capacity be expressed from the results of an exercise test?

5. What are cardiac output and stroke volume?

6. Give the mathematical expression for the relationship between cardiac output, systemic vascular resistance, and arterial blood pressure.

7. What is the significance of 1 mm depression of the S-T segment during exercise?

8. What are premature ventricular contractions?

9. What happens to left ventricular pressure during one cardiac cycle, and how does it change during exercise?

10. How is normal ventricular pressure altered in the presence of cardiac disease?

11. List the "coronary risk factors." Which ones are affected by exercise conditioning?

12. What is the principal physiological benefit of exercise conditioning in individuals who have coronary heart disease?

FURTHER READINGS

American Heart Association, The Committee on Exercise: *Exercise Testing and Training of Apparently Healthy Individuals. A Handbook for Physicians.* Dallas, Texas, American Heart Association, 1972.

American Heart Association, The Committee on Exercise: *Exercise Testing and Training of Individuals with Heart Disease or at High Risk for Its Development: A Handbook for Physicians.* Dallas, Texas, American Heart Association, 1975.

Hartley, L. H.: The value of clinical exercise testing. N. Engl. J. Med. *293*:400–401, 1975.

Hartley, L. H.: Exercise testing and conditioning programs for the heart patient. *In* Knuttgen, H. G. (ed): *Neuromuscular Mechanism for Developmental and Therapeutic Exercise.* Baltimore, University Park Press, 1976, pp. 119–133.

Fox, S. M., Naughton, J., and Gorman, P.: Physical activity and cardiovascular health. 1. Potential for prevention of coronary heart disease and possible mechanisms. Mod. Concepts Cardiovasc. Dis. *41*:17–20, 1972.

Fox, S. M., Naughton, J., and Gorman, P.: 2. The exercise prescription: intensity and duration. Mod. Concepts Cardiovasc. Dis. *41*:21–24, 1972.

Fox, S. M., Naughton, J., and Gorman, P.: 3. The exercise prescription: frequency and type of activity. Mod. Concepts Cardiovasc. Dis. *41*:25–30, 1972.

Bruce, R.: The benefits of physical training for patients with coronary heart disease. *In* Ingelfinger, F. J., Ebert, R. V., and Relman, A. S. (eds.): *Controversy in Internal Medicine II.* Philadelphia, W. B. Saunders Company, 1974, p. 145.

27

DRUG USE AND ABUSE

DANIEL F. HANLEY, M.D.

HISTORY

"The desire to take medicine is perhaps the greatest feature which distinguishes man from animals."

William Osler

Attempts to improve physical performance by the ingestion of special substances predate organized athletic competition. Drug use in sports derives from ancient and medieval times when warriors were given special potions thought to protect them and make them fight better. Scandinavian warriors, for example, used an extract of roots that produced hallucinations. These fierce people were called the "Berserkers" (Old Norse for "bear's skin"), and from this word came the expression "going berserk."

Throughout history, a great variety of drugs have been taken by athletes hoping to improve performance. Just before the end of the third century B.C., Greek athletes in the Olympic Games placed their faith in mushrooms that produced hallucinations — but no athletic records were broken. The first documented case of illicit drug use in sports occurred in 1865 among the canal swimmers of Amsterdam. This practice spread rapidly, and by 1879 the six-day bicycle racers of several nations were using caffeine, alcohol, nitroglycerine, ether dropped on sugar cubes, strychnine pills, cocaine, and opium. The Kaffirs of southeast Africa used a local brand of hard liquor called "dop" as a stimulant. This word reached the English language via the Boers, and "doping" first appeared in an English dictionary in 1889.[1]

Over the years, literally hundreds of ingredients have been used as "the magic potion": camphor, ephedrine, glycerine, gelatin, iron, oxygen, aspartic acid, amphetamines, tranquilizers, vitamins, steroids and red blood cells. The current fad is to use varying mixtures of these substances, vitamins, and the male hormone testosterone. Polypharmacy (the use of multiple drugs) reaches its most absurd proportions among athletes. The sad truth is that there is no substance or mixture of substances that will consistently improve performance in a normal, healthy, well-conditioned athlete. Improved performance comes from the hard work of intelligent practice.

GUIDELINES USED BY THE
INTERNATIONAL OLYMPIC COMMITTEE

*Definition of Doping**

A commission of experts convened by the Council of Europe in 1963 gave the following definition of doping: "Doping is defined as the administering or use of

396　*From the *I.O.C. Medical Commission Booklet.*[1]

substances in any form alien to the body, or of physiological substances in abnormal amounts and with abnormal methods, by health personnel with the exclusive aim of attaining an artificial and unfair increase of performance in competition. Furthermore, various psychological measures to increase performance in sport must be regarded as doping."[1]

This definition emphasized the intent of drug misuse. However, problems arise in the assessment of intent and in drawing the line between the therapeutic use of drugs and the use of drugs as doping agents. Some international federations of sports therefore drew up lists of forbidden drugs; proof that any of these drugs has been used by a competitor then constitutes proof that a doping agent has been used. The drawing up of a definite list, however, does not necessarily lead to the desired results because drugs (or chemicals) not on the list but producing effects similar to those on the list could be used. Also, the "pharmacologically sophisticated" countries could profit by substituting different substances and the competitors perhaps be placed in even greater danger than by using some of the drugs on the list.

From its commencement, the International Olympic Committee (I.O.C.) defined its policy as the attempt to prevent the use in sports of those drugs that were dangerous but to do so with minimal interference with the correct and necessary therapeutic use of drugs. Nevertheless, it was recognized that a firm and clear line had to be drawn and that even the therapeutic use of certain classes of drugs at sporting events could not be accepted without destroying the whole of the doping control system. The Committee also decided to ban only those compounds for which suitable analytical methods could be devised to detect the compounds unequivocally in urine (or blood) samples.

Contravention of the rules would be considered established only if a drug belonging to one of the forbidden classes of drugs could be detected in a urine sample obtained from the competitor under controlled conditions; accusations of using forbidden drugs would not be accepted as basis for any action.

The I.O.C. Medical Commission, in accordance with these principles, prepared a list of classes of agents that have been considered doping agents in sports. Examples of drugs in each class are recorded, but to indicate the extensiveness of the list, the words "and related compounds" are included at the end of the samples of each class.

List of Doping Substances*

Psychomotor Stimulant Drugs. Comment: Better known examples of this category are amphetamine (Benzedrine) and cocaine. These drugs stimulate the central nervous system. Effects include excitation, hyperactivity, euphoria, and insomnia. The sensation of fatigue may be decreased and appetite may be depressed. Judgment can be impaired. Pulse rate and blood pressure are increased.

Long-term use may produce confusion, delusions, hostility reactions, hallucinations, and toxic psychoses. These drugs are potentially addictive. A large fraction of the amphetamines produced in the United States goes into illicit "street drug" trade.

amphetamine
benzphetamine
cocaine

---

*The lists of doping substances are taken from the *I.O.C. Medical Commission Booklet.*[1] The *comments* have been added for the convenience of the reader.[2]

diethylpropion
dimethylamphetamine
ethylamphetamine
fencamfamine
methylamphetamine
methylphenidate
norpseudoephedrine
phendimetrazine
phenmetrazine
prolintane
and related compounds

Sympathomimetic Amines. Comment: Drugs of this category are frequently used as nasal decongestants and in the treatment of asthma. These stimulants mimic the effects of naturally occurring epinephrine (adrenalin). Their effects include increases in anxiety, jitteriness, pulse rate, blood pressure, and cardiac output. Peripheral blood vessels are constricted, as are certain sphincters, and bronchial muscles are relaxed.

ephedrine
methylephedrine
methoxyphenamine
and related compounds

Miscellaneous Central Nervous System Stimulants. Comment: These are stimulant drugs whose primary effect is on the central nervous system — the brain and spinal cord. Reflex excitability of the spinal cord is increased, and skeletal muscles respond in a coordinated manner. These drugs may produce muscle spasm and convulsions. They are poisons.

amiphenazole
bemegride
leptazol
nikethamide
strychnine
and related compounds

Narcotic Analgesics. Comment: These drugs produce decreased alertness and can lead to loss of consciousness. All are addictive.

heroin
morphine
methadone
dextromoramide
dipipanone
pethidine
and related compounds

Anabolic Steroids. Comment: These synthetically produced drugs (e.g., Dianabol) are associated with "tissue building."[3, 4] However, they also have masculinizing properties, decrease normal testosterone production, increase fluid retention, cause personality changes leading to psychoses, and increase the incidence of gastric ulcers and liver and kidney tumors. They should not be used by athletes and are especially harmful to diabetics.[2]

methandienone
stanozolol
oxymetholone
nandrolone decanoate
nandrolone phenpropionate
and related compounds

THERAPEUTIC DRUGS

Athletes, like everyone else, do contract some diseases. Fortunately, most of these infections (85 to 90 per cent) are of the minor self-limiting type, such as the common cold, vomiting, and diarrhea. These diseases are of short duration, and drugs do not appreciably change their course. Occasionally medicines are used for the relief of symptoms. However, the athlete and his physician must be aware that some common cold and antidiarrheal medicines contain drugs on the banned list. For example, Olympic athletes have been disqualified for treating a cold with "nose drops" that contain ephedrine. A common antidiarrheal preparation contains a banned narcotic (see page 260). The medications used in the treatment of chronic diseases such as epilepsy or diabetes do not fall in the category of banned drugs and may be used when prescribed by a physician. Officials of the Dope Control Team should be notified, in writing and before the event, of all medications taken by any athlete.

The healthy young adult who eats a normal diet does not need vitamins or dietary supplements. The benefits derived from these substances are tremendously overrated in athletic folklore. Vitamins do not contain energy. They are, of course, necessary for the maintenance of health but are present in adequate quantities in the average American diet. Megavitamin therapy (the ingestion of large quantities of vitamins by a healthy individual) does not improve athletic performance. Large doses of vitamins A and D, in fact, may be harmful. Vitamin E, a current favorite, is stored in the body as are other fat-soluble vitamins (A, D, K). Vitamin E no doubt has a toxic level, although that level has not yet been determined.

Athletes ingest protein supplements literally by the barrelful. There is no scientific justification for their use. They provide no significant benefit and sometimes have harmful effects. With large doses of protein, the blood level of uric acid may increase and damage the kidneys and joints of susceptible individuals. As for energy derived from protein, the reader burns up as much protein reading these words as he or she would by running around a track at top speed. Protein is an essential nutrient for health, and it is adequately supplied in the normal diet. The body burns protein for energy only in starvation.

Sedatives (sleeping pills, tranquilizers) are not on the "banned" list. Their use by athletes should be minimal and they should be administered by the physician, not by the trainer or the coach. Drugs of this type are fat-soluble and so have a biphasic excretion curve. The drug is absorbed through the intestine, processed through the liver, and circulated in the blood stream to the brain. Since it is fat-soluble, some of it is stored in the fat of the body and some is excreted immediately. That amount stored in body fat is slowly mobilized back into the blood stream and is excreted by the kidneys. Diazepam (Valium), one of today's most widely used drugs, has a biological half-life of about 48 hours. This means that the athlete may be under partial influence of this drug for several days, so its use should be carefully restricted. The effect of successive doses is cumulative, and the level of the drug in the body increases rapidly with daily doses.

ANABOLIC STEROIDS*

Steroid hormones are chemically related to cholesterol. Included in this group are the sex hormones such as testosterone, which is produced in the male by the

---

*See also the American College of Sports Medicine's position statement on "The Use and Abuse of Anabolic-Androgenic Steroids in Sports," page 411.

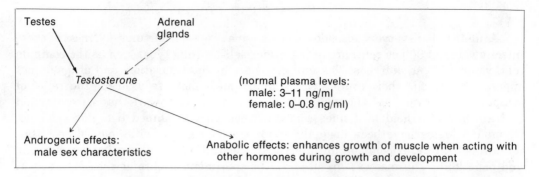

Figure 27–1. Testosterone is produced by the testis. It has both androgenic and anabolic effects.

testes. Also included are corticosteroid hormones (related to cortisone), which are produced by the adrenal gland and have a strong anti-inflammatory action. The corticosteroids are sometimes used in the treatment of athletic injuries.

The effects of testosterone can be separated into two components — anabolic and androgenic (Fig. 27–1). The anabolic effect is tissue-building; the androgenic effect is masculinizing. Synthetic anabolic hormones were created in an attempt to aid the rebuilding of tissue in starved or ill persons. Such hormones retain a masculinizing effect that is especially noticeable when they are given to females. Anabolic steroid hormones (e.g., Dianabol, Nilevar) have become widely used among athletes who hope to increase muscle bulk and strength.

Anabolic steroids can produce increased weight, but that weight is largely due to retained fluids rather than new muscle.[4] Increased muscle size comes from proper training and conditioning. In the adolescent, testosterone, working in conjunction with other naturally occurring hormones (pituitary, adrenal, etc.), does help to produce the male physique with its stronger muscles and heavier frame. However, the testes continue to produce testosterone from puberty to the late years of life, yet muscles do not increase in size and strength throughout life.

The body tends to keep a serum level of testosterone fairly constant. If testosterone or a synthetic anabolic steroid is administered to a male athlete, the individual's testes will secrete less of the natural hormone to preserve the normal balance in the body. If testosterone or synthetic anabolic steroids are taken for a long period of time and in large doses, the testes will cease to produce testosterone and the body will have to depend entirely upon the external source. In most young people, this is a reversible process.

Synthetic anabolic steroids produce other undesirable side effects. They tend to make the continued user irritable and difficult to get along with and have produced some true psychoses in borderline psychotics. Diabetics can also be affected adversely. The incidences of gastric ulcer and primary tumors of the liver and kidney are increased by prolonged use of steroid hormones. The administration of anabolic steroids before puberty and in early adolescence stunts growth by inducing early closure of the epiphyses (growth lines) of the bones.[5] It has been suggested that this effect may be exploited by some national teams to keep gymnasts tiny. Small people have a lower center of gravity, can do more somersaults in a shorter distance, and generally have greater "crowd appeal." When anabolic steroids are taken by women in large doses for a long period of time, secondary male sexual characteristics develop: male facial hair distribution, male type of skin, and deeper voice. When given to a young female, these drugs cause clitoral enlargement.

Laboratory tests have been developed for the identification of synthetic anabolic steroids in the urine. Thus, their use during international competition can be controlled. Eight urine samples from participants were positive for anabolic steroids in a recent set of international games. Such participants are disqualified. Some athletes now use the natural hormone testosterone, which is more difficult to identify in the laboratory because it cannot be distinguished from the testosterone produced by the testes.

BLOOD DOPING

In laboratory experiments,[6] blood was removed from athletes and was frozen and stored. Several weeks later, after the lost blood had been regenerated, the individual's red cells were reinfused to cause an unusually high hemoglobin level. The original investigators found that the endurance of these athletes was improved. However, other researchers studying the reinfusion of blood have not found increased endurance.[7, 8] (See also page 108.) High hemoglobin levels are not necessarily associated with high-endurance sports. Oarsmen and runners have been found to have relatively low hemoglobin levels. In contrast, rifle and pistol shooters, who are sedentary athletes, have hemoglobin levels that are higher than normal.

OTHER COMMONLY ABUSED DRUGS

Alcohol

Alcohol initially stimulates by interfering with the cerebral centers — "alcohol inhibits inhibitions." Subsequently, like a general anesthetic, it depresses the central nervous system. Problems occur when alcohol is used in quantities that exceed the body's capacity to metabolize it. Alcohol is absorbed directly from the stomach. A 170-pound adult can metabolize about ½ to ¾ ounce of pure alcohol per hour. Two ounces of 100-proof bourbon, for example, equal 1 ounce of pure alcohol, which will produce a blood level of 0.05 per cent in a 170-pound adult. Four ounces of pure alcohol produce a blood level of 0.20 per cent, causing severe intoxication. A blood level of 0.50 per cent produces coma and sometimes death.

Alcohol is a depressant. It interferes with coordination, vision, and judgment. It lowers alertness, slows reaction time, and can produce severe motor disturbances, staggering, impaired sensory perception, and even death. Long-term damage to brain and liver cells may result from its use. Alcohol is an addictive drug, particularly for certain types of people. It has no place in athletics.

Tobacco

"The control of cigarette smoking could do more to improve health, and probably life, than any other single action in the whole field of preventive medicine."

Report of World Health Organization, 1970

Tobacco smokers have a high incidence of emphysema, cancer of the mouth, throat, and lungs, and heart disease. In the early 1800's, nicotine, the active drug in tobacco, was used by athletes to improve their reaction time and thus improve their performance. It did not work, and for all practical purposes, nicotine is not used today. Even major league baseball players are switching from "burley" to bubble gum.

Street Drugs

Marijuana is a relaxant and impairs judgment. In high doses, it causes hallucinations.

Barbiturates are sedatives. They reduce anxiety and sometimes produce euphoria. They are addictive and may produce toxic psychoses. Withdrawal symptoms are severe.

Cocaine is a short-acting central nervous stimulant and a local anesthetic. It produces excitation and talkativeness. Convulsions can result. Severe depression may follow long-term use.

These drugs produce an initial high (euphoria) followed by a low — often a depression. The high is usually short-lived, and the depression generally lasts longer. Any discussion of these drugs tends to get bogged down in the question of whether the drug is physiologically or psychologically addictive. All have the potential to make the user dependent.[2]

DOPING CONTROL PROGRAM

The Russian chemist Bukowski was the first to find a method for detecting alkaloids in the saliva of racehorses that had been doped. Tests were conducted on horses in 1910. At that time, about 50 per cent of all racehorses were doped. Since then, laboratory testing has improved and become more widely used. It is estimated that now less than 1 per cent of racehorses are doped.

Since the early days of the modern Olympic Games, attempts have been made to control the use of drugs by athletes. At first, inspection of rooms and luggage was tried, but this was ineffective. Hazards of drug use were explained to athletes at the time of the Games, but this too proved unsuccessful. The deaths of the Danish athlete Knute Jennsen in the bicycle road race in Rome during the 1960 Olympic Games, and of Simpson, the British cyclist, during the Tour de France race in 1967, are two of the most widely publicized cases of doping. However, others have died, and hundreds of athletes have become severely ill after being doped.

France passed a federal law against doping in sports, and in 1977 the King of Belgium issued a royal decree against doping that follows the I.O.C. Medical Commission's list of banned drugs.[1]

Dope testing was first done at the Olympic Games of Grenoble and Mexico in 1968. The dope-detecting art has now improved to such a degree that nose drops containing ephedrine can be detected in the urine 48 hours after use. Since 1968 a strict protocol has been followed by the Medical Commission of the I.O.C. At the Olympic sites, special laboratories have been developed at which very small amounts of the banned drugs can be detected. Techniques of gas-liquid chromatography, mass spectrography, and radioimmunoassay are all utilized. Reliability is excellent. On each day of competition, samples that contain a known banned substance are included among the regular specimens so that the laboratory itself is checked by the I.O.C.

Dope control requires a large number of trained personnel to collect, record, and transport the specimens to the laboratory. It also requires another large group of highly skilled technicians and biochemists to operate the laboratory 24 hours a day so that results will be available as soon as possible after the event. The equipment and its maintenance are extremely expensive. A program of this type at one set of Olympic Games costs more than 2 million dollars. A drug control program should not be entered into lightly. It is fraught with the potential for disaster. Any laboratory can report negative results, but it takes an excellent laboratory to detect small quantities of drugs and to run an uncontestable drug control program.

CONCLUSION

We live in a drug-taking culture. Dr. S. R. Oakley says, "There are over 300 aspirin-containing products on the American market. Americans gobble down 44 million aspirin tablets (21 tons of acetylsalicylic acid) a day and eight billion doses of amphetamines a year."[2] For many drugs (tobacco, alcohol, thalidomide, pesticides, flu vaccine, steroids), major toxic effects will not be known for years. Thus, there is need for continuous reevaluation. There is growing evidence that every drug exacts its price for the biochemical changes it produces. In some instances, the "trade-off" is worth the action, but in many cases, this is not certain. Before any drug is used, its short-term and long-term potential for damage should be understood. Coaches, trainers, athletes, and sports physicians do not always assess drugs adequately. There is a great deal about drugs and their long-term effects that remains unknown. This much is known: in sports, there is no easy way and there is no magic potion. It is desire and hard work that produce improvement.

STUDY QUESTIONS

1. Is the use of drugs to improve the performance of an athlete a modern phenomenon?

2. Name three drugs that will consistently improve the performance of a well-trained, healthy, young adult athlete.

3. What is the difference between the therapeutic use of drugs and doping?

4. Do vitamins supply energy?

5. Are barbiturates and antihistamines on the I.O.C.'s banned list?

6. How long may tranquilizers remain in the body?

7. Should every school (college) have a dope control program?

8. Name three classes of drugs frequently abused by athletes.

9. Describe the effects of:
   (a) alcohol
   (b) cocaine
   (c) ephedrine
   (d) amphetamine
   (e) barbiturates

REFERENCES

1. Doping: *In* the *Medical Commission Booklet.* Published by the International Olympic Committee in cooperation with the Organizing Committee for the Olympic Games of Montreal, 1976.
2. Oakley, S. R.: *Drugs, Society and Human Behavior.* St. Louis, C. V. Mosby Company, 1972.
3. Fowler, W. M., Jr.: Effects of administering anabolic steroids in weight training. Paper presented at Track and Field Institute, University of Wisconsin, Madison, Wisconsin, June 29–30, 1966.

4. Golding, L. A., Greydinger, J. E., and Fishel, S. S.: The effect of an androgenic anabolic steroid and a protein supplement on size, strength, weight and body composition in athletes. Phys. Sportsmed., May, 1974.
5. Ruff, W. K.: Athletes warned about anabolic steroids. J. Natl. Athletic Trainers Assoc., Winter, 1965–66.
6. Ekblom, B., Goldberg, A. N., and Gullbring, B.: Response to exercise after blood loss and infusion. J. Appl. Physiol. *33*:175–180, 1972.
7. Rowell, L. B.: Human cardiovascular adjustments to exercise and thermal stress. Physiol. Rev. *54*:75–159, 1974.
8. Williams, M. H.: Blood doping—does it really help athletes? Phys. Sportsmed., January, 1975. p. 52.

FURTHER READINGS

Clarke, K. S. (ed.): *Drugs and the Coach.* Washington, D.C., American Association for Health and Physical Education and Recreation, 1976.
Connell, P. M.: Clinical manifestations and treatment of amphetamine type of dependence. J.A.M.A., *196*:718, 1966.
Golding, L. A., and Barnard, J. R.: The effect of d-amphetamine sulfate on physical performance. J. Sports Med. *3*:221, 1963.
Karpovich, P. V.: Effect of amphetamine sulfate on athletic performance. J.A.M.A., *170*:558, 1959.
Lovingwood, Blythe, Peacock, et al.: Effects of d-amphetamine sulfate, caffeine and high temperature on human performance. (Copy may be obtained by sending $1.25 for photoprint to Chief, Photoduplication Service, Library of Congress, Washington, D.C. 20540.)
Porritt, A.: Aims and perspectives: doping. J. Sports Med. *5*:166, 1965.
Ryan, A. J.: Athletics. *In* Born, G. V. R., et al. (eds.): *Handbook of Experimental Pharmacology.* Berlin, Springer-Verlag, 1976.
Talland, G. A., and Quarton, G. C.: The effects of drugs and familiarity on performance in continuous visual search. J. Nerv. Ment. Dis. *143*:266, 1966.
Weiss, B., and Laties, V. G.: Enhancement of human performance by caffeine and the amphetamines. Stanford Research Institute Project No. SU-3024, Life Sciences Division. "Drug Enhancement of Performance," prepared under contract Nonr-2993 (00) for the Physiological Psychology Branch, Psychological Sciences Division, Office of Naval Research.
Williams, M. H.: *Drugs and Athletic Performance.* Springfield, Ill., Charles C Thomas, 1974.
Wilson, L., Taylor, J. D., Nash, C. W., and Cameron, D. F.: The combined effects of ethanol and amphetamine sulfate on performance of human subjects. Can. Med. Assoc. J. *94*:478, 1966.

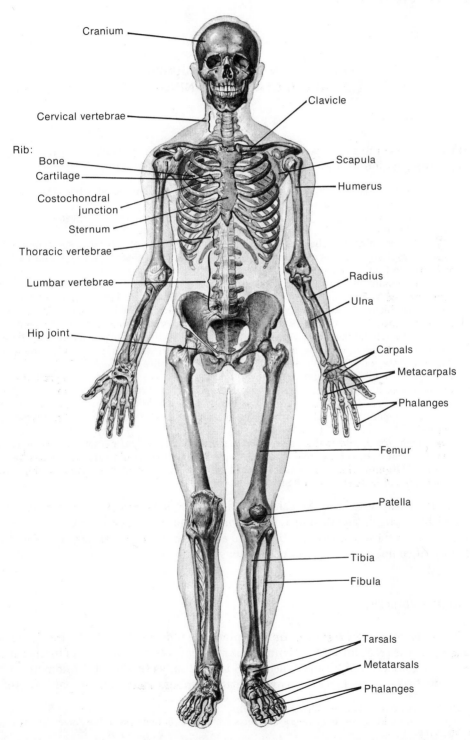

View of skeleton from the front. Certain ligaments are shown on one side. (Modified from Anson: *Atlas of Human Anatomy*.)

APPENDIX B

American College
of Sports Medicine*
Position Statements

PREVENTION OF HEAT INJURIES
DURING DISTANCE RUNNING**

Position Statement

Based on research findings and current rules governing distance running competition, it is the position of the American College of Sports Medicine that:

1. Distance races (> 16 km or 10 miles) should *not* be conducted when the wet bulb temperature–globe temperature† exceeds 28° C (82.4° F).[1, 2]
2. During periods of the year, when the daylight dry bulb temperature often exceeds 27° C (80° F), distance races should be conducted before 9:00 A.M. or after 4:00 P.M.[2, 7, 8, 9]
3. It is the responsibility of the race sponsors to provide fluids which contain small amounts of sugar (less than 2.5 gram glucose per 100 ml of water) and electrolytes (less than 10 mEq sodium and 5 mEq potassium per liter of solution.)[5, 6]
4. Runners should be encouraged to frequently ingest fluids during competition and to consume 400 to 500 ml (13 to 17 oz) of fluid 10 to 15 minutes before competition.[5, 6, 9]
5. Rules prohibiting the administration of fluids during the first 10 kilometers (6.2 miles) of a marathon race should be amended to permit fluid ingestion at frequent intervals along the race course. In light of the high sweat rates and body temperatures during distance running in the heat, race sponsors should provide "water stations" at 3 to 4 kilometer (2 to 2.5 mile) intervals for all races of 16 kilometers (10 miles) or more.[4, 8, 9]
6. Runners should be instructed in how to recognize the early warning symptoms that precede heat injury. Recognition of symptoms, cessation of running, and proper treatment can prevent heat injury. Early warning symptoms include the following: piloerection on chest and upper arms, chilling, throbbing pressure in the head, unsteadiness, nausea, and dry skin.[2, 9]
7. Race sponsors should make prior arrangements with medical personnel for the care of cases of heat injury. Responsible and informed personnel should supervise each "feeding station." Organizational personnel should reserve the right to stop runners who exhibit clear signs of heat stroke or heat exhaustion.

It is the position of the American College of Sports Medicine that policies established by local, national, and international sponsors of distance running events should adhere to these guidelines. Failure to adhere to these guidelines may jeopardize the health of competitors through heat injury.

Additional Information

The requirements of distance running place great demands on both circulation and body temperature regulation.[4, 8, 9] Numerous studies have reported rectal temperatures in excess of 40.6° C (105° F) after races of 6 to 26.2 miles (9.6 to 41.9 kilometers).[4, 8, 9] Attempting to counterbalance such overheating, runners incur large sweat losses of 0.8

*1440 Monroe Street, Madison, Wisconsin 53706

**Reprinted from Medicine and Science in Sports 7(1):vii, 1975. Courtesy of the American College of Sports Medicine.

†Adapted from Minard, D.: Prevention of heat casualties in Marine Corps Recruits. Milit. Med. *126*:261, 1961. WB-GT = 0.7 (WBT) + 0.2 (GT) + 0.1 (DBT).

to 1.1 liters/m²/hr.[4, 8, 9] The resulting body water deficit may total 6 to 10 per cent of the athlete's body weight. Dehydration of these proportions severely limits subsequent sweating, places dangerous demands on circulation, reduces exercise capacity and exposes the runner to the health hazards associated with hyperthermia (heat stroke, heat exhaustion and muscle cramps.)[2, 3, 9]

Under moderate thermal conditions, e.g., 65 to 70° F (18.5 to 21.3° C), no cloud cover, relative humidity 49 to 55 per cent, the risk of overheating is still a serious threat to highly motivated distance runners. Nevertheless, distance races are frequently conducted under more severe conditions than these. The air temperature at the 1967 U.S. Pan American Marathon Trial, for example, was 92 to 95° F (33.6 to 35.3° C). Many highly conditioned athletes failed to finish the race and several of the competitors demonstrated overt symptoms of heat stroke (no sweating, shivering, and lack of orientation).

The above consequences are compounded by the current popularity of distance running among middle-aged and aging men and women who may possess significantly less heat tolerance than their younger counterparts. In recent years, races of 10 to 26.2 miles (16 to 41.9 kilometers) have attracted several thousand runners. Since it is likely that distance running enthusiasts will continue to sponsor races under adverse heat conditions, specific steps should be taken to minimize the health threats which accompany such endurance events.

Fluid ingestion during prolonged running (two hours) has been shown to effectively reduce rectal temperature and minimize dehydration.[4] Although most competitors consume fluids during races that exceed 1 to 1.5 hours, current international distance running rules prohibit the administration of fluids until the runner has completed 10 miles (16 kilometers). Under such limitations, the competitor is certain to accumulate a large body water deficit (−3%) before any fluids would be ingested. To make the problem more complex, most runners are unable to judge the volume of fluids they consume during competition.[4] At the 1968 U.S. Olympic Marathon Trial, it was observed that there were body weight losses of 6.1 kg, with an average total fluid ingestion of only 0.14 to 0.35 liter.[4] It seems obvious that the rules and habits which prohibit fluid administration during distance running preclude any benefits which might be gained from this practice.

Runners who attempt to consume large volumes of sugar solution during competition complain of gastric discomfort (fullness) and an inability to consume fluids after the first few feedings.[4, 5, 6] Generally speaking, most runners drink solutions containing 5 to 20 grams of sugar per 100 milliliters of water. Although saline is rapidly emptied from the stomach (25 ml/min), the addition of even small amounts of sugar can drastically impair the rate of gastric emptying.[5] During exercise in the heat, carbohydrate supplementation is of secondary importance and the sugar content of the oral feedings should be minimized.

References

1. Adolph, E. F.: *Physiology of Man in the Desert.* New York Interscience, 1947.
2. Buskirk, E. R., and Grasley, W. C.: Heat injury and conduct of athletes. *In* Johnson, W. R., and Buskirk, E. R. (eds.): *Science and Medicine of Exercise and Sport,* 2nd ed. New York, Harper and Row, 1974.
3. Buskirk, E. R., Iampietro, P. F.: and Bass, D. E.: Work performance after dehydration: effects of physical conditioning and heat acclimatization. J. Appl. Physiol. *12*:189–194, 1958.
4. Costill, D. L., Kammer, W. F., and Fisher, A.: Fluid ingestion during distance running. Arch. Environ. Health *21*:520–525, 1970.
5. Costill, D. L., and Saltin, B.: Factors limiting gastric emptying during rest and exercise. J. Appl. Physiol. *37*(5):679–683, 1974.
6. Fordtran, J. A., and Saltin, B.: Gastric emptying and intestinal absorption during prolonged severe exercise. J. Appl. Physiol. *23*:331–335, 1967.

7. Myhre, L. G.: Shifts in blood volume during and following acute environmental and work stresses in man. (Doctoral Dissertation). Indiana University, Bloomington, Indiana, 1967.
8. Pugh, L. G. C., Corbett, J. I., and Johnson, R. H.: Rectal temperatures, weight losses and sweating rates in marathon running. J. Appl. Physiol. 23:347–353, 1957.
9. Wyndham. C. H., and Strydom, N. B.: The danger of an inadequate water intake during marathon running. S. Afr. Med. J. 43:893–896, 1969.

WEIGHT LOSS IN WRESTLERS*

Despite repeated admonitions by medical, educational, and athletic groups[2, 8, 17, 22, 33] most wrestlers have been inculcated by instruction or accepted tradition to lose weight in order to be certified for a class that is lower than their preseason weight.[34] Studies[34, 40] of weight losses in high-school and college wrestlers indicate that from 3 to 20 per cent of the preseason body weight is lost before certification or competition occurs. Of this weight loss, most of the decrease occurs in the final days or day before the official weigh-in[34, 40] with the youngest and/or lightest members of the team losing the highest percentage of their body weight.[34] Under existing rules and practices, it is not uncommon for an individual to repeat this weight losing process many times during the season because successful wrestlers compete in 15 to 30 matches per year.[13]

Contrary to existing beliefs, most wrestlers are not "fat" before the season starts.[35] In fact, the fat content of high-school and college wrestlers weighing less than 190 pounds has been shown to range from 1.6 to 15.1 per cent of their body weight with the majority possessing less than 8 per cent.[14, 28, 31] It is well known and documented that wrestlers lose body weight by a combination of food restriction, fluid deprivation, and sweating induced by thermal or exercise procedures.[20, 22, 34, 40] Of these methods, dehydration through sweating appears to be the method most frequently chosen.

Careful studies on the nature of the weight being lost show that water, fats, and proteins are lost when food restriction and fluid deprivation procedures are followed.[10] Moreover, the proportionality between these constituents will change with continued restriction and deprivation. For example, if food restriction is held constant when the volume of fluid being consumed is decreased, more water will be lost from the tissues of the body than before the fluid restriction occurred. The problem becomes more acute when thermal or exercise dehydration occurs because electrolyte losses will accompany the water losses.[16] Even when one to five hours are allowed for purposes of rehydration after the weigh-in, this time interval is insufficient for fluid and electrolyte homeostasis to be completely reestablished.[11, 37, 39, 40]

Since the "making of weight" occurs by combinations of food restriction, fluid deprivation, and dehydration, responsible officials should realize that the single or combined effects of these practices are generally associated with (1) a reduction in muscular strength[4, 15, 30]; (2) a decrease in work performance times[24, 26, 27, 30]; (3) lower plasma and blood volumes[6, 7, 24, 27]; (4) a reduction in cardiac functioning during submaximal work conditions which are associated with higher heart rates,[1, 19, 23, 24, 27] smaller stroke volumes[27] and reduced cardiac outputs[27]; (5) a lower oxygen consumption, especially with food restriction[15, 30]; (6) an impairment of thermoregulatory processes[3, 9, 24]; (7) a decrease in renal blood flow[21, 25] and in the volume of fluid being filtered by the kidney[21]; (8) a depletion of liver glycogen stores[12]; and (9) an increase in the amount of electrolytes being lost from the body.[6, 7, 16]

Since it is possible for these changes to impede normal growth and development, there is little physiological or medical justification for the use of the weight reduction

*Reprinted from Medicine and Science in Sports 8(2):xi, 1976. Courtesy of the American College of Sports Medicine.

methods currently followed by many wrestlers. These sentiments have been expressed in part within Rule 1, Section 3, Article 1 of the *Official Wrestling Rule Book*[18] published by the National Federation of State High School Associations, which states, "The Rules Committee recommends that individual state high school associations develop and utilize an effective weight control program which will discourage severe weight reduction and/or wide variations in weight, because this may be harmful to the competitor. . . ." However, until the National Federation of State High School Associations defines the meaning of the terms "severe" and "wide variations," this rule will be ineffective in reducing the abuses associated with the "making of weight."

Therefore, it is the position of the American College of Sports Medicine* that the potential health hazards created by the procedures used to "make weight" by wrestlers can be eliminated if state and national organizations will:

1. Assess the body composition of each wrestler several weeks in advance of the competitive season.[5, 14, 28, 31, 38] Individuals with a fat content less than 5 per cent of their certified body weight should receive medical clearance before being allowed to compete.
2. Emphasize the fact that the daily caloric requirements of wrestlers should be obtained from a balanced diet and determined on the basis of age, body surface area, growth and physical activity levels.[29] The minimal caloric needs of wrestlers in high schools and colleges will range from 1200 to 2400 kcal/day[32]; therefore, it is the responsibility of coaches, school officials, physicians, and parents to discourage wrestlers from securing less than their minimal needs without prior medical approval.
3. Discourage the practice of fluid deprivation and dehydration. This can be accomplished by:
   a. Educating the coaches and wrestlers on the physiological consequences and medical complications that can occur as a result of these practices.
   b. Prohibiting the single or combined use of rubber suits, steam rooms, hot boxes, saunas, laxatives, and diuretics to "make weight."
   c. Scheduling weigh-ins just prior to competition.
   d. Scheduling more official weigh-ins between team matches.
4. Permit more participants per team to compete in those weight classes (119 to 145 pounds) which have the highest percentages of wrestlers certified for competition.[36]
5. Standardize regulations concerning the eligibility rules at championship tournaments so that individuals can only participate in those weight classes in which they had the highest frequencies of matches throughout the season.
6. Encourage local and county organizations to systematically collect data on the hydration state[39, 40] of wrestlers and its relationship to growth and development.

References

1. Ahlman, K., and Karvonen, M. J.: Weight reduction by sweating in wrestlers and its effect on physical fitness. J. Sports Med. Phys. Fit. *1*:58-62, 1961.
2. AMA Committee on the Medical Aspects of Sports, Wrestling and Weight Control. J.A.M.A. *201*:541-543, 1967.
3. Bock, W. E., Fox, E. L., and Bowers, R.: The effect of acute dehydration upon cardiorespiratory endurance. J. Sports Med. Phys. Fit. *7*:62-72, 1967.
4. Bosco, J. S., Terjung, R. L., Greenleaf, J. E.: Effects of progressive hypohydration on maximal isometric muscular strength. J. Sports Med. Phys. Fit. *8*:81-86, 1968.
5. Clarke, K. S.: Predicting certified weight of young wrestlers: a field study of the Tcheng-Tipton method. Med. Sci. Sports *6*:52-57, 1974.
6. Costill, D. L., and Sparks, K. E.: Rapid fluid replacement following thermal dehydration. J. Appl. Physiol. *34*:299-303, 1973.
7. Costill, D. L., Cote, R., Miller, E., Miller, T., and Wynder, S.: Water and electrolyte replacement during repeated days of work in the heat. Aviat. Space Environ. Med. *46*:795-800. 1975.
8. Eriksen, F. G.: Interscholastic wrestling and weight control: current plans and their loopholes. *Proceedings of the Eighth National Conference on The Medical Aspects of Sports*. Chicago, AMA, 1967, pp. 34-39.
9. Grande, F. J., Monagle, E., Buskirk, E. R., and Taylor, H. L.: Body temperature responses to exercise in man on restricted food and water intake. J. Appl. Physiol. *14*:194-198, 1959.

---

*The services of the American College of Sports Medicine are available to assist local and national organizations in implementing these recommendations.

10. Grande, F.: Nutrition and energy balance in body composition studies. *In* Brôzek, J., and Henschel, A. (eds.): *Techniques for Measuring Body Composition.* Washington, D.C., National Acad. Sci. & Nat. Res. Council, pp. 168–188, 1961.
11. Herbert, W. G., and Ribisl, P. M.: Effects of dehydration upon physical work capacity of wrestlers under competitive conditions. Res. Quart. *43*:416–422, 1972.
12. Hultman, E., and Nilsson, L.: Liver glycogen as glucose-supplying source during exercise. *In* Keul, J. (ed.): *Limiting Factors of Physical Performance,* Stuttgart, Georg Thieme, 1973, pp. 179–189.
13. *1975 Program for the 55th State Wrestling Tournament.* Iowa High School Athletic Association, pp. 7–9.
14. Katch, F. I., and Michael, E. D., Jr.: Body composition of high school wrestlers according to age and wrestling weight category. Med. Sci. Sports *3*:190–194, 1971.
15. Keys, A. L., Brôzek, J., Henschel, A., Mickelsen, O., and Taylor, H. L.: *The Biology of Human Starvation,* Vol. 1. Minneapolis, University of Minnesota Press, 1950, pp. 718–748.
16. Kozlowski, S. and Saltin, B.: Effect of sweat loss on body fluids. J. Appl. Physiol. *19*:1119–1124, 1964.
17. Kroll, W.: Guidelines for rules and practices. *Proceedings of the Eighth National Conference on the Medical Aspects of Sports.* Chicago, AMA, pp. 40–44, 1967.
18. *The National Federation 1974–75 Wrestling Rule Book.* Elgin, Ill. The National Federation Publications, p. 6.
19. Palmer, W.: Selected physiological responses of normal young men following dehydration and rehydration. Res. Quart. *39*:1054–1059, 1968.
20. Paul, W. D.: Crash diets in wrestling. J. Iowa Med. Soc. *56*:835–840, 1966.
21. Radigan, L. R., and Robinson, S.: Effect of environmental heat stress and exercise on renal blood flow and filtration rate. J. Appl. Physiol. *2*:185–191, 1949.
22. Rasch, P. G., and Kroll, W.: *What Research Tells the Coach About Wrestling.* Washington, AAHPER, 1964, pp. 41–50.
23. Ribisl, P. M., and Herbert, W. G.: Effect of rapid weight reduction and subsequent rehydration upon the physical working capacity of wrestlers. Res. Quart. *41*:536–541, 1970.
24. Robinson, S.: The effect of dehydration on performance. *In Football Injuries.* Washington, Nat. Acad. Sci., pp. 191–197, 1970.
25. Rowell, L. B.: Human cardiovascular adjustments to exercise and thermal stress. Physiol. Rev. *54*:75–159, 1974.
26. Saltin, B.: Aerobic and anaerobic work capacity after dehydration. J. Appl. Physiol. *19*:1114–1118, 1964.
27. Saltin, B.: Circulatory response to submaximal and maximal exercise after thermal dehydration. J. Appl. Physiol. *19*:1125–1132, 1964.
28. Sinning, W. E.: Body composition assessment of college wrestlers. Med. Sci. Sports *6*:139–145, 1974.
29. Suggested Daily Dietary Requirements. National Research Council Data. *In* Oser, B. O.: *Hawk's Physiological Chemistry,* 14th ed. New York, McGraw-Hill, pp. 1370–1371, 1965.
30. Taylor, H. L., Buskirk, E. R., Brôzek, J., Anderson, J. T., and Grande, F.: Performance capacity and effects of caloric restriction with hard physical work on young men. J. Appl. Physiol. *10*:421–429, 1957.
31. Tcheng, T. K., and Tipton, C. M.: Iowa wrestling study: anthropometric measurements and the prediction of a "minimal" body weight for high school wrestlers. Med. Sci. Sports *5*:1–10, 1973.
32. Tipton, C. M.: Unpublished calculations on Iowa High School Wrestlers using a height and weight surface area nomogram. (Consalazio, C. F., Johnson, R. E., and Pecora, L. J.: *Physiological Measurements of Metabolic Functions in Man.* New York, McGraw-Hill, 1963, p. 27, which was constructed from the Dubois-Meech formula published in Arch. Intern. Med. *17*:863–871, 1916), plus the metabolic standards for age used by the Mayo Foundation Standards that were published by Boothby, Berkson and Dunn in Am. J. Physiol. *116*:467–484, 1936.
33. Tipton, C. M., Tcheng, T. K., and Paul, W. D.: Evaluation of the Hall Method for determining minimum wrestling weights. J. Iowa Med. Soc. *59*:571–574, 1969.
34. Tipton, C. M., and Tcheng, T. K.: Iowa wrestling study: weight loss in high school students. J.A.M.A. *214*:1269–1274, 1970.
35. Tipton, C. M.: Current status of the Iowa Wrestling Study. *The Predicament,* Dec. 30, 1973, p. 7.
36. Tipton, C. M., Tcheng, T. K., and Zambraski, E. J.: Iowa Wrestling Study: weight classification systems. Med. Sci. Sports *8*:101–104, 1976.
37. Vaccaro, P., Zauner, C. W., and Cade, J. R.: Changes in body weight, hematocrit and plasma protein concentration due to dehydration and rehydration in wrestlers. Med. Sci. Sports *7*:76, 1975.
38. Wilmore, J. H., and Behnke, A.: An anthropometric estimation of body density and lean body weight in young men. J. Appl. Physiol. *27*:25–31, 1969.
39. Zambraski, E. J., Tipton, C. M., Tcheng, T. K., Jordan, H. R., Vailas, A. C., and Callahan, A. K.: Changes in the urinary profiles of wrestlers prior to and after competition. Med. Sci. Sports *7*:217–220, 1975.
40. Zambraski, E. J., Foster, D. T., Gross, P. M., and Tipton, C. M.: Iowa wrestling study: Weight loss and urinary profiles of collegiate wrestlers. Med. Sci. Sports *8*:105–108, 1976.

THE USE AND ABUSE OF ANABOLIC-ANDROGENIC STEROIDS IN SPORTS*

Based on a comprehensive survey of the world literature and a careful analysis of the claims made for and against the efficacy of anabolic-androgenic steroids in improving human physical performance, it is the position of the American College of Sports Medicine that:

1. The administration of anabolic-androgenic steroids to healthy humans below age 50 in medically approved therapeutic doses often does not of itself bring about any significant improvements in strength, aerobic endurance, lean body mass, or body weight.
2. There is no conclusive scientific evidence that extremely large doses of anabolic-androgenic steroids either aid or hinder athletic performance.
3. The prolonged use of oral anabolic-androgenic steroids (C_{17}-alkylated derivatives of testosterone) has resulted in liver disorders in some persons. Some of these disorders are apparently reversible with the cessation of drug usage, but others are not.
4. The administration of anabolic-androgenic steroids to male humans may result in a decrease in testicular size and function and a decrease in sperm production. Although these effects appear to be reversible when small doses of steroids are used for short periods of time, the reversibility of the effects of large doses over extended periods of time is unclear.
5. Serious and continuing effort should be made to educate male and female athletes, coaches, physical educators, physicians, trainers, and the general public regarding the inconsistent effects of anabolic-androgenic steroids on improvement of human physical performance and the potential dangers of taking certain forms of these substances, especially in large doses, for prolonged periods.

Research Background for the Position Statement

This position stand has been developed from an extensive survey and analysis of the world literature in the fields of medicine, physiology, endocrinology, and physical education. Although the reactions of humans to the use of drugs, including hormones or drugs which simulate the actions of natural hormones, are individual and not entirely predictable, some conclusions can nevertheless be drawn with regard to what desirable and what undesirable effects may be achieved. Accordingly, whereas positive effects of drugs may sometimes arise because persons have been led to expect such changes ("placebo" effect),[8] repeated experiments of a similar nature often fail to support the initial positive effects and lead to the conclusion that any positive effect that does exist may not be substantial.

1. Administration of testosterone-like synthetic drugs which have anabolic (tissue building) and androgenic (development of male secondary sex characteristics) properties in amounts up to twice those normally prescribed for medical use has been associated with increased strength, lean body mass and/or body weight in some studies[6, 19, 20, 26, 27, 33, 34, 36] but not in others.[9, 10, 12, 13, 21, 35, 36] One study[13] reported an increase in the amount of weight the steroid group could lift compared to controls but found no difference in isometric strength which suggests a placebo effect in the drug group, a learning effect or possibly a differential drug effect on isotonic compared to isometric strength. An initial report of enhanced aerobic endurance after administration of an anabolic-androgenic steroid[20] has not been confirmed.[6, 9, 21, 27] Because of the lack of adequate control groups in many studies it seems likely that some of the positive effects on strength that have been reported are due to "placebo" effects,[3, 8] but a few apparently well-designed studies have

*Reprinted from Medicine and Science in Sports 9(4):xi, 1977. Courtesy of the American College of Sports Medicine.

also shown beneficial effects of steroid administration on muscular strength and lean body mass. Some of the discrepancies in results may also be due to differences in the type of drug administered, the method of drug administration, the nature of the exercise programs involved, the duration of the experiment, and individual differences in sensitivity to the administered drug. High-protein dietary supplements do not insure the effectiveness of the steroids.[13, 21, 36] Because of the many failures to show improved muscular strength, lean body mass, or body weight after therapeutic doses of anabolic-androgenic steroids, it is obvious that for many individuals any benefits are likely to be small and not worth the health risks involved.

2. Testimonial evidence by individual athletes suggests that athletes often use much larger doses of steroids than those oridinarily prescribed by physicians and those evaluated in published research. Because of the health risks involved with the long-term use of high doses and requirements for informed consent it is unlikely that scientifically acceptable evidence will be forthcoming to evaluate the effectiveness of such large doses of drugs on athletic performance.

3. Alterations of normal liver function have been found in as many as 80 per cent of one series of 69 patients treated with C_{17}-alkylated testosterone derivatives (oral anabolic-androgenic steroids).[29] Cholestasis has been observed histologically in the livers of persons taking these substances.[31] These changes appear to be benign and reversible.[30] Five reports[4, 7, 23, 31, 39] document the occurrence of peliosis hepatitis in 17 patients without evidence of significant liver disease who were treated with C_{17}-alkylated androgenic steroids. Seven of these patients died of liver failure. The first case of hepato-cellular carcinoma associated with taking an androgenic-anabolic steroid was reported in 1965.[28] Since then at least 13 other patients taking C_{17}-alkylated androgenic steroids have developed hepato-cellular carcinoma.[5, 11, 14, 15, 16, 17, 18, 25] In some cases dosages as low as 10-15 mg/day taken for only three or four months have caused liver complications.[13, 25]

4. Administration of therapeutic doses of androgenic-anabolic steroids in men often[15, 22] but not always,[1, 10, 19] reduces the output of testosterone and gonadotropins and reduces spermatogenesis. Some steroids are less potent than others in causing these effects.[1] Although these effects on the reproductive system appear to be reversible in animals, the long-term results of taking large doses by humans is unknown.

5. Precise information concerning the abuse of anabolic steroids by female athletes is unavailable. Nevertheless, there is no reason to believe females will not be tempted to adopt the use of these medicines. The use of anabolic steroids by females, particularly those who are either prepubertal or have not attained full growth, is especially dangerous. The undesired side effects include masculinization,[2, 29, 30] disruption of normal growth pattern,[30] voice changes,[2, 30, 32] acne,[2, 29, 30, 32] hirsutism,[29, 30, 32] and enlargement of the clitoris.[29] The long-term effects on reproductive function are unknown, but anabolic steroids may be harmful in this area. Their ability to interfere with the menstrual cycle has been well documented.[29]

For these reasons, all concerned with advising, training, coaching, and providing medical care for female athletes should exercise all persuasions available to prevent the use of anabolic steroids by female athetes.

References

1. Aakvaag, A., and Stromme, S. B.: The effect of mesterolone administration to normal men on the pituitary-testicular function. Acta Endocrinol. 77:380–386, 1974.
2. Allen, D. M., Fine, M. H., Necheles, T. F., and Dameshek, W.: Oxymetholone therapy in aplastic anemia. Blood 32:83–89, 1968.
3. Ariel, G., and Saville, W.: Anabolic steroids: the physiological effects of placebos. Med. Sci. Sport 4:124–126, 1972.
4. Bagheri, S. A., and Boyer, J. L.: Peliosis hepatitis associated with androgenic-anabolic steroid therapy. Ann. Intern. Med. 81:610–618, 1974.
5. Bernstein, M. S., Hunter, R. L., and Yachrin, S.: Hepatoma and peliosis hepatitis developing in a patient with Fanconi's anemia. N. Engl. J. Med., 284:1135–1136, 1971.
6. Bowers, R., and Reardon, J.: Effects of methandro-stenolone (Dianabol) on strength development and aerobic capacity. Med. Sci. Sports 4:54, 1972.
7. Burger, R. A., and Marcuse, P. M.: Peliosis hepatitis, report of a case. Am. J. Clin. Path. 22:569–573, 1952.
8. Byerly, H.: Explaining and exploiting placebo effects. Prosp. Biol. Med. 19:423–436, 1976.

9. Casner, S., Early, R., and Carlson, B. R.: Anabolic steroid effects on body composition in normal young men. J. Sports Med. Phys. Fit. *11*:98–103, 1971.
10. Fahey, T. D., and Brown, C. H.: The effects of an anabolic steroid on the strength, body composition, and endurance of college males when accompanied by a weight training program. Med. Sci. Sports *5*:272–276, 1973.
11. Farrell, G. C., Joshua, D. E., Uren, R. F., Baird, P. J., Perkins, K. W., and Kraienberg, H.: Androgen-induced hepatoma. Lancet *1*:430–431, 1975.
12. Fowler, W. M., Jr., Gardner, G. W., and Egstrom, G. H.: Effect of an anabolic steroid on physical performance of young men. J. Appl. Physiol. *20*:1038–1040, 1065.
13. Golding, L. A., Freydinger, J. E., and Fishel, S. S.: Weight, size and strength unchanged by steroids. Phys. Sports Med. *2*:39–45, 1974.
14. Guy, J. T., and Auxlander, M. O.: Androgenic steroids and hepato-cellular carcinoma. Lancet *1*:148, 1973.
15. Harkness, R. A., Kalshaw, B. H., and Hobson, B. M.: Effects of large doses of anabolic steroids. Brit. J. Sport Med. *9*:70–73, 1975.
16. Henderson, J. T., Richmond, J. and Sumerling, M. D.: Androgenic-anabolic steroid therapy and hepato-cellular carcinoma. Lancet *1*:934, 1972.
17. Johnson, F. L.: The association of oral androgenic-anabolic steroids and life threatening disease. Med. Sci. Sports *7*:284–286, 1975.
18. Johnson, F. L., Feagler, J. R., Lerner, K. G., Majems, P. W., Siegel, M., Hartman, J. R., and Thomas, E. D.: Association of androgenic-anabolic steroid therapy with development of hepato-cellular carcinoma. Lancet *2*:1273–1276, 1972.
19. Johnson, L. C., Fisher, G., Sylvester, L. J. and Hofheins, C. C.: Anabolic steroid: effects on strength, body weight, O₂ uptake and spermatogenesis in mature males. Med. Sci. Sports *4*:43–45, 1972.
20. Johnson, L. C., and O'Shea., P. P.: Anabolic steroid: effects on strength development. Science *164*:957–959, 1969.
21. Johnson, L. C., Roundy, E. S., Allsen, P., Fisher, A. G., and Sylvester, L. J.: Effect of anabolic steroid treatment on endurance. Med. Sci. Sports, *7*:287–289, 1975.
22. Kilshaw, B. H., Harkness, R. A., Hobson, B. M., and Smith, A. W. M.: The effects of large doses of the anabolic steroid, methandrostenolone, on an athlete. Clin. Endocr. *4*:537–541, 1975.
23. Kantzen, W., and Silny, J.: Peliosis hepatitis after administration of fluoxymesterone. Can. Med. Assoc. J. *83*:860–862, 1960.
24. McCredie, K. B.: Oxymetholone in refractory anaemia. Brit. J. Haematology. *17*:265–273, 1969.
25. Meadows, A. T., Naiman, J. L., and Valdes-Dapena, M. V.: Hepatoma associated with androgen therapy for aplastic anemia. J. Pediatr. *84*:109–110, 1974.
26. O'Shea, J. P.: The effects of an anabolic steroid on dynamic strength levels of weight lifters. Nutr. Report Internat. *4*:363–370, 1971.
27. O'Shea, J. P., and Winkler, W.: Biochemical and physical effects of an anabolic steroid in competitive swimmers and weight lifters. Nutr. Report Internat. *2*:351–362, 1970.
28. Recant, L., and Lacy, P.: Fanconi's anemia and hepatic cirrhosis. Clinicopathologic Conference. Am. J. Med. *39*:464–475, 1965.
29. Sanchez-Medal, L., Gomez-Leal, A., Duarte, L., and Guadalupe-Rico, M.: Anabolic-androgenic steroids in the treatment of acquired aplastic anemia. Blood *34*:283–300, 1969.
30. Shahidi, N. T.: Androgens and erythropoiesis. N. Engl. J. Med. *289*:72–79, 1973.
31. Sherlock, S.: *Disease of the Liver and Biliary System,* 4th ed. Philadelphia, F. A. Davis, 1968, p. 371.
32. Silink, J., and Firkin, B. G.: An analysis of hypoplastic anaemia with special reference to the use of oxymetholone ("Adroyd") in its therapy. Australian Ann. Med. *17*:224–235, 1968.
33. Stanford, B. A., and Moffat, R.: Anabolic steroid: effectiveness as an ergogenic aid to experienced weight trainers. J. Sports Med. Phys. Fit. *14*:191–197, 1974.
34. Steinbach, M.: Uber den Einfluss anabolen Wirkstoffe und Korpergewicht Muskelkraft und Muskeltraining. Sportarzt und Sport-medizin *11*:485–492, 1968.
35. Samuels, L. T., Henschel, A. F., and Kays, A.: Influence of methyltestosterone on muscular work and creatine metabolism in normal young men. J. Clin. Endocrinol. Metab. *2*:649–654, 1942.
36. Stromme, S. B., Meen, H. D., and Aakvaag, A.: Effects of an androgenic-anabolic steroid on strength development and plasma testosterone levels in normal males. Med. Sci. Sports. *6*:203–208, 1974.
37. Ward, P.: The effect of an anabolic steroid on strength and lean body mass. Med. Sci. Sports *5*:277–282, 1973.
38. Zak, F. G.: Peliosis hepatitis. Am. J. Pathol. *26*:1–15, 1950.
39. Ziegenfuss, J., and Carabasi, R.: Androgens and hepato-cellular carcinoma. Lancet *1*:262, 1973.

THE RECOMMENDED QUANTITY AND
QUALITY OF EXERCISE FOR
DEVELOPING AND MAINTAINING
FITNESS IN HEALTHY ADULTS*

Increasing numbers of persons are becoming involved in endurance training activities, and thus the need for guidelines for exercise prescription is apparent.

Based on the existing evidence concerning exercise prescription for healthy adults and the need for guidelines, the American College of Sports Medicine makes the following recommendations for the quantity and quality of training for developing and maintaining cardiorespiratory fitness and body composition in the healthy adult:

1. Frequency of training: 3 to 5 days per week.
2. Intensity of training: 60 per cent to 90 per cent of maximum heart rate reserve or 50 per cent to 85 per cent of maximum oxygen uptake ($\dot{V}o_{2\ max}$).
3. Duration of training: 15 to 60 minutes of continuous aerobic activity. Duration is dependent on the intensity of the activity, thus lower intensity activity should be conducted over a longer period of time. Because of the importance of the "total fitness" effect and the fact that it is more readily attained in longer duration programs, and because of the potential hazards and compliance problems associated with high-intensity activity, lower to moderate intensity activity of longer duration is recommended for the nonathletic adult.
4. Mode of activity: Any activity that uses large muscle groups, that can be maintained continuously, and is rhythmical and aerobic in nature, e.g. running-jogging, walking-hiking, swimming, skating, bicycling, rowing, cross-country skiing, rope skipping, and various endurance game activities.

Rationale and Research Background

The questions "How much exercise is enough and what type of exercise is best for developing and maintaining fitness?" are frequently asked. It is recognized that the term "physical fitness" is composed of a wide variety of variables included in the broad categories of cardiovascular-respiratory fitness, physique and structure, motor function, and many histochemical and biochemical factors. It is also recognized that the adaptive response to training is complex and includes peripheral, central, structural, and functional factors. Although many such variables and their adaptative response to training have been documented, the lack of sufficient in-depth and comparative data relative to frequency, intensity, and duration of training make them inadequate to use as comparative models. Thus, in respect to the above questions, fitness will be limited to changes in $\dot{V}o_{2\ max}$, total body mass, fat weight (FW), and lean body weight (LBW) factors.

Exercise prescription is based upon the frequency, intensity, and duration of training, the mode of activity (aerobic in nature, e.g., listed under No. 4 above), and the initial level of fitness. In evaluating these factors, the following observations have been derived from studies conducted with endurance training programs.

1. Improvement in $\dot{V}o_{2max}$ is directly related to frequency,[2, 23, 32, 58, 59, 65, 77, 79] intensity,[2, 10, 13, 26, 33, 37, 42, 56, 77] and duration [3, 14, 29, 49, 56, 77, 86] of training. Depending upon the quantity and quality of training, improvement in $\dot{V}o_{2\ max}$ ranges from 5 per cent to 25 per cent.[4, 13, 27, 31, 35, 36, 43, 45, 52, 53, 62, 71, 77, 78, 82, 86] Although changes in $\dot{V}o_{2\ max}$ greater than 25 per cent have been shown, they are usually associated with large total body mass and FW loss, or a low initial level of fitness. Also, as a result of leg fatigue or a lack of

---

*Reprinted from Medicine and Science in Sports *10*(3):vii, 1978. Courtesy of the American College of Sports Medicine.

motivation, persons with low initial fitness may have spuriously low initial $Vo_{2\ max}$ values.

2. The amount of improvement in $Vo_{2\ max}$ tends to plateau when frequency of training is increased above 3 days per week.[23, 62, 65] For the nonathlete, there is not enough information available at this time to speculate on the value of added improvement found in programs that are conducted more than 5 days per week. Participation of less than two days per week does not show an adequate change in $Vo_{2\ max}$.[24, 56, 62]

3. Total body mass and FW are centrally reduced with endurance training programs,[67] while LBW remains constant[62, 67, 87] or increases slightly.[34] Programs that are conducted at least 3 days per week,[58, 59, 61, 62, 87] of at least 20 minutes duration[48, 62, 87] and of sufficient intensity and duration to expend approximately 300 kilocalories (kcal) per exercise session are suggested as a threshold level for total body mass and FW loss.[12, 29, 62, 67] An expenditure of 200 kcal per session has also been shown to be useful in weight reduction if the exercise frequency is at least 4 days per week.[80] Programs with less participation generally show little or no change in body composition.[19, 25, 42, 62, 67, 84, 85, 87] Significant increases in $Vo_{2\ max}$ have been shown with 10 to 15 minutes of high intensity training.[34, 49, 56, 62, 77, 78] Thus, if total body mass and FW reduction is not a consideration, then short duration, high-intensity programs may be recommended for healthy, low-risk (cardiovascular disease) persons.

4. The minimal threshold level for improvement in Vo_{2max} is approximately 60 per cent of the maximum heart rate reserve (50 per cent of $Vo_{2\ max}$).[33, 37] Maximum heart rate reserve represents the per cent difference between resting and maximum heart rate, added to the resting heart rate. The technique is described by Karvonen, Kentala, and Mustala,[37] was validated by Davis and Convertino,[14] and represents a heart rate of approximately 130 to 135 beats/minute for young persons. As a result of the aging curve for maximum heart rate, the absolute heart rate value (threshold level) is inversely related to age, and can be as low as 110 to 120 beats/minute for older persons. Initial level of fitness is another important consideration in prescribing exercise.[10, 40, 46, 75, 77] The person with a low fitness level can get a significant training effect with a sustained training heart rate as low as 110 to 120 beats/minute, while persons of higher fitness levels need a higher threshold of stimulation.[26]

5. Intensity and duration of training are interrelated, with the total amount of work accomplished being an important factor in improvement in fitness.[2, 7, 12, 40, 61, 76, 78] Although more comprehensive inquiry is necessary, present evidence suggests that when exercise is performed above the minimal threshold of intensity, the total amount of work accomplished is the important factor in fitness development[2, 7, 12, 61, 62, 76, 79] and maintenance.[68] That is, improvement will be similar for activities performed at a lower intensity–longer duration compared to higher intensity–shorter duration if the total energy cost of the activities is equal.

   If frequency, intensity, and duration of training are similar (total kcal expenditure), the training result appears to be independent of the mode of arobic activity.[56, 60, 62, 64] Therefore, a variety of endurance activities, e.g., listed above, may be used to derive the same training effect.

6. In order to maintain the training effect, exercise must be continued on a regular basis.[2, 6, 11, 21, 44, 73, 74] A significant reduction in working capacity occurs after two weeks of detraining[73] with participants returning to near pretraining levels of fitness after 10 weeks[21] to 8 months of detraining.[44] Fifty per cent reduction in improvement of cardiorespiratory fitness has been shown after 4 to 12 weeks of detraining.[21, 41, 73] More investigation is necessary to evaluate the rate of increase and decrease of fitness with varying training loads and reduction in training in relation to level of fitness, age, and length of time in training. Also, more information is needed to better identify the minimal level of work necessary to maintain fitness.

7. Endurance activities that require running and jumping generally cause significantly more debilitating injuries to beginning exercisers than other non–weight bearing activities.[42, 55, 69] One study showed that beginning joggers had increased foot, leg, and knee injuries when training was performed more than 3 days per week and longer than 30 minutes duration per exercise session.[69] Thus, caution should be taken when recommending the type of activity and exercise prescription for the beginning exerciser. Also, the increase of orthopedic injuries as related to overuse (marathon training) with chronic jogger-runners is apparent. Thus, there is a need for more inquiry into the effect that different types of activities and the quantity and quality of training has on short-term and long-term participation.

8. Most of the information concerning training described in this position statement has been conducted on men. The lack of information on women is apparent, but the available evidence indicates that women tend to adapt to endurance training in the same manner as men.[8, 22, 89]

9. Age in itself does not appear to be a deterrent to endurance training. Although some earlier studies showed a lower training effect with middle-aged or elderly participants,[4, 17, 34, 83, 86] more recent study shows the relative change in $\dot{V}_{O_2 \, max}$ to be similar to that in younger age groups.[3, 52, 66, 75, 86] Although more investigation is necessary concerning the rate of improvement in $\dot{V}_{O_{2max}}$ with age, at present it appears that elderly participants need longer periods of time to adapt to training.[17, 66] Earlier studies showing moderate to no improvement in $\dot{V}_{O_{2max}}$ were conducted over a short time-span[4] or exercise was conducted at a moderate to low kcal expenditure,[17] thus making the interpretation of the results difficult.

Although $\dot{V}_{O_2 \, max}$ decreases with age, and total body mass and FW increase with age, evidence suggests that this trend can be altered with endurance training.[9, 12, 38, 62] Also, 5 to 10 year follow-up studies where participants continued their training at a similar level showed maintenance of fitness.[39, 70] A study of older competitive runners showed decreases in $\dot{V}_{O_2 \, max}$ from the fourth to seventh decade of life, but also showed reductions in their training load.[63] More inquiry into the relationship of long-term training (quantity and quality) for both competitors and noncompetitors and physiological function with increasing age is necessary before more definitive statements can be made.

10. An activity such as weight training should not be considered as a means of training for developing $\dot{V}_{O_2 \, max}$, but has significant value for increasing muscular strength and endurance, and LBW.[16, 24, 47, 88] Recent studies evaluating circuit weight training (weight training conducted almost continuously with moderate weights, using 10 to 15 repetitions per exercise session with 15 to 30 seconds rest between bouts of activity) showed little to no improvements in working capacity and $\dot{V}_{O_2 \, max}$.[1, 24, 90]

Despite an abundance of information available concerning the training of the human organism, the lack of standardization of testing protocols and procedures, methodology in relation to training procedures and experimental design, a preciseness in the documentation and reporting of the quantity and quality of training prescribed make interpretation difficult.[62, 67] Interpretation and comparison of results are also dependent on the initial level of fitness,[18, 74-76, 81] length of time of the training experiment,[20, 57, 58, 61, 62] and specificity of the testing and training.[64] For example, data from training studies using subjects with varied levels of $\dot{V}_{O_2 \, max}$, total body mass and FW have found changes to occur in relation to their initial values,[5, 15, 48, 50, 51] i.e., the lower the initial $\dot{V}_{O_2 \, max}$ the larger the per cent of improvement found, and the higher the FW the greater the reduction. Also, data evaluating trainability with age, comparison of the different magnitudes and quantities of effort, and comparison of the trainability of men and women may have been influenced by the initial fitness levels.

In view of the fact that improvement in the fitness variables discussed in this position statement continues over many months of training,[12, 38, 39, 62] it is reasonable to believe that short-term studies conducted over a few weeks have certain limitations. Middle-aged sedentary and older participants may take several weeks to adapt to the initial rigors of training, and thus need a longer adaptation period to get the full benefit from a program. How long a training experiment should be conducted is difficult to determine, but 15 to 20 weeks may be a good minimum standard. For example, two investigations conducted with middle-aged men who jogged either 2 or 4 days per week found both groups to improve in $\dot{V}_{O_2 \, max}$. Midtest results of the 16- and 20-week programs showed no difference between groups, while subsequent final testing found the 4 day per week group to improve significantly more.[58, 59] In a similar study with young college men, no differences in $\dot{V}_{O_2 \, max}$ were found among groups after 7 and 13 weeks of interval training.[20] These latter findings and those of other investigators point to the limitations in interpreting results from investigations conducted over a short time-span[62, 67]

In summary, frequency, intensity, and duration of training have been found to be effective stimuli for producing a training effect. In general, the lower the stimuli, the lower the training effect,[2, 12, 13, 27, 35, 46, 77, 78, 90] and the greater the stimuli, the greater the effect.[2, 12, 13, 27, 58, 77, 78] It has also been shown that endurance training less than two days per week, less than 50 per cent of maximum oxygen uptake, and less than 10 minutes per day is inadequate for developing and maintaining fitness for healthy adults.

For references, see Medicine and Science in Sports *10*(3):vii, 1978.

APPENDIX C

Cardiopulmonary Resuscitation

Editor's Note: All persons with responsibility related to sports (physicians, trainers, coaches, physical educators) should be trained in cardiopulmonary resuscitation. As a partial review for persons who have been so trained, the following guidelines are excerpted from the Journal of the American Medical Association.*

In cases of collapsed or unconscious persons, the adequacy or absence of breathing and circulation must be determined immediately. If breathing alone is inadequate or absent, rescue breathing may be all that is necessary. If circulation is also absent, artificial circulation must be started in combination with rescue breathing. The methods of recognizing adequacy or absence of breathing or circulation and the recommended techniques for performing artificial ventilation and artificial circulation are presented below.

ARTIFICIAL VENTILATION

Opening the airway and restoring breathing are the basic steps of artificial ventilation. The steps can be performed quickly under almost any circumstance and without adjunctive equipment or help from another person. They constitute emergency first aid for airway obstruction and respiratory inadequacy or arrest.

Respiratory inadequacy may result from an obstruction of the airway or from respiratory failure. An obstructed airway is sometimes difficult to recognize until the airway is opened. At other times, a partially obstructed airway is recognized by labored breathing or excessive respiratory efforts, often involving accessory muscles of respiration, and by soft tissue retractions of the intercostal, supraclavicular, and suprasternal spaces. Respiratory failure is characterized by minimal or absent respiratory effort, failure of the chest or upper abdomen to move, and inability to detect air movement through the nose or mouth.

Airway

The most important factor for successful resuscitation is immediate opening of the airway. This can be accomplished easily and quickly by tilting the victim's head backward as far as possible. Sometimes this simple maneuver is all that is required for breathing to resume spontaneously. To perform the head tilt, the victim must be lying on his back. The rescuer places one hand beneath the victim's neck and the other hand on his forehead. He then lifts the neck with one hand and tilts the head backward by pressure with his other hand on the forehead. This maneuver extends the neck and lifts the tongue away from the back of the throat. Anatomical obstruction of the airway caused by the tongue dropping against the back of the throat thereby is relieved. The head must be maintained in this position at all times. (See Figure 1.)

The head tilt method is effective in most cases. If head tilt is unsuccessful in opening the air passage adequately, additional forward displacement of the lower jaw — jaw

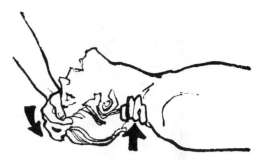

thrust — may be required. This can be accomplished by a triple airway maneuver in which the rescuer places his fingers behind the angles of the victim's jaw and (1) forcefully displaces the mandible forward while (2) tilting the head backward and (3) using his thumbs to retract the lower lip to allow breathing through the mouth as well as through the nose. The jaw thrust is performed best from a position at the top of the victim's head.

However, if the victim does not resume spontaneous breathing, the rescuer must move to the victim's side to perform mouth-to-mouth or mouth-to-nose ventilation. Several variations of the jaw thrust may be used. When using jaw thrust for mouth-to-mouth ventilation, the rescuer must keep the victim's mouth open with his thumbs and seal the nose by placing his cheek against it. However, this is more difficult to teach and practice on manikins, and more difficult and tiring to perform on victims than the head tilt method. For mouth-to-nose ventilation with jaw thrust, the rescuer uses his cheek to seal the victim's mouth and does not retract the lower lip with his thumbs. Such special details of performance and the problems associated with manikin practice limit use of jaw thrust techniques to specially trained personnel.

Breathing

If the victim does not promptly resume adequate spontaneous breathing after the airway is opened, artificial ventilation, sometimes called rescue breathing, must be started. Mouth-to-mouth breathing and mouth-to-nose breathing are both types of artificial ventilation.

To perform mouth-to-mouth ventilation, the rescuer uses his hand behind the victim's neck to maintain the head in a position of maximum backward tilt. He pinches the victim's nostrils together with the thumb and index finger of his other hand, which also continues to exert pressure on the forehead to maintain the backward head tilt. The rescuer then opens his mouth widely, takes a deep breath, makes a tight seal with his mouth around the victim's mouth and blows into the victim's mouth. He then removes his mouth and allows the victim to exhale passively, watching the victim's chest fall. This cycle is repeated *once every five seconds* as long as respiratory inadequacy persists.

Adequate ventilation is ensured on every breath by the rescuer

1. Seeing the chest rise and fall.
2. Feeling in his own airway the resistance and compliance of the victim's lungs as they expand.
3. Hearing and feeling the air escape during exhalation. The initial ventilatory maneuver should be *four quick, full, breaths* without allowing time for full lung deflation between breaths. (See Figure 2.)

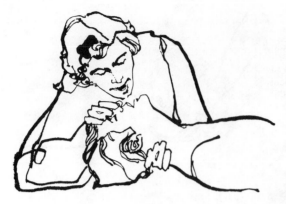

Figure 2. Mouth-to-mouth resuscitation. (From *Standards for Cardiopulmonary Resuscitation (CPR) and Emergency Cardiac Care (ECC)*. Reprinted from the Supplement to Journal of the American Medical Association, February 18, 1974. Copyright, 1974, the American Medical Association. Reprinted with permission from the American Heart Association.)

In some cases, mouth-to-nose ventilation is more effective than mouth-to-mouth ventilation. The former is recommended when it is impossible to open the victim's mouth, when it is impossible to ventilate through his mouth, when the victim's mouth is seriously injured, when it is difficult to achieve a tight seal around his mouth, and when, for some other reason, the rescuer prefers the nasal route.

For the mouth-to-nose technique, the rescuer keeps the victim's head tilted back with one hand on the forehead and uses the other hand to lift the victim's lower jaw. This seals the lips. The rescuer then takes a deep breath, seals his lips around the victim's nose and blows in until he feels the lungs expand. The rescuer removes his mouth and the victim is allowed to exhale passively. The rescuer can see the chest fall when the victim exhales. When mouth to-nose ventilation is used, it may be necessary to open the victim's mouth or separate his lips to allow the air to escape during exhalation because the soft palate may cause nasopharyngeal obstruction. This cycle should be repeated approximately every five seconds.

No adjuncts are required for effective rescue breathing; so artificial ventilation should never be delayed to obtain or apply adjunctive devices.

Infants and Children. Opening the airway and performing artificial ventilation are essentially the same for children as for adults. There are some differences, however. For infants and small children, the rescuer covers both the mouth and nose of the child with his mouth and uses small breaths with less volume to inflate the lungs *once every three seconds*. The neck of an infant is so pliable that forceful backward tilting of the head may obstruct breathing passages. Therefore, the tilted position should not be exaggerated.

Accident Cases. In accident cases, it is imperative that caution be used to avoid extension of the neck when there is a possibility of neck fracture. A fractured neck should be suspected in diving or automobile accidents when the victim has lacerations of the face and forehead. If a fracture is suspected, all forward, backward, lateral, or turning movement should be avoided. To open the airway, a modification of the jaw thrust maneuver described above should be used. In this variation, the rescuer places his hands on either side of the victim's head so the head is maintained in a fixed, neutral position without the head extended. The index fingers should then be used to displace the mandible forward without tilting the head backward or turning it to either side (modified jaw thrust). If required, artificial ventilation usually can be provided in this position. If this is unsuccessful, the head should be tilted back very slightly and another attempt made to ventilate, using the modified jaw thrust maneuver.

Foreign Bodies. The rescuer should not look for foreign bodies in the upper airway unless their presence is known or strongly suspected. The first effort to ventilate the lungs will determine whether an airway obstruction is present. If the first attempts to ventilate are unsuccessful despite properly opening the airway and providing an airtight seal around the mouth, an attempt should be made immediately to clear the airway with the fingers. The victim should be rolled onto his side, with the rescuer's knee placed under his shoulder. The victim's mouth then is forced open with the thumb and index crossed-finger technique. The rescuer runs his index finger or index and middle fingers down the inside of the victim's cheek toward the base of the tongue, deep into his throat. The rescuer's fingers are moved across the back of the victim's throat with a sweeping motion. Repeated attempts may be required. Where skilled, advanced life support personnel and equipment are available, direct laryngoscopy may permit the foreign body to be removed.

Larger foreign bodies frequently can be extricated by these finger maneuvers. If the rescuer is unable to dislodge the foreign body, or if it is impacted below the epiglottis, the victim should be rolled onto his side toward the rescuer, who then delivers sharp blows with the heel of his hand between the victim's shoulder blades. Further attempts at clearing the airway then should be made. If unsuccessful, there should be repeated efforts at mouth-to-mouth resuscitation, blows to the back, and probing the upper airway with the fingers. A small child having airway obstruction should be quickly picked up and inverted over the arm of the rescuer while the blows are being delivered between the child's shoulder blades.

If all of these maneuvers fail, emergency cricothyroid puncture and insertion of a 6 mm tube have been recommended for adults. However, this requires appropriate instruments and training and must be regarded as an advanced life support technique.

Gastric Distension.   Artificial ventilation frequently causes distension of the stomach. This occurs most often in children, but it is not uncommon in adults. It is most likely to occur when excessive pressures are used for inflation or if the airway is obstructed. Slight gastric distension may be disregarded. However, marked distension of the stomach may be dangerous because it promotes regurgitation, and it reduces lung volume by elevating the diaphragm. Several cases of gastric rupture resulting from overdistension have been reported. Obvious gross distension should be relieved whenever possible. In the unconscious victim, this can be accomplished without adjuncts by using one hand to exert moderate pressure over the victim's epigastrium between the umbilicus and the rib cage. To prevent aspiration of gastric contents during this maneuver, the victim's head and shoulders should be turned to one side.

ARTIFICIAL CIRCULATION (EXTERNAL CARDIAC COMPRESSION)

When sudden, unexpected cardiac arrest occurs, all of the A B C's of basic life support are required in rapid succession. This includes both artificial ventilation and artificial circulation (external cardiac compression). Cardiac arrest is recognized by pulselessness in large arteries in an unconscious victim having a deathlike appearance and absent breathing. The status of the carotid pulse should be checked as quickly as possible when cardiac arrest is suspected. In an unwitnessed cardiac arrest, the rescuer first opens the airway and quickly ventilates the lungs four times. He then maintains the head tilt with one hand on the forehead, and with the tips of the index and middle fingers of the other hand, gently locates the victim's larynx and slides his fingers laterally into the groove between the trachea and the muscles at the side of the neck where the carotid pulse can be felt. The pulse area must be felt gently, not compressed.

There are a number of reasons for recommending palpation of the carotid pulse rather than other pulses. First, the rescuer already is at the victim's head to perform artificial ventilation and the carotid pulse is in the same area. Second, the neck area generally is accessible immediately, without removal of any clothing. Third, the carotid arteries are central and sometimes these pulses will persist when more peripheral pulses are no longer palpable. Trainees should practice palpation of the carotid pulse during classes. In hospital situations, palpation of the femoral artery is an acceptable option to use instead of the carotid artery. It is not practical to feel the carotid pulse in infants and small children. Instead, the rescuer's hand should be placed gently over the precordium to feel the apical beat.

Absence or questionable presence of the pulse is the indication for starting artificial circulation by means of external cardiac compression. External cardiac compression consists of the rhythmic application of pressure over the lower one half of the sternum, but *not over the xiphoid process*. The heart lies slightly to the left of the middle of the chest between the lower sternum and the spine. Intermittent pressure applied to the sternum compresses the heart and produces a pulsatile artificial circulation. During cardiac arrest, properly performed external cardiac compression can produce systolic blood pressure peaks of over 100 mm Hg, but the diastolic pressure is zero and the mean pressure seldom exceeds 40 mm Hg in the carotid arteries. The carotid artery blood flow resulting from external cardiac compression on a cardiac arrest victim usually is only one quarter to one third of normal.

External cardiac compression always must be accompanied by artificial ventilation. Compression of the sternum produces some ventilation, but the volumes are insufficient for adequate oxygenation of the blood. Therefore, artificial ventilation is *always* required when external cardiac compression is used.

Technique for External Cardiac Compression

The patient always must be in the horizontal position when external cardiac compression is performed since, during cardiac arrest, there is no blood flow to the brain when the body is in the vertical position, even during properly performed external cardiac compression. It is imperative, therefore, to get the cardiac arrest victim into a horizontal position as quickly as possible in situations where he is vertical, such as in a dental chair, trapped in a vehicle, stricken on a telephone pole, while in a stadium seat, or in any similar situation. Elevation of the lower extremities, while keeping the rest of the body horizontal, may promote venous return and augment artificial circulation during external cardiac compression.

Effective external cardiac compression requires sufficient pressure to depress an adult's lower sternum a minimum of 1½ to 2 inches. For external cardiac compression to be effective, the victim must be on a firm surface. This may be the ground, floor, or a spineboard on a wheeled litter. If the victim is in bed, a board, preferably the full width of the bed, should be placed under his back. However, chest compression must not be delayed while this support is awaited.

The rescuer positions himself close to the victim's side and places the long axis of the heel of one hand parallel to and over the long axis of the lower one half of the sternum. Great care must be exercised not to place the hand over the lower tip of the sternum (xiphoid process) that extends downward over the upper abdomen. To avoid this the rescuer feels the tip of the xiphoid and places the heel of his hand on the lower one half of the sternum about 1 to 1½ inches away from the tip of the xiphoid and toward the victim's head. He then places the other hand on top of the first one (and may interlock the fingers), brings his shoulders directly over the victim's sternum, keeps his arms straight, and exerts pressure almost vertically downward to depress the lower sternum a minimum of 1½ to 2 inches. The compressions must be regular, smooth, and uninterrupted. Relaxation must immediately follow compression and be of equal duration. The heel of the rescuer's hand should not be removed from the chest during relaxation but pressure on the sternum should be completely released so that it returns to its normal resting position between compressions. (See Figure 3.)

Since artificial circulation always must be combined with artificial ventilation, it is preferable to have two rescuers. One rescuer positions himself at the victim's side and performs external cardiac compression while the other one remains at the victim's head, keeping it tilted back, and continues rescue breathing. *The compression rate for two rescuers is 60 per minute.* When performed without interruption, this rate can maintain adequate blood flow and pressure and will allow cardiac refill. This rate is practical because it avoids fatigue, facilitates timing on the basis of one compression per second, and allows optimum ventilation and circulation to be achieved by quickly interposing one inflation after each five chest compressions without any pause in compressions (5:1 ratio). The rate of 60 compressions per minute allows breaths to be interposed without any pauses. Interposing the breaths without any pauses in compression is important, since any interruption in cardiac compression results in a drop in blood flow and blood pressure to zero. (See Figure 3.)

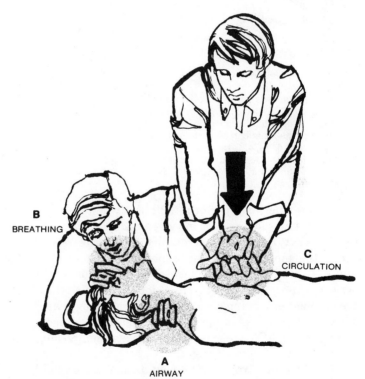

B
BREATHING

C
CIRCULATION

A
AIRWAY

Figure 3. Two-rescuer cardiopulmonary resuscitation.
5 chest compressions
Rate of 60/minute
No pause for ventilation
1 lung inflation
After each 5 compressions
Interposed between compressions
(From *Standards for Cardiopulmonary Resuscitation (CPR) and Emergency Cardiac Care (ECC).* Reprinted from the Supplement to Journal of the American Medical Association, February 18, 1974. Copyright 1974, the American Medical Association. Reprinted with permission from the American Heart Association.)

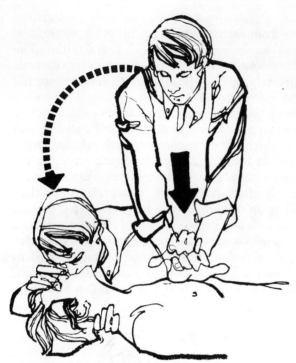

Figure 4. One-rescuer cardiopulmonary resuscitation.
  15 chest compressions (rate of 80/minute)
  2 quick lung inflations
   (From *Standards for Cardiopulmonary
Resuscitation (CPR) and Emergency Cardiac
Care (ECC)*. Reprinted from the Supplement
to Journal of the American Medical Association, February 18, 1974. Copyright 1974, the
American Medical Association. Reprinted
with permission from the American Heart
Association.)

Two rescuers can perform CPR best when they are on opposite sides of the victim. They can then switch positions when necessary without any significant interruption in the 5:1 rhythm. This is accomplished by the rescuer who is performing artificial ventilation moving to the side of the victim's chest immediately after he has inflated the lungs. He places his hands in the air next to those of the other rescuer who continues to perform external cardiac compression. As soon as the other hands are properly placed, the rescuer performing chest compression removes his hands (usually after the third or fourth in the series of compressions) and the other rescuer then continues with the series of compressions. The rescuer who had been compressing then moves to the victim's head and interposes the next breath.

If the victim's trachea has been intubated, lung inflation is easier and compression rates up to 80 per minute can be used since breaths can be either interposed or superimposed following endotracheal intubation.

When there is only one rescuer, he must perform both artificial ventilation and artificial circulation using a 15:2 ratio. This consists of *two very quick lung inflations after each 15 chest compressions* (Fig. 4.) Because of the interruptions for lung inflation, the single rescuer must perform each series of 15 chest compressions at the faster rate of *80 compressions per minute* in order to achieve an actual compression rate of 60 per minute. The two full lung inflations must be delivered in rapid succession, within a period of five to six seconds, without allowing full exhalation between the breaths. If time for full exhalation were allowed, the additional time required would reduce the number of compressions and ventilations that could be achieved in a one-minute period.

Infants and Children.   With a few exceptions,the cardiac compression technique is similar for children. For small children, only the heel of one hand is used, and, for infants, only the tips of the index and middle fingers are used. The ventricles of infants and small children *lie higher in the chest* and the external pressure should be exerted over the midsternum. The danger of lacerating the liver is greater in children because of the pliability of the chest and the higher position of the liver under the lower sternum and xiphoid. Infants require a ½- to ¾- inch compression of the sternum; young children require ¾ to 1½ inches. The compression rate should be 80 to 100 per minute with breaths delivered as quickly as possible after each five compressions.

In infants and small children, backward tilt of the head lifts the back. A firm support beneath the back is therefore required for external cardiac compression and can be provided by the rescuer slipping one hand beneath the child's back while using the other hand to compress the chest. A folded blanket or other adjunct can also be used beneath the shoulders to provide support. For small infants, an alternate method is to encircle the chest with the hands and compress the midsternum with both thumbs.

Checking Effectiveness of CPR.   The reaction of the pupils should be checked periodically during cardiopulmonary resuscitation, since this provides the best indication of delivery of oxygenated blood to the victim's brain. Pupils that constrict when exposed to light indicate adequate oxygenation and blood flow to the brain. If the pupils remain widely dilated and do not react to light, serious brain damage is imminent or has occurred. Dilated but reactive pupils are less ominous. Normal pupillary reactions may be altered in the aged and frequently are altered, in any individual, by the administration of drugs.

The carotid pulse should be palpated periodically during CPR in order to check the effectiveness of external cardiac compression or the return of a spontaneous effective heartbeat. This should be done after the first mintue of CPR and every few minutes thereafter, when additional rescuers are present and interruptions can be minimized. It should be checked particularly at the time of change of rescuers.

PITFALLS IN PERFORMANCE OF CPR

When CPR is performed improperly or inadequately, artificial ventilation and artificial circulation may be ineffective in providing basic life support. Enumerated below are important points to remember in performing external cardiac compression and artificial ventilation.

1. Do not interrupt CPR for more than five seconds for any reason, except in the following circumstances.
    a. Under emergency conditions, endotracheal intubation usually cannot be accomplished in five seconds. However, it is an advanced life support measure and should be performed only by those who are well trained and well practiced in the technique and *only* after the victim has been properly positioned and all preparations made. Even under these circumstances, interruptions in CPR for endotracheal intubation should never exceed 15 seconds.
    b. When moving a victim up or down a stairway, it is difficult to continue effective CPR. Under these circumstances, it is best to perform effective CPR at the head or foot of the stairs, then interrupt CPR at a given signal and move quickly to the next level where effective CPR is resumed. Such interruptions usually should not exceed 15 seconds.

2. Do not move the patient to a more convenient site until he has been stabilized and is ready for transportation or until arrangements have been made for uninterrupted CPR during movement.
3. Never compress the xiphoid process at the tip of the sternum. The xiphoid extends downward over the abdomen. Pressure on it may cause laceration of the liver, which can lead to severe internal bleeding.
4. Between compressions, the heel of the hand must completely release its pressure but should remain in constant contact with the chest wall over the lower one half of the sternum.
5. The rescuer's fingers should not rest on the victim's ribs during compression. Interlocking the fingers of the two hands may help avoid this. Pressure with fingers on the ribs or lateral pressure increases the possibility of rib fractures and costochondral separation.
6. Sudden or jerking movements should be avoided when compressing the chest. The compression should be smooth, regular and uninterrupted (50 per cent of the cycle should be compression and 50 per cent should be relaxation). Quick jabs increase the possibility of injury and produce quick jets of flow; they do not enhance stroke volume or mean flow and pressure.
7. Do not maintain continuous pressure on the abdomen to decompress the stomach while performing external cardiac compression. This may trap the liver and could cause it to rupture.
8. The shoulders of the rescuer should be directly over the victim's sternum. The elbows should be straight. Pressure is applied vertically downward on the lower sternum. This provides a maximally effective thrust, minimal fatigue for the rescuer, and reduced hazard of complications for the victim. When the victim is on the ground or floor, the rescuer can kneel or stand at his side. When he is on a bed or high-wheeled litter, the rescuer must be on a step or chair or kneeling on the bed or litter. With a low-wheeled litter, the rescuer can stand at the victim's side. Problems arise with the use of low-wheeled litters in ambulances. Special arrangements must be made for proper positioning of the rescuer based on the design of the ambulance.
9. The lower sternum of an adult must be depressed 1½ to 2 inches by external cardiac compression. Lesser amounts of compression are ineffectual since even properly performed cardiac compression provides only about one quarter to one third of the normal blood flow.
10. While complications may result from improperly performed external cardiac compression and precordial thumps, even properly performed external cardiac compression may cause rib fractures in some patients. Other complications that may occur with properly performed CPR include fracture of the sternum, costochondral separation, pneumothorax, hemothorax, lung contusions, lacerations of the liver, and fat emboli. These complications can be minimized by careful attention to details of performance. It must be remembered, however, that during cardiac arrest, effective cardiopulmonary resuscitation is required even if it results in complications, since the alternative to effective CPR is death.

DROWNING

Extensive research has delineated the events and mechanisms of drowning and the detailed physiological variations between fresh water and sea water submersion. However, basic life support resuscitation procedures following drowning are the same as basic life support principles presented above, and CPR should be performed as quickly as possible. There are a few special considerations, given below:

1. When attempting to rescue a drowning victim, the rescuer should get to him as quickly as possible, preferably with some conveyance, such as a boat or surfboard. If a conveyance is not available, a flotation device should be carried by the rescuer. The rescuer always must exercise care not to endanger himself while trying to aid a drowning person.
2. External cardiac compression should never be attempted in the water because it is impossible to perform it there effectively.
3. Mouth-to-mouth or mouth-to-nose ventilation may be performed in the water, although it is difficult and often impossible in deep water unless the rescuer has some type of flotation device to support the victim's head.

4. Artificial ventilation always should be started as soon as possible, even before the victim is moved out of the water, into a boat or onto a surfboard. As soon as the rescuer can stand in shallow water he should begin artificial ventilation.
5. In cases of suspected neck injury, the victim must be floated onto a back support before being removed from the water. If artificial respiration is required, the routine head tilt or jaw thrust maneuvers should not be used. Artificial ventilation should be accomplished with the head maintained in a neutral position and using a modified jaw thrust maneuver (as described under "Accident Cases," p. 420).
6. When removed from the water, the victim should have standard artificial ventilation or cardiopulmonary resuscitation performed according to the standards previously described.
7. Drowning victims swallow large volumes of water and their stomachs usually become distended. This impairs ventilation and circulation and should be alleviated as soon as possible. To relieve the distension, the victim may be turned on his side and his upper abdomen compressed or he may be turned over quickly into the prone position and lifted with the rescuer's hands under the stomach to force water out. This is referred to as "breaking" the victim.
8. There should be no delay in moving the victim to a life support unit where advanced life support capabilities are available. Every submersion victim, even one who requires only minimal resuscitation, should be transferred to a medical facility for follow-up care.

BEGINNING AND TERMINATING BASIC LIFE SUPPORT

CPR is most effective when started immediately after cardiac arrest. If cardiac arrest has persisted for more than 10 minutes, cardiopulmonary resuscitation is unlikely to restore the victim to his prearrest central nervous system status. If there is any question of the exact duration of the arrest, the victim should be given the benefit of the doubt and resuscitation started.

Basic life support is not indicated for a victim who is known to be in the terminal stages of an incurable condition. When resuscitation is indicated and started in the absence of a physician, it should be continued until one of the following occurs:

1. Effective spontaneous circulation and ventilation have been restored.
2. Resuscitation efforts have been transferred to another responsible person who continues basic life support.
3. A physician assumes responsibility.
4. The victim is transferred to properly trained and designated professional medical or allied health personnel charged with responsibilities for emergency medical services.
5. The rescuer is exhausted and unable to continue resuscitation.

The decision to stop resuscitative efforts is a medical one.

INDEX